Michael D. Shankle, MPH
Editor

The Handbook of Lesbian, Gay, Bisexual, and Transgender Public Health

A Practitioner's Guide to Service

Pre-publication
REVIEWS,
COMMENTARIES,
EVALUATIONS . . .

"It's about time that a book on LGBT health care has been written. This book is more than just a how-to guide. It takes you inside the world of the LGBT community, exploring myths, revealing much of its history, and providing insights about our society.

The chapters are written by some of the best-known LGBT health professionals and are devoted to many aspects of providing optimal care, including cultural competency training, access to care, drug treatments, and men and women's health. Gay and straight alike will find it helpful and those who care for the LGBT community will find it an invaluable reference."

Walter Tsou, MD, MPH
President, American Public Health Association

"This is the first handbook to address public health issues of LGBT populations. For too long, LGBT health meant HIV/AIDS. In recent years, without abandoning their important role in the AIDS epidemic, public health professionals have begun to recognize the complex problems that comprise LGBT health, including the need to address a wide range of public health concerns and to design programs tailored to diverse LGBT populations. This collection provides an indispensable resource for public health practitioners and community health activists who heed the call to eliminate health disparities and need the knowledge and professional tools to be effective in promoting the health of LGBT individuals."

Ilan H. Meyer, PhD
Associate Professor of Clinical Sociomedical Sciences, and Deputy Chair for Master's Programs, Department of Sociomedical Sciences, Columbia University

More pre-publication
REVIEWS, COMMENTARIES, EVALUATIONS . . .

"This is a breakthrough book—it boldly addresses significant health disparities and would interest a broad range of public health practitioners.

This excellent book contains discussions of topics rarely addressed in the public health community but which certainly deserve broader recognition. It addresses common problems in the LGBT community, including substance abuse, health access, hate crime violence, and teen suicide. Moving beyond deficits in the field and focusing on effective methods, the book provides practical theories and solutions.

Both comprehensive and well organized, this book looks at the influences of health research, health care, government, and the media on major issues affecting the LGBT community. It contains some of the clearest, most easily accessible discussions of strategies to achieve equal health outcomes for the LGBT community. It is more than a reference book; it is a well-reasoned strategy for health equality with a unique focus on LGBT health.

This book will provide a solid foundation for public health practitioners to address LGBT health disparities and serves the purpose of being a better provider of public health to the LGBT community."

Charles B. Collins, PhD
Science Application Section Chief,
Division of HIV/AIDS Prevention,
Centers for Disease Control and Prevention

"This is the first comprehensive guide that I am aware of that looks at the health care needs and concerns of the LGBT community as a *community*. It explicates the sometimes murky—for this clinician anyway—discipline of public health in a way that makes the health of societies as lucid and as vital as the care of the individual patient.

Editor Michael Shankle has assembled a panel of contributors comprising a who's who of providers, researchers, and policymakers dedicated to improving the health of the LGBT community. I would urge anyone who works in LGBT health to read this book cover to cover. It is crisply written and accessible for professionals and laypersons concerned about LGBT health. It is also passionate without being strident and political without being partisan. In short, this handbook is essential reading for anyone concerned with the health of LGBT persons and the LGBT community."

Ken Haller, MD, FAAP
Former President, Gay and Lesbian
Medical Association;
Assistant Professor of Pediatrics,
Saint Louis University
School of Medicine

HPP

Harrington Park Press®
An imprints of The Haworth Press, Inc.
New York • London • Oxford

The Handbook
of Lesbian, Gay, Bisexual,
and Transgender
Public Health
A Practitioner's Guide to Service

HARRINGTON PARK PRESS®
Titles of Related Interest

The Handbook
of Lesbian, Gay, Bisexual,
and Transgender
Public Health
A Practitioner's Guide to Service

Michael D. Shankle, MPH
Editor

HPP

Harrington Park Press®
An imprint of The Haworth Press, Inc.
New York • London • Oxford

For more information on this book or to order, visit
http://www.haworthpress.com/store/product.asp?sku=5557

or call 1-800-HAWORTH (800-429-6784) in the United States and Canada
or (607) 722-5857 outside the United States and Canada

or contact orders@HaworthPress.com

Published by

Harrington Park Press®, an imprint of The Haworth Press, Inc., 10 Alice Street, Binghamton, NY 13904-1580.

PUBLISHER'S NOTE
The development, preparation, and publication of this work has been undertaken with great care. However, the Publisher, employees, editors, and agents of The Haworth Press are not responsible for any errors contained herein or for consequences that may ensue from use of materials or information contained in this work. The Haworth Press is committed to the dissemination of ideas and information according to the highest standards of intellectual freedom and the free exchange of ideas. Statements made and opinions expressed in this publication do not necessarily reflect the views of the Publisher, Directors, management, or staff of The Haworth Press, Inc., or an endorsement by them.

Cover design by Kerry E. Mack.

Library of Congress Cataloging-in-Publication Data

The handbook of lesbian, gay, bisexual, and transgender public health : a practitioner's guide to service / Michael D. Shankle, editor.
    p. cm.
    Includes bibliographical references and index.
    ISBN-13: 978-1-56023-495-1 (hc. : alk. paper)
    ISBN-10: 1-56023-495-4 (hc. : alk. paper)
    ISBN-13: 978-1-56023-496-8 (pbk. : alk. paper)
    ISBN-10: 1-56023-496-2 (pbk. : alk. paper)
    1. Gays—Medical care—United States. 2. Bisexuals—Medical care—United States. 3. Transsexuals—Medical care—United States. 4. Health services accessibility—United States. 5. Discrimination in medical care—United States. I. Shankle, Michael D.
    [DNLM: 1. Homosexuality—United States. 2. Public Health—United States. 3. Bisexuality—United States. 4. Community Health Services—United States. 5. Health Services Accessibility—United States. 6. Transsexualism—United States. WA 300 H2365 2005]

RA564.9.H65H36 2005
362.1'086'60973—dc22

                           2005010626

To all my lesbian, gay, bisexual, and transgender
brothers and sisters who struggle each and every day
to overcome barriers to better health and a better life

and for all our lesbian, gay, bisexual, and transgender allies
for your dedication and support
in our struggle for equal and civil rights

and for all those who have provided us strong foundations
to advance our causes

and for those who have lost their lives
in the struggle along the way.

Whoever saves one life, saves the world entire.

Itzhak Stern

First they came for the
socialists, and I did not speak out
because I was not a socialist.

Then they came for the
trade unionists, and I did not speak out
because I was not a trade unionist.

Then they came for the Jews,
and I did not speak out
because I was not a Jew.

Then they came for me,
and there was no one left
to speak for me.

Pastor Martin Niemöller*

*Pastor Niemöller's quote is used by permission of Syracuse Cultural Workers. A poster, notecard, and bookmark are available with this quote from www. syrculturalworkers.com.

CONTENTS

ABOUT THE EDITOR

Michael D. Shankle, MPH, is a research specialist at the University of Pittsburgh, Graduate School of Public Health, Department of Infectious Diseases and Microbiology. He holds a master of public health degree from the University of Pittsburgh. From November 2001 to November 2003, Mr. Shankle served as chair of the Lesbian, Gay, Bisexual, Transgender (LGBT) Caucus of Public Health Workers, in official relations with the American Public Health Association. He is also a member of the University of Pittsburgh's Center for Research on Health and Sexual Orientation. Mr. Shankle's research interests include LGBT health issues, HIV prevention and young adults, and public health technology integration. He is committed to advancing research knowledge related to sexual minorities and is a founding board member of Lesbian, Gay, Bisexual, and Transgender Health, Education and Research Trust, Inc.

CONTRIBUTORS

Scott H. Arrowood, MSW, is a social worker with practice in family and children services, public health research, and community organization. His work in family services has included direct practice in foster care, foster parent recruitment and training, and supervision of case managers. His current practice in public health research includes HIV prevention planning, needs assessment, program development, and evaluation. He is on staff at the Department of Infectious Diseases and Microbiology at the Graduate School of Public Health, University of Pittsburgh.

Amy Baernstein, MD, is an assistant professor in the department of Medicine at the University of Washington. She attended Cornell University Medical College and completed her residency in Internal Medicine at the University of Washington. She is an attending physician in the Emergency Trauma Center, Harborview Medical Center, Seattle, Washington, and is a teacher in the University of Washington School of Medicine College Faculty. Her research interests include medical education and professionalism.

Rodger L. Beatty, PhD, LSW, is an assistant professor at the University of Pittsburgh Graduate School of Public Health, Department of Infectious Diseases and Microbiology, Communicable Diseases and Behavioral Health Sciences Program. Dr. Beatty served as president of the National Association of Addiction Professionals (NALGAP) for five years and is a founding faculty member of the Center for Research on Health and Sexual Orientation (CRHSO) and the Behavioral Health Sciences MPH Program. He has written book chapters and peer reviewed articles on LGBT substance use and HIV as well as facilitating the writing of Chapter 26, "Substance Abuse," for the *Healthy People 2010 Companion Document on LGBT Health.* In addition, he assisted in securing writers for and was a field reviewer of the Center for Substance Abuse Treatment's (CSAT) "Providers Introduction to Substance Abuse Treatment for LGBT Individuals." He is a member of the Steering Committee for the Institute for Research, Education and Training in Addictions (IRETA) and the CSAT contractor for the Northeast Addiction Technology Transfer Center. Dr. Beatty also is the chair of the Community Advisory Board for the University of Pittsburgh Pitt Treatment Evaluation Unit (PTEU) Adult AIDS Clinical Trials Group (AACTG).

Wendy B. Bostwick, PhD, MPH, just completed her doctorate in public health from the University of Illinois at Chicago. Her research interests include bisexual women's health, sexual identity stigma and its relationship to substance use and mental health outcomes, and the measurement of sexual orientation and sexual identity. She is currently a NIDA postdoctoral fellow at the University of Michigan Substance Abuse Research Center.

Kathleen R. Carrick, MSW, is currently a member of the Center for Research on Health and Sexual Orientation at the University of Pittsburgh. Ms. Carrick has completed the requirements for a PhD from the University of Pittsburgh School for Social Work. She is an adjunct instructor at Chatham College and believes that improving our understanding of diversity is a key component in preparing future health care professionals to meet the challenging demands of our health care system. She has worked in all aspects of direct service delivery, from grassroots activism to community mental health, to foster care, to inpatient psychiatric and hospital social work. Her focus for the past fourteen years has been primarily in trauma work. Ms. Carrick received her MSW in clinical social work from Smith College, and a BA in psychology from Chatham College in 1987.

Alwyn T. Cohall, MD, is an associate professor of Clinical Public Health and Pediatrics at Columbia University's Mailman School of Public Health and New York Presbyterian Hospital, where he is the director of the Harlem Health Promotion Center, one of thirty-three Prevention Research Centers funded by the Centers for Disease Control and Prevention. In addition, Dr. Cohall is the director of Project STAY (Services to Assist Youth), a clinical program, funded by the New York State Department of Health's AIDS Institute, that provides comprehensive medical and psychosocial services to high-risk and HIV-infected youth. He received his BA degree from Wesleyan University (1976), and his MD degree from the University of Medicine and Dentistry in New Jersey (1980). Following the completion of his pediatric residency at Montefiore Hospital (1983), Dr. Cohall completed a fellowship in adolescent medicine at Mt. Sinai Hospital (1984). He is board certified in both pediatrics and adolescent medicine, and during his professional career, has been instrumental in developing clinical care programs for youth in community centers, runaway/homeless shelters, and substance abuse residential treatment facilities. In particular, he has worked extensively with LGBTQ youth both as a service provider and as a member of various community advocacy groups.

Laurie Drabble, PhD, MSW, MPH, is an assistant professor at San Jose State University College of Social Work and is an affiliate associate scientist with the Alcohol Research Group (ARG) in Berkeley, California. Dr. Drabble has extensive experience as a researcher, consultant, and trainer in the alcohol and drug field, specializing in women's and LGBT issues. Among other projects, she is working with the Alcohol Research Group on studies related to alcohol, tobacco, and other drug consumption among lesbian, gay, and bisexual populations based on data from the National Alcohol Survey. Dr. Drabble has also served as cofacilitator for the Center for Substance Abuse Treatment (CSAT) national LGBT Workgroup and, over the past twenty years, has provided numerous trainings and conference presentations on culturally competent prevention and treatment services for LGBT communities. Dr. Drabble was co-coordinator for the first regional conference on "Prevention of Tabacco and Alcohol Problems in LGBT Communities" and has provided consultation in the development of several LGBT-specific substance abuse prevention programs in California. She has also authored several book chapters and journal articles related to alcohol, tobacco, and other drug use prevention and treatment in LGBT communities.

Patricia M. Dunn, JD, MSW, received a juris doctorate from the University of California at Davis and a master of social work with an emphasis in social policy, administration, and community development from Washington University in St. Louis, where she was a National Institute of Mental Health Primary Prevention fellow. She has worked for over fifteen years in policy and programmatic positions in public health. She has wide-ranging experience in research, analysis, and writing on health policy issues, as well as in program planning and development. Dunn has worked on behalf of diverse and marginalized communities, including lesbian, gay, bisexual, and transgender (LGBT) populations; immigrants; people living with HIV/AIDS; women; and low-income populations. Prior to starting her health policy consulting business, Ms. Dunn served as policy and program director for the Gay and Lesbian Medical Association. In this position, Patricia coordinated the collaborative development of the *Healthy People 2010 Companion Document for LGBT Health,* and worked on other LGBT health issues such as prevention and cessation of LGBT smoking, policy development, survey design and administration, health communication campaigns, and smoking cessation counseling training for providers. She was a member of the American Legacy Foundation's Priority Populations LGBT Experts Panel and consulted with the Tobacco Technical Assistance Consortium, including coordinating, writing, and editing the *National LGBTI Community Action Plan: Research, Prevention, and Cessation.* She worked with the CDC Office on Smoking and Health (CDC/OSH) on several projects, including coordination of the CDC/OSH Experts Panel on LGBT Smoking.

Joshua L. Ferris received his BA from the University of Pittsburgh in 2004. Josh was a lead organizer in the fight for domestic partner benefits at the University of Pittsburgh, with a victory in the fall of 2004. His is currently employed by the Service Employees International Union District 1199P. His research interests include the use of sexual identity in contemporary politics and the demonization of nonheterosexual practices in the ancient world. He is currently interested in documenting the history of queer people in Pittsburgh, Pennsylvania. Mr. Ferris is the former president of the Rainbow Alliance, and has been affiliated with League of Gay & Lesbian Voters; State of Pennsylvania Rights Coalition; Steel-City Stonewall Democrats; the Lambda Foundation; and America Votes. He was also a Lambda Foundation scholarship recipient in 2002.

Rob J. Fredericksen, MPH, is a lecturer at the Boston University School of Public Health, Department of International Health, where he teaches social and behavioral science, as well as courses in public health research and writing. Mr. Fredericksen received his master of public health in May 2000, concentrating in international health. He is also a PhD candidate at Boston University in the field of medical anthropology. Rob's areas of research interest include mental health, substance abuse prevention and treatment among the economically and/or socially marginalized, occupational health, and HIV/STD prevention and control. Areas of expertise include behavioral science, medical anthropology, study and intervention design, policy analysis, coalition building, and engaging hard-to-reach populations. Rob has social work experience with adults with chronic and acute psychiatric disabilities, sex workers, and youth living with HIV. He has acted as a development consultant for Massachusetts gay youth organizations, and currently serves on the executive committee of the Boston University Program for Lesbian, Gay, Bisexual, and Transgender Public Health Research.

Shawn L. Fultz, MD, MPH, is an assistant professor of medicine at Yale University School of Medicine, New Haven, Connecticut, and the VA Connecticut Healthcare System, West Haven. Dr. Fultz completed his undergraduate degree at Pennsylvania State University. He then went on to the University of Pittsburgh where he completed his medical degree (master of public health), internship and residency in internal medicine, and a general internal medicine fellowship. Dr. Fultz is a health services researcher whose primary focus is on the management of comorbid diseases in patients with HIV, particularly liver disease and anemia. Dr. Fultz is a former board member of the Gay and Lesbian Medical Associaltion and has lectured on the health care needs of sexual minority patients.

Kim W. Goodman, MSW, LCSW-C, earned her master of social work from Virginia Commonwealth University. She joined the University of Southern California's School of Social Work Field Education Faculty in 2004. She serves as the field education coordinator for the health concentration and first-year students at the University Park Campus. In addition to her coordinating duties, she teaches a first-year integrative seminar. Prior to joining the USC Field Education Faculty, Ms. Goodman spent four years serving as the director of client service at the Mautner Project, a national organization that serves women who partner with women (WPW) with cancer, their partners, and caregivers. In addition to providing direct client care, Ms. Goodman developed, implemented, and evaluated an LGBT smoking cessation program and a weekend health and healing retreat for WPW cancer survivors. She has presented at national conferences on topics such as LGBT smoking cessation, barriers to health care for WPW, and mind-body-spirit medicine. Ms. Goodman continues to educate MSW students on LGBT issues and is an active advocate for LGBT rights and equal access to health care.

Manuel Hernandez, MD, is the chairman of the Department of Emergency Medicine at Parkway Regional Medical Center in North Miami Beach, Florida, and serves as an area medical officer for Sterling Healthcare Corporation. Dr. Hernandez is board certified in emergency medicine and an assistant professor of family medicine at NOVA Southeastern University College of Osteopathic Medicine in Fort Lauderdale, Florida. He also serves as president of the Lesbian, Gay, Bisexual and Transgender Health, Education and Research Trust (LGBT HEART), a national nonprofit dedicated to promoting LGBT health through the advancement of scholarship and research. Dr. Hernandez's primary interests in LGBT health focus on advanced planning, LGBT consumer satisfaction with health care systems, and recreational drug use by the LGBT community. He frequently provides talks nationwide to medical students, residents, and other health care professionals about LGBT health. A graduate of the University of Pittsburgh School of Medicine, Dr. Hernandez is currently pursuing an MBA at the University of California at Irvine.

Daryl Herrschaft, the deputy director of the Human Rights Campaign's WorkNet, has overseen HRC WorkNet, the workplace project of the Human Rights Campaign Foundation since 1998. In this capacity, he monitors and evaluates corporate policies surrounding gay, lesbian, bisexual, and transgender employees, consumers, and investors. In 2002, he launched HRC's annual Corporate Equality Index, a simple and effective tool that rates corporate policies and practices on several key criteria that impact LGBT people. He is also lead author of the HRC Foundation's annual report, "The State of the Workplace for Lesbian, Gay, Bisexual and Transgender Americans." Herrschaft has directly consulted with dozens of major corporations seeking to implement domestic partner benefits and/or nondiscrimination policies. He has presented HRC findings to diverse audiences including the Conference Board, the Society for Human Resource Management, and the New York City Council. He is frequently called upon by national and local media and has appeared on CNN and CNBC. He is a member of the Massachusetts-based Linkage Inc.'s Diversity Summit Advisory Board and the board of the San Francisco–based Out & Equal Workplace Advocates. Before joining HRC, he was a research associate at the Urban Institute. He holds a bachelor's degree from George Washington University.

Tonda L. Hughes, PhD, is an associate professor at the University of Illinois at Chicago (UIC) College of Nursing and School of Public Health, and the research director for the UIC National Center of Excellence in Women's Health. Dr. Hughes received her master's degree in community mental health from the University of Kentucky and her PhD from the University of Illinois at Chicago, College of Nursing. She was awarded individual National Research Service Awards for both her doctoral and her postdoctoral research focusing on women's use of alcohol and other drugs. Her funded research over the past ten years has focused on issues related to mental health and substance use among lesbians. She has published extensively on these issues and has addressed numerous local, national, and international audiences. Her current study, Sexual Identity and Drinking, is a longitudinal project funded by the National Institute of Alcohol Abuse and Alcoholism. Dr. Hughes provided expert testimony to the Institute of Medicine's Committee on Lesbian Health Research Priorities in 1997 and has served on several national workgroup or consensus panels, including Substance Abuse Treatment: Addressing the Specific Needs of Women; Center for Substance Abuse Treatment (CSAT); Substance Abuse and Mental Health Services Administration; Cultural Competence in Substance Abuse Treatment; and Lesbian, Gay, Bisexual, and Transgender Substance Abuse Treatment, CSAT.

Joyce Hunter, DSW, a research scientist at the HIV Center for Clinical & Behavioral Studies/New York State Psychiatric Institute and Columbia University, is codirector fo the Community Collaborative Core and Principal Investigator of "Working It Out," an intervention program for LGB adolescents. Dr. Hunter is an assistant clinical professor at Columbia University's Schools of Psychiatry and Public Health. Dr. Hunter has been a clinician and human rights activist for over thirty years, specializing in issues of youth, women, the LGBT communities, and HIV/AIDS. She is a founding member of the Hetrick-Martin Institute Board and cofounder of its Harvey Milk High School. In 1979, she co-coordinated the first National Lesbian/Gay March on Washington and is the former president of the National Lesbian & Gay Health Association (1991-1996). Dr. Hunter served on the Human Rights Commission of New York City, 1983 to 1988, and the New York State Governor's Task Force on Lesbian and Gay Concerns. A former Governing Council member of the International AIDS Society, Dr. Hunter is a founding member of the IAS Women's Caucus and is IAS Liaison to the Caucus. She has co-coordinated symposiums at several World AIDS Conferences. She is also cochair of Global AIDS Action Network. Dr. Hunter has conducted clinical training for professionals and students in health care, mental health, and education. She serves on the editorial board of the *Journal of Gay and Lesbian Social Services,* is a reviewer for *Families in Society Journal,* and consulting editor of *The Encyclopedia of AIDS.*

JoAnne G. Keatley, MSW, received her master of social welfare degree from the University of California, Berkeley. She is the project director at Health Studies for People of Color, where she directs multiple NIDA and SAMHSA transgender projects and manages a diverse transgender staff of fourteen. She is proud to be a Latina woman and is bilingual in English and

Spanish. JoAnne served as a member of the Ryan White HIV Planning Council Santa Clara County from 1995-1998. Currently she is a board member of New Leaf and SalvaSIDA. JoAnne is chair and a founding member of San Francisco Transgender Empowerment Advocacy and Mentorship (SFTEAM). JoAnne is also an active committee member of the CSAT Cultural Competency and Diversity Network, the CSAT National Latino Coalition, the UCSF Chancellor's Advisory committee on LGBT issues, TransPRIDE, and the CDC working group on Transgender Health. JoAnne received the CAPS International Women's Day Award in 2000, the UCSF Chancellor's Award for LGBT Leadership in 2001, and the American Immigration Law Foundation Community Service Award in 2004. JoAnne lives with her nine-year-old boxer, Twiggers, in Oakland. They both enjoy hiking in the Oakland Hills, camping, and fun times at home.

Nancy J. Kennedy, DrPH, has over thirty years of professional and personal experience in the fields of substance abuse and mental health. Her work experiences have included state government, nonprofit organizations, academia, and the federal government. When Dr. Kennedy worked at the Health Resources and Services Administration in the Department of Health and Human Services (HHS), she was the first HHS employee to work full-time on LGBT issues. Her main accomplishment was writing and editing *Healthy People 2010: A Companion Document for LGBT Health.* She is an active board member of the Association of the Clinicians for the Underserved (ACU). Dr. Kennedy has a doctorate in public health from the Department of Mental Hygiene, Bloomberg School of Public Health, Johns Hopkins University in Baltimore, Maryland, and also a master of public health degree from the University of North Carolina. Her multiple publications span a quarter of a century, including both peer-review journals as well as popular press, and she is passionate about preventing and treating behavioral health issues, especially for LGBT populations.

Sheila C. Kirk, MD, the director of research for Persad Center, Pittsburgh, Pennsylvania, is a board-certified gynecologic surgeon and endocrinologist. Her clinical experience in transgender care includes GRS and related surgeries; HIV diagnosis and management; endocrinologic concerns of the MTF and FTM individual, and sexually transmitted disease management. Her unique position as the only transsexual surgeon who is experienced in trans-related surgeries and who has developed and directed a full-service transgender surgical and medical facility provides her with valuable insight into the health care needs of the transgender population. As an author and lecturer, she has written numerous books and articles on transgender medical and surgical care and has lectured extensively at both professional and transgender venues. Dr. Kirk was the first transsexual surgeon elected to the Harry Benjamin International Gender Dysphoria Association (HBIGDA) Board of Directors. She also serves on their Standards of Care Committee, HIV and AIDS Committee, and the Advocacy and Liaison Committee. Dr.

Kirk is currently serving her second term as secretary/treasurer for the organization. She also serves on the editorial board of the *International Journal of Transgenderism* and is a member of GLMA (Gay and Lesbian Medical Association).

Claudette Kulkarni, PhD, is a Jungian psychotherapist in private practice and at the Women's Center of Beaver County, Beaver, Pennsylvania, working with victims of domestic violence and adult survivors of childhood abuse. She spent nearly fifteen years as a clinical therapist at Persad Center, Pittsburgh, Pennsylvania, a mental health center serving the LGBT community, where she had responsibility for the Transgender Team. She was awarded her PhD in depth psychology from The Union Institute and is a member of the Association of Women in Psychology. Among her publications are *Lesbians and Lesbianisms: A Post-Jungian Perspective* (Routledge, 1997) and "Radicalizing Jungian Theory," a chapter in *Contemporary Perspectives on Psychotherapy and Homosexualities* (London: Free Association Press, 1998).

Walter J. Lear, MD, MS, is the president of the Institute of Social Medicine and Community Health. For more than twenty years before he founded the institute in 1970 and became a medical historian, he served as a public health and medial services administrator and as a health and community advocate. His history research and writing focus was on the U.S. Health Left—its people, organizations, publications, movements, and issues. His political activism began in 1945 as a medial student and has included substantial work in the peace movement, the civil rights movement, and the gay and lesbian liberation movement. Lear received his bachelor of science degree from Harvard College in 1943 and his MD from the Long Island College of Medicine in 1946. In 1948, he recieved his MS in hospital administration from the Columbia University School of Public Health. In 1975, while serving as Pennsylvania's Southeast Regional commissioner for Health Services, Lear came out publicly as a gay man. That year, he became involved in campaigns to promote a proposed Philadelphia law banning discrimination against people because of their sexual orientation. He remained active in that fight until the city council's passage of the Gay Rights Bill in 1982. He has cofounded, cochaired, served on the board of directors, or played other key leadership roles in dozens of national and local lesbian and gay, medical, peace/antiwar, and socialist-left organizations.

Rosemary Madl-Young, PhD, CRNS, has been in human services for over thirty years. Currently, she is the director of continuous quality improvement and staff development for Gaudenzia, Inc. Dr. Madl-Young has trained nationally in the areas of women in treatment, lesbian issues in treatment, addictions, co-occurring disorders, and cultural diversity. She served on the American Nurses' Association, Advisory Board of the Center for Ethics and Human Rights, Washington, DC. She has been on the Pennsylvania Department of Health Task Force addressing Sexual Minorities in

Treatment, Women in Treatment, and HIV/AIDS. She has been involved with the issues of HIV/AIDS for the past twenty-five years, both in clinical work and in community building and advocacy. Dr. Madl-Young has been an assistant professor at the Lincoln University Master in Human Services Program for the past twenty-seven years. She is the past recipient of the Woman of the Year Award, AA/EEO Program–U.S. Postal Services, the Mayor's Award for Distinguished Public Services, and the Phi Gamma Mu Distinguished Professor award from the Graduate Chapter–Lincoln University, Master in Human Services Award.

Patricia D. Mail, PhD, MPH, is a graduate of the Yale School of Public Health and holds degrees in physical education (Arizona, Smith College), cultural anthropology (Arizona), and community health (Maryland). She served as a commissioned officer in the U.S. Public Health Service for twenty-seven years, working with American Indians, health manpower shortages, HIV/AIDS programs, and in research focusing on alcohol and substance misuse while assigned to the National Insitutes of Health. A forty-year member of the American Public Health Association, she has served in various Section and Caucus capacities, as a member of the executive board, and as president of APHA. She has been active in a variety of other professional associations. She has held teaching positions at Seattle University and the Puyallup Tribe's Medicine Creek College. She has also worked on Indian health issues at Oregon Health and Sciences University and the Addictive Behaviors Research Center, University of Washington. She volunteers for work with gay and lesbian organizations in communities where she lives, including political office candidate interviews. While in Maryland, she and her partner helped build an MCC church in suburban Maryland for LGBT worship.

Gerald P. Mallon, MSW, DSW, is an associate professor and the executive director of the National Resource Center for Family Centered Practice and Permanency Planning at the Hunter College School of Social Work in New York City. He is also the former associate executive director of Green Chimneys Children's Services in New York City, the first mainstream child welfare agency in the country to develop specialized residential programs for lesbian, gay, bisexual, transgender, and questioning youth. For more than twenty-nine years, Dr. Mallon has been a child welfare practitioner, advocate, and researcher. He is the author or editor of seventeen books and numerous peer-reviewed publications in professional journals. His most recent publications are the book *Gay Men Choosing Parenthood,* published by Columbia University Press, and the book *Facilitating Permanency for Youth: A Toolbox for Child Welfare Professionals,* from the Child Welfare League of America.

George Marcelle is an information, communications, and social marketing professional with more than thirty years of experience in substance abuse. He is the communications director for ORC Macro/Social & Health Ser-

xxvi   THE HANDBOOK OF LGBT PUBLIC HEALTH

vices, Ltd., and for its Materials Development and Marketing Support contract with the Substance Abuse and Mental Health Services Administration's Center for Substance Abuse Prevention. Since 2003 he has chaired the California Alcohol and Drug Programs Department's LGBT Constituent Committe and coordinated the committee's May 2004 report to the state, *Invisible Californians*. George has been an active member of the National Association of Lesbian and Gay Addiction Professionsals throughout its twenty-five-year history, has held offices on its board of directors, and cochaired several of its annual conferences. He has written numerous articles, presentations, chapters, and online informational pieces on LGBT substance abuse topics, is a past chair of the Substance Abuse Librarians and Information Specialists, and a member of the European Association of Libraries and Information Services on Alcohol and Drugs. In 1987, NALGAP honored him as a "national pioneer" in LGBT substance abuse; SALIS honored him at its 1998 conference; and in 2003 the National Prevention Network presented him with its annual Award of Excellence.

Nina Markovic, PhD, is an associate professor at the University of Pittsburgh. Dr. Markovic is an epidemiologist and investigator on the ESTHER Project, a clinical study of cardiovascular risk factors among lesbian women. She is also codirector of the Center for Research on Health and Sexual Orientation at the University of Pittsburgh.

Jeanne M. Marrazzo, MD, MPH, is an associate professor in the Division of Allergy and Infectious Diseases at the University of Washington in Seattle, and the medical director of the Seattle STD/HIV Prevention Training Center. She has led several studies on health outcomes of interest to lesbian and bisexual women, including infection with human papillomavirus, genital herpes, and bacterial vaginosis, and barriers to STD-related risk assessment and routine pap smear screening. Her current research interests include etiology and management of bacterial vaginosis, diagnosis of chlamydial infection, and efficacy of vaginal microbicides in preventing women's acquisition of HIV and STDs. Dr. Marrazzo is a fellow of the American College of Physicians and serves on several national advisory boards relevant to women's health.

Matthew B. Moyer, MPH, is the director and principal investigator of the Youth Empowerment Project and a researcher at the University of Pittsburgh, Graduate School of Public Health, Department of Infectious Diseases and Microbiology. At the University of Pittsburgh, Mr. Moyer worked on several HIV/STD prevention programs reaching gay men in the Pitt Men's Sudy, as well as working with adolescent and young adult populations throughout the state of Pennsylvania, involving them in both research and evaluation. Mr. Moyer has served on several community boards and special LGBT advocate groups, and continues his membership on the Lesbian, Gay, Bisexual, Transgender Caucus of Public Health Workers in official relations with the American Public Health Association. Mr. Moyer continues working in public health at Children's Hospital Los Angeles, coordinating an adolescent pregnancy prevention program reaching high school youth in south Los Angeles.

Robert C. Preston Jr., MBA, holds a master's of business administration in management degree as well as a bachelor's in marketing. He has spent the past seven years in human resources roles as both a staff and contract recruiter. This has allowed him to bring to the project a unique perspective across industries on employment and attrition. His research pursuits are in the areas of employment best practices and work/life balance. He resides with his life partner of six years in a small community near Palm Springs, California.

Scott D. Rhodes, PhD, MPH, CHES, is a behavioral scientist whose research focuses on the integration of community development and health promotion and disease prevention in rural and urban communities. He is an assistant professor in the Department of Public Health Sciences, with an adjunct faculty appointment in the Maya Angelou Research Center on Minority Health, at Wake Forest University School of Medicine in Winston-Salem, North Carolina. His research explores sexual health, HIV and sexually transmitted disease (STD) prevention, and other health disparities among vulnerable communities. Dr. Rhodes has extensive experience working with self-identifying gay and bisexual men; men who have sex with men (MSM); Latino communities; urban African-American adolescents; persons living with HIV and AIDS; and men of color. He has experience in quantitative and qualitative data collection and analysis techniques; the design, implementation, and evaluation of multiple-level interventions for improved health outcomes; community-capacity development; community-based participatory research (CBPR); the application of behavioral theory; community-campus partnerships; photovoice as a methodology of participatory action research (PAR); lay health advisor approaches; the exploration of sociocultural determinants of health; and Internet research, including data collection, intervention delivery, and evaluation.

James P. Riddel Jr., RN, MS, CPNP, is a registered nurse and board-certified pediatric nurse practitioner. He has been in practice for the past fifteen years. Currently Mr. Riddel is in his third year of doctoral study at the University of California, San Francisco. The topic of his research is the genetics of von Willebrand disease. Mr. Riddel's clinical experience has included pediatric emergency nursing, clinical research coordinator for the pediatric HIV program, and presently he is the program coordinator for the Hempohilia Treatment Center at Children's Hospital & Research Center at Oakland.

Randall L. Sell, ScD, is an assistant professor at Columbia University's Mailman School of Public Health. Dr. Sell's research focuses on defining and measuring sexual orientations, and sampling sexual minorities for public health research. Dr. Sell has researched and published on the history and best practices of sampling homosexuality, has created an assessment of sexual orientation, and was one of the first to estimate the prevalence of lesbians, gays, and bisexuals in a probability sample of the United States, United Kingdom, and France. Dr. Sell has also examined and reported on the importance of routinely including sexual orientation variables in public health data collection activities, and he serves as a consultant to an ever-increasing number of surveys and programs that have begun to collect sexual orientation data.

M. Kate Shirah, MPH, an instructor in the Department of Health Behavior and Health Education (HBHE) at the School of Public Health at the University of North Carolina at Chapel Hill (UNC–CH), coteaches two core courses for HBHE master's students: Foundations of Health Behavior & Health Education Practice and Action-Oriented Community Diagnosis. In addition, Ms. Shirah serves as the field coordinator, assisting master's students in fulfilling their practicum requirements, and project manager of Men as Navigators (MAN) for Health, a community-based participatory research project to improve the health and well-being of African-American and Latino men in Chatham, Orange, and Wake counties. She also is the faculty advisor for the School of Public Health Lesbian, Gay, Bisexual, and Transgender (LGBT) Caucus. Ms. Shirah currently sits on the board of directors of the Lesbian Resource Center of Durham, North Carolina, and the Advisory Council for Project Rainbow Net, a program of the NC Coalition Against Domestic Violence, to address domestic violence issues in the LGBT community, Ms. Shirah regularly conducts community presentations and trainings on LGBT health issues. Ms. Shirah received her bachelor's of science in public health in health policy and administration and her master's of public health in health behavior and health education from UNC–CH. Her primary public health interests include health disparities, with a focus on community-level practice and research, and community, organizational, and social change in addressing LGBT health issues.

Vincent Michael Bernard Silenzio, MD, MPH, holds joint appointments as an assistant professor in the Departments of Family Medicine, Psychiatry, and Community and Preventive Medicine at the University of Rochester, and Sociomedical Sciences at Columbia University. He is an honors graduate of the University of Pennsylvania, received his MD/MPH from the UMDNJ–Robert Wood Johnson Medical School, and completed residency and fellowship training at the Jefferson University Hospital in Philadelphia. Dr. Silenzio has been nationally active in the area of LGBT health research. He is a founding member of the Columbia Program in Lesbian, Gay, Bisexual, and Transgender Health Research in the Mailman School of Public Health. He also served as co–editor in chief of the *Journal of the Gay and Lesbian Medical Association,* and as a member of the GLMA board of directors. He was co-author and editor of the White Paper on LGBT Health for the Department of Health and Human Services, which helped lead to the *Healthy People 2010 Companion Document on LGBT Health*. Dr. Silenzio is a practicing academic physician, medical ethnographer, and medical educator. In addition to his full-time academic responsibilities, he practices full-spectrum primary care, with an emphasis on sexual minority families and with a special interest in transgender health. His research interests center on the medical anthropology and health effects of same-sex sexual expression among ethnic, racial, and other social groups in the United States and abroad. His current research focuses on the prevention of suicide and related phenomena in sexual minority adolescents and young adults.

Anthony J. Silvestre, PhD, is a social worker whose practice is research and community organizing. He is an associate professor in the Department of Infectious Diseases and Microbiology at the Graduate School of Public Health at the University of Pittsburgh and is the director of the University's Center for Research on Health and Sexual Orientation. Dr. Silvestre is a coinvestigator of the Pitt Men's Study, part of the Multicenter AIDS Cohort Study (MACS), a twenty-year-old study of HIV among MSM. He is the principal investigator of the PA Prevention Project, an HIV-related program that includes needs assessment, evaluation, community capacity building among racial/ethnic and LGBT communities, and prevention planning and implementation in rural and urban Pennsylvania, excluding Philadelphia. Dr. Silvestre is also a coinvestigator on EXPORT and leads the HIV core where he works closely with African-American community members to design and implement an HIV prevention research project. He has published articles on marketing HIV education and research, health and prevention capacity building in communities, evaluating HIV programs and public counseling and test sites, and LGBT issues. He has founded and served with many national, state, and local community organizations including HIV service organizations, LGBT mental health and youth services, and advocacy organizations. He also chaired the Governor's Council for Sexual Minorities, created in Pennsylvania in 1976.

Helen A. Smith is currently finishing a master's degree in human sexuality studies from San Francisco State University and working toward a master's degree in public health at the University of Pittsburgh. She completed her undergraduate degree in anthropology at Pennsylvania State University. Helen is currently a graduate student researcher for the ESTHER (Epidemiologic **ST**udy of **HE**alth **R**isk in Women) study. Her research interests include women's health, LGBT health, maternal child health, and rural health.

Jodi B. Sperber, MSW, MPH, is a manager of client analytics and operations for Health Dialog Services Corporation, a leading provider of telephonic health coaching and data analytic services that help health plans and employers improve health care quality and reduce health care costs. Ms. Sperber previously served as the director of the Gay, Lesbian, Bisexual, and

Transgender Health Access Project, the nation's only statewide, state-funded program dedicated to eradicating disparities in access to health care and social services for LGBT populations, and John Snow, Inc., an internationally recognized public health consulting firm. She has more than ten years of experience in conducting and managing a range of research and technical assistant projects related to health care and public policy, lesbian, gay, bisexual, and transgender health, and related issues. Her areas of technical expertise include needs assessment, technical assistance, survey instrument design, evaluation, and qualitative research methodology and analysis. Ms. Sperber is involved in a wide range of activities, including the LGBT Caucus of Health Workers (a part of the American Public Health Association), sitting on the board of the Hesed Foundation, and serving on the LGBT Advisory Board of the American Cancer Society. Ms. Sperber earned both her MSW and MPH at Boston University. She completed undergraduate work at the State University of New York at Geneseo.

Katherine (Kat) L. Turner, MPH, is a senior training and services advisor at Ipas, an international nongovernmental organization working to advance women's sexual and reproductive health and rights. At Ipas, she leads the development of organizational training vision, strategies, curricula, and networks and organizes international capacity-building workshops for staff, consultants, and lead trainers. She provides technical assistance to other units and national teams on training design, methodologies and tools, service delivery improvement strategies, adolescent and STI/HIV initiatives, and reproductive health counseling. Ms. Turner earned a bachelor of arts in psychology, a certificate with honors in women's studies, a certificate in nonprofit management from Duke University, and a master of public health (MPH) from the University of North Carolina at Chapel Hill (UNC–CH). She remains active in the Duke University women's studies program and serves as an adjunct instructor in the School of Public Health at UNC–CH, where she mentors and trains master's students in the Department of Health Behavior and Health Education (HBHE). Ms. Turner was a founding member of the board of directors of the Lesbian Resource Center of Durham, North Carolina, and has served on the board of directors of several North Carolina–based nonprofit organizations addressing LGBT and women's health. Ms. Turner has been working since 1986 in the United States and internationally as a sexual and reproductive health educator, counselor, trainer, program manager, and community leader. She has developed, implemented, and evaluated numerous health education, training, and research programs and published training curricula and articles on her work. She has received awards for her leadership and public health service.

Wayne L. Wilson, MPH, is the program coordinator for HealthWorks, a program of Triangle Community Works (Raleigh, North Carolina, www.tcworks.org), an all-volunteer community-based organization promoting healthy LGBT communities. HealthWorks provides resources, referrals, and training to health care providers, health office staff, and LGBT communities and their allies. Since 2000 he has worked at Family Health International, most recently as senior advisor for site identification and development supporting global HIV-prevention clinical trials, and previously as community program manager for the HIV Prevention Trial Network (HPTN), where he coordinated the HPTN community involvement program and assisted the development and maintenance of international community advisory boards (CABs) for HIV-prevention clinical trials. Wayne's areas of expertise include behavioral epidemiology, behavior change theory, human sexuality issues, STI issues, popular education techniques, community mobilization, research ethics, and training development/implementation and evaluation. He co-authored "Research Ethics Training Curriculum for Community Representatives." He holds a public health master's degree from the University of North Carolina at Chapel Hill with a focus on health behavior and health education. His previous work experience includes the U.S. National AIDS and STD Hotlines as shift manager, and North Carolina State government as a community health educator and the state's first coordinator for HIV Prevention Community Planning. He also worked for PPD International as project manager, coordinating patient recruitment and Phase III/IV pharmaceutical clinical trials. Wayne's international work has solidified his passion for creating healthy LGBT environments, and he commits his volunteer work to support efforts locally and abroad.

Leland J. Yee, PhD, MPH, is an infectious desease epidemiologist at the University of Pittsburgh, where the main focus of his research concerns viral hepatitis infections. In addition to clinical aspects of viral hepatitis infections, such as identifying ways to improve treatment outcomes in hepatitis B and hepatitis C, he has an interest in the public health prevention of viral hepatitis and has worked to identify ways to improve hepatitis A and hepatitis B vaccination uptake, particularly in communities that are adversely affected by these infections. Much of his research has been conducted in the context of understanding and improving the health disparities that surround these infections. Dr. Yee is actively involved in trying to identify mechanisms that account for racial differences in treatment outcomes for hepatitis C virus infection. As an epidemiologist, Dr. Yee also has an interest in the application of new methods, such as the use of electronic media, including the Internet, to epidemiologic research.

Foreword

I am pleased to contribute this foreword for the first ever *Handbook of LGBT Public Health: A Practitioner's Guide to Service*. In order to achieve equal health outcomes for our community we will need to not only do more in the twenty-first century but also to proceed quite differently. For many, LGBT health refers only to HIV and AIDS; however, nothing could be further from the truth. Although HIV and AIDS continue to be of major concern, improving LGBT health is hampered at all levels by a general lack of knowledge and appreciation for the extent of the problems facing this population.

It is an established fact that members of the LGBT community have significant health disparities in areas such as substance abuse and teen suicide, to cite just two examples. In many other areas, such as transsexual health, information is either sparse or completely absent. Although Healthy People 2010, the federal government's roadmap for prevention, included several health objectives that address LGBT health, virtually none of these objectives included strategies to collect data that might be used in measuring progress toward accomplishment of these goals. Consequently, we may still find ourselves without critical information in future years.

In order to address barriers to better health, a broader recognition must develop that differences in health status do exist. The "White Paper on LGBT Health," commissioned by the Health Resources and Services Administration (HRSA) and precursor to the Healthy People Companion Document on LGBT Health, identified numerous areas (including health access, hate-crime violence, substance abuse, and others) where it appears the LGBT community suffers disparities in health outcomes in comparison to the general population. One major system disparity identified is the lack of research and survey findings to clearly document what is known. Much of the funding for research by the National Institutes of Health and other federal agencies is viewed only through the prism of HIV and AIDS. Also, most federal- and state-level surveys, such as the National Health and Nutrition Examination Survey (NHANES), the National Health Interview Survey (NHIS), and the Behavioral Risk Factor Survey, currently collect few if any data that inform us about LGBT health.

Another systemic problem is that when we do have information that informs public health and individual patient practices, translation is slow to occur. An example would be medical evidence on human papilloma virus and the increasing incidence of rectal cancer, with the resultant recommendation for rectal pap smears in sexually active gay men. Despite this information, the number of practitioners who now incorporate this recommendation into their practice is estimated to be still quite small.

Despite these and other shortcomings, opportunities abound for us to address and improve LGBT health. The United States Public Health Service agencies, as well as state and local public health departments, could with few or no additional resources place LGBT health on the public roadmap to better health. Government at all levels could create offices of LGBT health, similar to what has been done in women's health, to focus efforts on reducing the health disparities. These efforts could catalyze a more systematic look at what we do and do not know and what can be done about it. Efforts in data collection by the National Institutes of Health, the National Center for Health Statistics, and state and local health departments could incorporate questions on LGBT health in studies and surveys and greatly enhance our body of knowledge. Public health agencies could take these actions with minimal reallocation of resources and help us leap decades forward in acknowledging and beginning to solve LGBT disparities. Such moves would also give license and creditability to look at other factors that affect LGBT health, such as cultural competency, and to address issues too long in the proverbial closet, such as teen suicide among gay or questioning youth.

While I was administrator of HRSA, the agency identified immediate and concrete ways that many of its programs, from rural health to maternal and child health, could take positive steps to not only put LGBT health on the radar screen but to empower "straight colleagues" to focus more of their interest and effort on these issues. LGBT health, although initially eliminated from an agency health disparities report, was included in the final document. Other agencies could take similar steps within their current activities. For example, the Agency for Health Care Research and Quality could make LGBT health an integral part of the "Clinical Guide to Preventive Services," and the Centers for Disease Control and Prevention could incorporate LGBT health into their "Community Guide to Preventive Services." These are just a few examples of current vehicles that could be used to promote better LGBT health.

Public health is about populations and, I believe, about equality. The LGBT population has in many ways been invisible and, I would argue, never equal when measured in health access and health outcomes. I encourage all who read this publication to think of LGBT health when you consider issues of health access, outcomes, and disparities, and to search for ways to make these issues not a separate effort but an integral part of the public campaign for a healthier global society and a healthier America.

Claude Earl Fox, MD, MPH
Director, Johns Hopkins Urban Health Institute;
Professor, Johns Hopkins Bloomberg School of Public Health

Preface

This publication is designed to provide readers with a unique focus on lesbian, gay, bisexual, and transgender (LGBT) public health. In recent years, LGBT health has emerged as a vibrant area of research and practice. Books and journals have flooded the literary market in an effort to increase our knowledge of this underserved and often unrecognized community. Our design is to assist individuals to integrate fragmented LGBT research into their practices and services. A primary goal is to assist individuals in moving beyond the current deficits afflicting this minority community and begin focusing on effective methods to overcome these shortcomings. We will examine the resiliency and protective factors that have assisted this disenfranchised community in surviving and emerging from the closet of isolation and inadequate services.

The contributors and I share the common goals of offering positive direction for practitioners (clinicians, medical doctors, nurses, dentists, public health professionals, community-based agencies and organizations, social workers) who are desperate for guidance in methods to assure a healthy community for all individuals. In these pages we will attempt to provide practical theories and solutions for overcoming the problems and disparities experienced by the LGBT community on a daily basis in this country.

The structure of the publication follows the Institute of Medicine's (2002) *Future of the Public's Health in the 21st Century* model for assuring conditions for population health. This model is crafted around the idea that to achieve or assure conditions of health for any population requires the collaborative efforts of public and private agencies, as well as many community-based organizations and individuals. Although public health is often thought of as being the responsibility only of governmental infrastructure, we must ensure the health of our communities by stepping up to the plate and taking an active role in moving beyond minimal standards and practices. The model indicates that in order to achieve true conditions for population health, we must look at the influences of academia, the community, our health care delivery system, governmental and public health infrastructure, our employers and businesses, and the media. All of these groups play an important role in the determinants of LGBT health. Academic institutions train practitioners; the health care delivery system maintains our health and well-being and provides access to our complex health care system; governmental and public health infrastructures create laws, policies, and procedures that affect health and access to health-related services; employers and businesses influence our economics, workplace environments, and health-promotion activities; the media assists in shaping public opinion, health knowledge, and behaviors; and, finally, the community plays a multitude of roles in promoting and assuring health (IOM, 2002).

The book begins with providing readers with a context in which to better understand the relationship between LGBT health and public health (Part I). The materials describe the LGBT community, provide a historical framework for LGBT public health, and outline the current status of LGBT research. The remaining sections utilize the model outline in the IOM publication but focus on what we know about the particular target areas and provide readers with the practical solutions for altering the system to make services more LGBT friendly and supportive. Part II utilizes the experience of researchers in improving academic institutions and continuing education programs by incorporating LGBT cultural competency. Part III targets the specific segments of the LGBT community (lesbian and bisexual women, gay and bisexual men, and transgender individuals). These chapters highlight the major health issues afflicting these broad segments of the community. Part IV is dedicated to the health care delivery system and provides practitioners with guidance in overcoming barriers to health care access while highlighting the special health needs of LGBT substance users, youth and young adults, and the aging community. Part V provides readers with strategies for improving city, county, state, and national public health infrastructures. This section also outlines how many policies affect the LGBT community and its health. Part VI focuses on how to influence employers and businesses in creating safer, more productive work environments for LGBT individuals while illustrating many issues that may affect the business community. Finally, Part VII addresses the many dimensions of media and its intersections with LGBT health, including influencing mainstream media, addressing health in LGBT media, challenging target marketing, and navigating through the evolving world of LGBT Internet resources.

This book outlines many of the major issues affecting the health of the LGBT community, provides vignettes of actual situations experienced by members of the community, highlights case studies that can be adapted to make a medical practice more accepting and welcoming, and identifies resources and community partners to assist agencies in becoming better providers of public health to the LGBT community. This publication is not intended to be an all-encompassing resource. Instead, it is just a starting point, as entire books could be written on the topic of any single chapter.

REFERENCE

Institute of Medicine. (2002). *The future of the public's health in the 21st century.* Washington, DC: The National Academies Press.

Acknowledgments

I express my sincerest appreciation to

The contributors for their time and dedication to this project;
Drs. Anthony J. Silvestre and Rodger L. Beatty for their tremendous support and mentoring;
Regina Yuhaniak and Nicole Pirain for their technical support; and
Matthew Allen Scruggs, my partner, for his continued encouragement and love.

PART I:
INTRODUCTORY MATERIALS

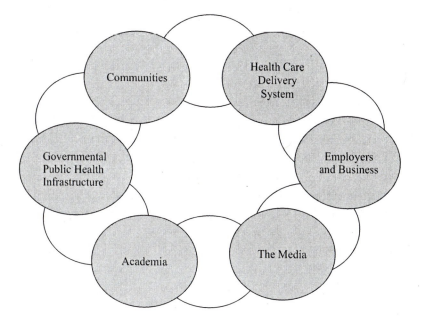

1

Chapter 1

The Nomenclature of the Community: An Activist's Perspective

Joshua L. Ferris

INTRODUCTION

The lesbian, gay, bisexual, and transgender community is an extraordinarily diverse group of people. Along with the community comes an alphabet soup of names and terms. Terms such as *LGBT, GLBT, queer, homosexual,* and *gay and lesbian* can be used interchangeably. The importance of this nomenclature rests on the individual addressing the community and his or her personal identity and politics. Likewise, one should not assume that these terms completely capture everyone who identifies as LGBT. Recently, while attending a conference concerning this population, I overheard the term GLBTQQCSI (gay, lesbian, bisexual, transgender, queer, questioning, confused, supportive, and intersexed). This acronym was clearly alarming, but it should not frighten people from attempting to learn and use much of the jargon associated with the LGBT community at present. This term was merely a way for the conference official to include a very diverse group of individuals. Terms are not the foundation of any community, but nonetheless vocabulary is quite relevant when attempting to address and target a community for disease prevention and health promotion.

For effective health advocates, terminology is an essential part of their ability to connect with the community. It is a matter of personal opinion for an individual to decide for himself or herself whether to use the newest and freshest terms or whether the terms he or she is using are the most effective to address the targeted population. Those working with the community tend to use LGBT or GLBT. For the sake of writing, LGBT will be consistently used henceforth, because it is a commonly recognized term and it is the preferred parlance of this book.

What is the LGBT community?
Who are its members?
What is its function in the greater societal model?

3

These are a few very broad and complex questions that arise for health officials when they begin to work with the LGBT community. Currently, almost everyone is familiar with the idea of someone identifying as LGBT. It may not be a personal or close relationship, but most people have heard of NBC's *Will & Grace,* Ellen DeGeneres, or MTV's *The Real World.* LGBT people are all over the airwaves and are part of most families' television-watching lineup.

It could be argued that media exposure has been one of the most beneficial changes for the LGBT rights movement. People are now more comfortable with the LGBT community than they were twenty years ago. As great as this is, an unheard disclaimer accompanies all of this mainstream attention. Television is not the flagship for the LGBT community (or any group, for that matter). The fact that all of the television programs have a consistent character type only narrows the public's actual experience of the queer community. Not everyone is an upper-middle-class white man, secure with his sexual identity, who has both accepting family and friends. We must realize that these programs are for entertainment purposes and, for the most part, represent only the characters in the show, displaying very little of the true diversity of the LGBT community.

People from every race, nationality, gender, class, and political and religious affiliation are represented in the LGBT community. Gay and bisexual men tend to be categorically stereotyped as flamboyant and meticulously dressed. Lesbian and bisexual women tend to be categorically stereotyped as "butch," flannel-shirt-wearing with short hair. These stereotypes, of course, are not at all accurate. Gay and bisexual men and lesbian and bisexual women are as different and unique as heterosexual men and women. Reducing any people to a base stereotype is incorrect and potentially dangerous. It is important to note, however, that some men and women fit very neatly into the gay and lesbian stereotype, and this is perfectly acceptable. It is just as acceptable as a gay man who plays rugby or works construction. Stereotypes, though sometimes accurate, represent only a small piece of the community.

Being part of the community is a matter of self-identification. To identify as a gay man or lesbian woman is a choice made when a person is comfortable with his or her affectional preference. To be LGBT is not to be understood as a choice; the choice lies in one's decision to *identify* as LGBT. There are people who choose to have sex with people of the same gender or have same-gender attractions but who do not identify as a part of the LGBT community. Conversely, there are people who identify with the LGBT community whose primary means of identification is neither sexual nor affectional preference. Identifying with the LGBT community is not limited to identities based on sexual attraction, but rather, because of an emotional attraction or mental alignment. From my interaction with parents of LGBT children, these parents feel very much a part of the gay and lesbian community.

COMING OUT

"Coming out of the closet" is a buzz phrase that most people have heard. This is the process by which LGBT people acknowledge that they are not exclusively heterosexual. Many people self-identify as lesbian, gay, or bisexual based upon their sexual attraction. Others identify with the LGBT community. Two very important phases characterize the coming-out process. The first is coming out to oneself. This is the time in which many people realize that their personal attractions and fantasies are valid and that it is acceptable to express these attractions. For many, it is the first time a person says, "I'm gay." This moment is a very serious one, because for many people it drastically changes their world. This is because most people live in a society where heterosexuality is considered the norm.

Most of us have been raised in a severely heterosexist world. Heterosexism is the assumption that society by default is heterosexual and that heterosexuality is superior to any other identity. Our culture presupposes that humans are naturally heterosexual. Heterosexuals do not have to come out the way LGBT people do. Heterosexism derives itself from the assumption of heteronormativism. Heteronormative is loosely defined as the idea that heterosexuality is normal and anything else is not normal or natural. This of course sallies forth many scientific, political, and philosophical questions, such as "what is normal?" Michael Warner, in his book *The Trouble with Normal* (1999), looked at American heteronormative culture. Warner is witnessing LGBT people's fight for inclusion in what society considers normal. Normalization for Warner includes the legal right to get married, the fight against the stereotype of promiscuity, and the greater idea that LGBT people are trying to assimilate into normal society.

This view stands apart from the debate on assimilation versus separation. Is heterosexuality normal or is it merely the pronounced norm in society? It can be assumed that the majority of LGBT people are inclined toward assimilation. People in general want to be part of the society they are familiar with and do not want to be categorically stereotyped and stigmatized. A few people who fall along the lines of Warner's thesis believe normal society should not be the goal for which to strive. They believe LGBT people have a unique opportunity to redefine society's present relation with the entire spectrum of sexuality. Of course, this is by no means a definitive argument that all people take sides in, but rather one reserved for theorists and activists.

The second phase is coming out to people the person encounters. This process is unfortunately lifelong, and it rarely gets easier. For many people this is an extremely difficult process. Questions such as "Will my sexuality be an issue with this person?" and "Is this portion of my life relevant to the relationship I have with this person?" are prevalent. LGBT people answer these and similar questions differently all of the time. For many, it is important for people to know that they identify as LGBT, while others consider it part of their private lives. This is a matter of personal preference and should not be subjected to outside judgments.

The coming-out process is very self-empowering. It gives many people a new sense of self-confidence and personal control that they may not have felt before. Once people come out to themselves, they wonder if it will completely turn their worlds upside down. Many people feel as though they are turning their backs on the world. This varies from person to person, but it is an extraordinarily important moment in a person's life. If someone comes out to you, it is because he or she trusts you. You should try to be supportive. Realize that he or she is not a different person, but that you are now privileged to know the same person in more depth.

The period for coming out is ongoing and has no age boundaries. People will identify as LGBT when they are elderly and as early as preadolescence. The younger end of the spectrum has been something of tremendous research and focus in recent years. As the LGBT community has become more mainstream, the coming-out age has gotten younger. Adolescents for the first time are experiencing LGBT people during the time when they first start to think about sexuality. They are not so isolated as previous generations.

For those of us privileged enough to attend a university after high school, this is a moment when many people begin to realize that they are not heterosexual. It is the first time many young adults have freedom in their daily routines. This freedom allows some students to act on feelings or interests that may have been suppressed when they were in high school. Along with this freedom comes the opportunity to experience a diverse academic environment. People from all lifestyles, places, and cultures are confronting one another all of the time. This is for many LGBT students the first time they may meet other LGBT students.

Many unique factors are at work for people of color who are going through the coming-out process. When people identify as LGBT, they have then subscribed to a personalized label. Does this mean that this is one's only label? Is it the primary label? Many LGBT people of color battle this with themselves and with their communities every day. These questions are never easily answered but have become the basis of much writing and research in current years. A move in the public health sector is attempting to reconcile some of these differences. These differences are tremendously complicated by the multitude of stereotypes that follow any marginalized community.

STEREOTYPICAL LIFESTYLES

Bars and Clubs

The idea that members of the LGBT community live fast-paced and extraordinary lifestyles is pervasive. Socializing seems to revolve around bars and dance clubs, where life is everything but boring. This stereotype is present in both the heterosexual and LGBT community. For those members of the LGBT community who do enjoy going to bars and clubs, many times this becomes the community norm to them. Those people who do not enjoy crowded dance clubs or the typical bar scene are many times forgotten. A portion of this can be attributed to the media; successful television rarely reflects the lifestyle of the average person—LGBT people included.

This being said, something can be recognized about bars and clubs within the LGBT community. From the 1950s through the 1970s there were very few places to meet other LGBT people other than bars. Bars provided a safe space for LGBT people to be open about their sexuality and to meet other LGBT people. Bars, though seemingly prominent, play no different role than they do in the heterosexual community. Bars are everywhere, and some people choose to go and some people do not. Some LGBT people choose to go to heterosexual bars, and some heterosexual people like to hang out in LGBT bars. There are no standards here, and bars by no means stand as a foundation of the LGBT community.

The Gay Ghettos

In many cities you will find a neighborhood where the population density of LGBT is higher than it is in other parts of the city. Many times you will hear these areas called "gayborhoods" or "gay ghettos." These will most commonly be found in large metropolitan areas. Most people find comfort in numbers. Many people would rather live in a neighborhood where their sexuality is not a cause for concern or question. Not every urban area in the world has a strongly defined LGBT area, but many do. The Castro in San Francisco, Soho in New York, and West Hollywood in Los Angeles are some of the most famous LGBT neighborhoods.

Politics

This population density has been one of the major factors in the development of the LGBT community as a political base in America. As LGBT people began to move closer together and form their own neighborhoods, they gained political power to elect local officials. The stereotype of LGBT people as liberal Democrats may be one of the largest misunderstandings that the community deals with. This is a stereotype inside and outside the borders of the community. With the rise of groups such as the Log Cabin Republicans, the Republican Unity Coalition, and the Lavender Greens one can easily see that LGBT people are not exclusively Democrats. One can never assume that LGBT people are diehard liberals with total allegiance to the Democratic Party.

Affluence

Another stereotype associated with the LGBT community is affluence. This has been perpetuated by the public knowledge that the LGBT community has become a very prominent target for marketing strategists. It is true the LGBT community has become a specific market for most industries, but this does not mean that every LGBT person has disposable income. In the past LGBT people typically did not have the usual expenses associated with parenthood. This allowed more disposable income for home improvement, lifestyle events, and entertainment. However, in recent years the phenomena of gay adoptions have become more frequent, and there are many studies right now about LGBT people in economically depressed communities. In the near future, the stereotype of affluence may be the first to be put to rest.

GENDER IDENTITY

Although sexual orientation and identifying with the community are important, many issues of gender arise. Some people in the community challenge the typical gender roles constructed by society. This challenge of gender has seeped into the mainstream, especially in fashion. Transgender is a word that describes people who express their gender differently from established stereotypes. This term is relatively new in the English lexicon and does not exist in *The Encyclopedia of Homosexuality* (Dynes, 1990). It is something of an umbrella term that tends to include people who cross-dress or anyone who displays gender characteristics different from what may be expected and considered normal by society. Transgender is part of the concept of gender identity.

For many people this idea is very difficult to understand. Gender is a very interesting idea that has been confused for a very long time with sex. Sex and gender are very different terms that describe very different concepts. Sex is determined by our genetic and physical makeup at birth. This is a scientific and medical definition. Gender, since the 1970s, has distinguished itself from biological sex as the social distinctions between masculine and feminine behavior. Generally, our society raises children in a fashion specific to the assumed characteristics of the sex of the child. Some people may have been born biologically male but they feel female. These people have the right to express themselves as who they are, and this expression should not be hindered because of their biological sex.

It is important for people to realize that gender identity is not related to sexual orientation. Sexual orientation is, as described, about the biological sex to which we are attracted. Gender identity is how we express our gender. Dealing with transgender issues is sometimes very different from dealing with LGBT issues. Many transgender people are attracted to people of the opposite gender. Not all LGBT issues are relevant to the transgender community. The issue of transgenderism will be explored in more detail in Chapter 7.

CONCLUSION

In conclusion, here are a few stone-cold facts that define the LGBT community. The community is composed of people who feel that their gender and sexuality are different from that of mainstream society. It is most important to realize that all people are extremely complex, and respecting diversity is of the utmost importance. The LGBT community has no clear boundaries and is being redefined every day. Terms are changing and definitions are constantly evolving.

QUESTIONS TO CONSIDER

1. How do LGBT people that you know self-identify?
2. What are terms and acronyms used in your community to address the LGBT community?
3. Are these terms descriptive, empowering, marginalizing, community building, political, slang, or destructive to the LGBT community?
4. Are there terms used in your agency or by the agency's staff that LGBT people may think are negative or offensive?

5. What practices has your agency implemented that have, consciously or unconsciously, constructed terminology barriers that may prevent members of the LGBT community from accessing services?
6. The best method to identify a population is to ask them how they wish to be identified and use those terms. How does your agency use terminology to include members of the LGBT community?
7. How can your agency use terminology to facilitate the LGBT community's comfort while accessing services?

REFERENCES

Dynes, W.R. (Ed.). (1990). *The encyclopedia of homosexuality.* New York: Garland Publ.
Warner, M. (1999). *The trouble with normal: Sex, politics, and the ethics of queer life.* New York: Free Press.

Chapter 2

The Role of Public Health in Lesbian, Gay, Bisexual, and Transgender Health

Patricia D. Mail
Walter J. Lear

INTRODUCTION

"Public health" is thought of by many individuals, regardless of their sexual orientation, as combating contagious epidemics, educating about cancer and heart disease, providing HIV and AIDS services, and controlling health hazards in our food, water, air, soil, and work environments. It is all that and much more. Within these public health activities are both specific benefits and problems for lesbian, gay, bisexual, transgender, and questioning individuals of all ages, geographical locations, and racial/ethnic/cultural backgrounds.

Public health is not a well-known profession, either to the general public or to clinicians. This may be due to the fact that public health programs and services, when they are effective, are taken for granted. The goals of this host of programs and services are to promote health and prevent disease, injury, and disability. When public health functions in accord with these goals, nothing adverse is likely to happen and it benefits every individual, every community, the nation as a whole, as well as people worldwide. When public health is marginalized, distorted by unscientific pressures, or even totally absent, large numbers of people can become diseased, injured, disabled, or killed.

Even when public health services for individuals are presumably available to everyone, they are often denied to LGBT persons because of homophobia, miscommunication, or fear. Such improper denial of service is compounded by attitudes and conduct derived from the sexism, racism, and classism still so widespread in the United States.

For those who work on LGBT health matters, knowing the basics about public health in this country and about the experiences that LGBT people have had in addressing their health needs will make public health practitioners' work more effective and the LGBT community's difficulties more understandable.

WHAT IS "PUBLIC HEALTH"?

"Public health" is defined by the Institute of Medicine as "what we, as a society, do collectively to assure the conditions in which people can be healthy. This requires that continuing and emerging threats to the health of the public can be successfully countered" (Committee for the Study of Public Health, 1988, p. 1). The report goes on to observe that these threats include immediate crises such as the AIDS epidemic, enduring problems such as injuries and chronic illnesses, and impending crises such as those that can develop from the toxic by-products of modern society (Committee for the Study of Public Health, 1988).

Definitions of public health have expanded over the past centuries, beginning with governmental efforts (quarantine) to stop the importation and spread of epidemic contagious diseases, and today different versions of the definition are used. Some define public health as all the health activities of government, including in more recent decades health care for pregnant women and infants, evaluations/licensing of prescribed medicines to assure their safety and efficacy, family medical care centers, financial support for health care students, research on occupational health problems, required standards for hospitals and nursing homes, and therapy for substance abusers. Other definitions include the work of nongovernmental programs and services that also have the goals of health promotion and disease/injury/disability prevention.

Public health, whether provided by government agencies or private organizations, is intended for everyone. This means that LGBT people and their children should have public health as their primary resource for preventive care and health promotion. However, this is not the case for many LGBT people, intimidated by known or anticipated homophobia of providers or, like much of the population, thinking such clinics and programs are available only to those who are indigent (as is the case with Medicaid). A few health departments have actively reached out to LGBT people, providing essential scientific information in a manner customized for LGBT people. Examples of this outreach include the Public Health Department of Seattle and King County, Washington, which has specific LGBT Web pages (www.metrokc.gov/health/glbt/index.htm), and a 1975 Pennsylvania Department of Health booklet about sexually transmitted diseases and gay men, written by an out gay medical student and appropriately illustrated.

RESEARCH AND PUBLIC HEALTH

Research is a major activity of public health. This research deals with a wide range of areas and topics, especially the health status of people, the causes of their health problems, and the best ways to solve these problems. The leading government research player in the United States is the National Institutes of Health (NIH), part of the U.S. Public Health Service (PHS). The NIH conducts extensive research and provides substantial financial support for research done by academic institutions, health departments, community organizations, and medical services of all kinds. In some of this research, information about LGBT people is separately identified and analyzed. Relatively few health research projects specifically address LGBT health issues. Therefore, limited scientific information is being accumulated about the LGBT population. A great deal of information is still not known, and much more research on LGBT health issues remains to be done.

A major aspect of public health research is based on government-required data about births, deaths, certain diseases, injuries, and disabilities. These data, called vital statistics, are analyzed and disseminated by government health agencies. These data enable comparisons from year to year, among different geographical areas, and according to gender, age, economic/class status, and racial/ethnic backgrounds of the nation's population. Such analyses are crucial for determining the most significant current health issues and promptly detecting emerging health problems.

Epidemiology is defined as "the study of the distribution and determinants of health-related states or events in specific populations, and the application of this study to control of health problem" (Last, 1995, p. 55).

Information from research makes possible the identification of behavioral and environmental risks to health and, thereby, appropriate planning of educational interventions, medical services, and environmental control improvements. Such research benefits are well illustrated in a few examples of recent LGBT research work. A study of lesbian health behavior in the greater Pittsburgh area showed that lesbians smoked tobacco more than other women (35.5 percent versus 25.5 percent), used alcohol to a greater extent (57.5 percent versus 44.6 percent), were heavy alcohol drinkers (4.7 percent versus 1.1 percent), were more sedentary (34.2 percent versus 31.4 percent), and were more overweight (47.8 percent versus 31.6 percent). However, these same lesbians reported a higher frequency of pap tests than other women (94.2 percent versus 93.8 percent) and had mammograms done more frequently (93.3 percent versus 85.1 percent) (Aaron et al.,

2001). Furthermore, using data from public health departments, surveys, and other studies, it was possible to identify those LGBT populations with higher prevalence of certain conditions such as hepatitis B (MacKellar et al., 2001), gonorrhea (Fox et al., 2001), human papilloma virus (Marrazzo, Koutsky, Kiviat, Kuypers, & Stine, 2001), and substance abuse (Gruskin, Hart, Gordon, & Ackerson, 2001). In addition, LGBT individuals are susceptible to other conditions that are frequent in the population at large: obesity, diabetes, smoking-induced illnesses, and others associated with a sedentary lifestyle.

THE LGBT HEALTH MOVEMENT EMERGES AND THRIVES

The LGBT health movement in the United States was inspired and energized by several important political and social forces—the civil rights movement of the 1950s and 1960s, the modern feminist movement of the 1960s and 1970s, and the out-front gay and lesbian movement following the 1969 Stonewall riots. In addition, the struggles for better health services, particularly for racial/ethnic minorities, low- and no-income people, and others grossly underserved because of limited resources, were relevant, as these populations included many LGBT individuals.

In the 1970s, the most significant aspect of the country's political/social environment for LGBT individuals was the longstanding, pervasive, and intense hostility in society at large, including mainstream health services and practitioners, toward homosexuality in general and toward homosexual men and women in particular (homophobia).

Homophobia "now means both irrational fear of and hatred and contempt for homosexuals and homosexuality and indeed any sexual orientation that varies from heterosexuality" (Finnegan & McNally, 2002, p. 225).

As a result, LGBT issues were rarely discussed publicly. This hostility induced a necessary but detrimental-to-health secrecy and disregard of sexual orientation and practices when LGBT people utilized mainstream health services. LGBT health issues seemed, therefore, nonexistent. To politically conscious homosexuals in a period of great social ferment, homophobia in the health field was no longer tolerable; an appropriate response was mandatory, and so emerged the LGBT health movement (see Table 2.1).

Two political occurrences complemented and reinforced the gestating LGBT health movement, helping to move LGBT health out of the closet and into clinical settings, health professional circles, and public health

TABLE 2.1. Significant Dates in the Gay and Lesbian Public Health Movement

Date	Event	Source
1956	Dr. Evelyn Hooker reports her study of nonpatient homosexual men (i.e., healthy) compared to a similar sample of nonpatient heterosexual men matched by age and profession. The results show no mental health differences in the groups other than their sexual orientation	Deyton & Lear, 1988
1973	Dr. Howard J. Brown, commissioner of public health for New York City, publicly "comes out" as a gay man	Deyton & Lear, 1988
December 15, 1973	The board of trustees of the American Psychiatric Association adopts the recommendation that the nomenclature of homosexuality be removed from the *Diagnostic and Statistical Manual of Mental Disorders*	Deyton & Lear, 1988
1974	The American Psychological Association follows suit in adopting resolutions that normalize homosexuality	Rubinstein, 1995
1975	The Gay Nurses' Alliance, an adjunct to the American Nurses Association, is founded by David Waldren and E. Carolyn Innes	Deyton & Lear, 1988
November 1975	The Caucus of Gay Public Health Workers (now known as the Lesbian, Gay, Bisexual, and Transgender Caucus of Public Health Workers) of the American Public Health Association (APHA) is granted official relations with the APHA by a vote of the Governing Council	Deyton & Lear, 1988
1975-1976	The American Academy of Physician Assistants; American Association of Sex Educators, Counselors and Therapists; American Medical Association; American Psychological Association; American Psychiatric Association; and the National Association of Social Workers, among others, establish gay and lesbian caucuses or committees as a means of recognizing the specific health needs of gay and lesbian people	Deyton & Lear, 1988
May 1976	The National Gay Health Coalition is founded (in 1985, the name was changed to the National Gay Health Education Foundation)	Deyton & Lear, 1988

TABLE 2.1 *(continued)*

Date	Event	Source
1978	The American Nurses Association adopts a resolution that endorses civil rights at the local, state, and federal levels that would provide the same protection to all people, regardless of sexual and affectional preference	APHA, 1978
1980	National Gay Health Coalition sends recommendations for strengthening services and research with gay and lesbian people to the Department of Health and Human Services and the U.S. Public Heath Service	Lear, 1980
1981	American Association of Physicians for Human Rights founded; changes name to The Gay and Lesbian Medical Association in 1994	GLMA (http://www.glma.org)

agencies. These occurrences were the nationally publicized coming out of a prominent physician and the removal of homosexuality from the professional list of mental health disorders.

In 1973, Howard J. Brown, a former czar of New York City governmental health functions, deliberately "came out" in a very public fashion. This unprecedented act, unusually courageous for that time (and even now thirty years later), was an inspiring model to many in and out of the health field (including this chapter's physician co-author). Moreover, Brown was a white, Protestant, male specialist with the highest professional standing and wide public recognition. After coming out he appeared on national talk shows, was featured on the cover of *Time* magazine, spoke extensively throughout the country to public and physician groups, and gave comforting responses to thousands of letters and calls from LGBT individuals. He was one of the two principal founders of the first national homosexual education and advocacy organization, the National Gay Task Force (NGTF) (now called the Gay and Lesbian Task Force), and served as its first board chairperson. This grueling schedule, followed against doctor's orders, resulted in his death from a second coronary infarct after one year (Brown, 1976; Deyton & Lear, 1988).

Until this time almost all psychiatric literature about homosexuality was based on dysfunctional and very unhappy persons who sought therapeutic help from psychiatrists. What the psychiatrists did not understand was that most of the "illness" they saw was a natural reaction to the social stigmatization, discrimination, and violence inflicted on LGBT individuals by a homophobic society. Of course, psychiatrists did not *knowingly* come in contact with healthy homosexuals, even fellow psychiatrists, who were all closeted. The exception to this knowledge deficiency was the well-designed, properly controlled studies of homosexuality that had been done as early as 1956 by Dr. Evelyn Hooker, a psychotherapist. She compared nonpatient homosexual men with straight men matched by age and profession. Her studies showed there were no differences in the groups other than their sexual orientation. Psychiatrists ignored these studies because they were not conducted by a fellow psychiatrist (Rubinstein, 1995).

The "illness" concept of homosexuality was the prevailing thought in the health, legal, and religious fields, as well as in the part of the public that had rejected the moralistic "sin" concept of homosexuality. It was a principal root of the social stigma experienced by all LGBT people and, therefore, a logical and essential target of the earliest gay rights advocates. A sophisticated, energetic, and multiyear campaign to remove homosexuality from the American Psychiatric Association's (APA) official *Diagnostic and Statistical Manual of Mental Disorders* was designed and successfully implemented. The campaign's remarkable leaders were two pre-Stonewall, militant, nonhealth LGBT activists, Barbara Gittings of Philadelphia and Franklin Kameny of Washington, DC. For key roles in the campaign they recruited several psychiatrists, some straight people, and some closeted gays, including Judd Marmor, a former APA president, Richard Pillard of Boston, and John E. Fryer of Philadelphia.

In December 1973, the APA's board of trustees adopted the recommendation of their committee on nomenclature to remove homosexuality from the list of "mental disorders." However, this act was so controversial that an unprecedented vote of APA members was demanded and held, which confirmed the board's pro-gay-rights decision. For an excellent, comprehensive account and analysis of this critical political highlight in the LGBT health movement's history, see *Homosexuality and American Psychiatry: The Politics of Diagnosis,* by the eminent medical ethicist Ronald Bayer. Bayer concludes, "The status of homosexuality is a political question, representing an historically rooted, socially determined choice regarding the ends of human sexuality" (Bayer, 1981, p. 5). Howard Brown comments in more practical terms: "The Board's vote made millions of Americans who had been officially ill that morning officially well that afternoon. Never in history had so many people been cured in so little time" (Brown, 1976, pp. 200-201).

By the end of 1973, a few LGBT professionals in the major health disciplines were courageous enough to come out at their workplaces and in their respective professional circles, join together in professional support and political action groups, or create gay health services. The first health professional group was the Gay Nurses' Alliance, associated with the American Nurses Association, founded by Philadelphia nurses E. Carolyn Innes and David Waldron with encouragement and help from their friend Barbara Gittings. The psychiatrists and the psychologists also formed professional groups in their national associations. These groups were conceived by their assertive founders as agents of change for LGBT health and began with the preparation and advocacy of pro-gay-rights policy statements and implementation plans for their respective national associations. For example, the American Psychiatric Association policy stated,

> Whereas homosexuality per se implies no impairment of judgment, stability, reliability, or general vocational capabilities, . . . therefore, be it resolved that the APA supports and urges the repeal of all legislation making criminal offenses of sexual acts performed by consenting adults in private. (Brown, 1976, p. 200)

Shortly afterward, LGBT caucuses and committees having similar goals and functions were formed within nearly all national health-profession organizations: medical students, social workers, physician assistants, health educators, counseling and guidance personnel, gerontologists, alcoholism therapists, and public health workers. The national organizations yielded to this LGBT militancy, adopting the proposed policy statements and recognizing the caucuses or even creating new relevant structures. The (nonpsychiatrist) LGBT physicians were the last to establish their group, but when they did it was totally independent and unrelated to the unfriendly American Medical Association.

In response to the need and demand of LGBT people for LGBT providers or, at least, LGBT-friendly services, LGBT health services were established in a number of cities, beginning in Boston, Chicago, Los Angeles, New York City, and Philadelphia. Many dealt with sexually transmitted diseases in gay men; some were counseling and mental health agencies, including care of alcoholics and other substance abusers; and all undertook health-promotion and disease-prevention education. By 1986 the National Gay Task Force listed almost 100 clinics and medical service programs and over 300 counseling and mental health programs that were LGBT friendly and accepting. Another major priority of these first, out LGBT health professionals was pressuring local clinics, hospitals, and health departments to employ openly gay and lesbian staff and to educate their staffs about LGBT lifestyles and special health care needs.

The Caucus of Gay Public Health Workers (currently called the Lesbian, Gay, Bisexual, and Transgender Caucus of Public Health Workers [LGBTC]) made its debut at the 1975 Annual Meeting of the American Public Health

Association in Chicago. The overall objective of the Caucus was clear: to bring out of the closet the serious and wide-ranging problems encountered by gay persons in receiving and providing health care. The Caucus founder, then a Pennsylvania public health official who is co-author of this chapter, was helped in the planning by a friend, Barbara Gittings, and during the convention itself by about thirty young volunteers (one-third women), who, though naive about APHA, were determined, resourceful, and engaging. The debut consisted of an eye-catching booth, a professionally toned brochure (2,000 copies distributed), a three-room hospitality suite, and a forthright and comprehensive gay rights resolution. Following three suspenseful days of intensive lobbying, and with the crucial support of several straight APHA leaders, past presidents, and others, the entire resolution was overwhelmingly adopted without change by APHA's governing council.

At the 1976 APHA Annual Meeting, the Caucus presented three scientific sessions, the first ever at a major scientific meeting by open lesbian and gay health workers about lesbian and gay health issues and services. The education of the APHA family had a lighter touch (bordering on the outrageous)—same-gender couples dancing flamboyantly together at the convention's formal dinner-dance. The Caucus concluded its activities with its own dinner at a fine gay restaurant. This pattern of scientific sessions, education of and networking with straight peers, and delightful social events has continued at all subsequent APHA annual meetings.

In keeping with its "gay" sensibilities, the Caucus prepared a provocative educational pamphlet mocking mainstream homophobia for APHA's 1977 annual meeting. The pamphlet was titled, *Heterosexuality: Can It Be Cured?* It discussed the causes of heterosexuality, the hazards of heterosexual behavior, and treatments and possible cures for the condition. Such humorous reversal of the frequent assumptions and questions about homosexuality proved to be an effective stimulus for rethinking social, political, and professional understanding of the subject (APHA, 1977).

The Caucus was invited to participate in a January 1978 workshop on sexually transmitted diseases (STDs) organized by the deputy assistant secretary of health. Among the many comments and recommendations of the Caucus were the importance of having openly gay persons on the staffs of the Centers for Disease Control (CDC) and STD clinics, and improving information about homosexuality in the public health field, including having one of the proposed regional research centers focused on STDs in gay men.

A very special highlight of APHA's 1981 annual meeting was the celebration of the election of a Caucus member, Stan Matex, as the president-elect of APHA—probably the first open gay president of any national health organization. At several other conventions the Caucus prepared policy resolutions for APHA's governing council, which received sympathetic attention.

By 1976 it was already obvious to the leaders of the LGBT health-profession and health-service groups that they had important interests in common, that they would benefit from sharing experiences, and that they should cooperate on particular tasks that cut across their various disciplines. Therefore, the founding chairperson of Gay Public Health Workers convened a meeting of what shortly became the National Gay Health Coalition (NGHC). This was a rather informal, unfunded effort which held meetings twice a year.

The NGHC's first major project was the first National Gay Health Conference. This was organized by a volunteer committee in Philadelphia under the leadership of Frances Hanckel, a hospital administrator, and Jack Doren, a psychologist. It was held May 19-21, 1978, in a church basement in Washington, DC, and was attended by 400 gay and lesbian health workers from all parts of the country. The climax of the conference was the presentation of the first award for "outstanding contributions to the health and welfare of gay people." The award, named the Jane Addams-Howard Brown Award, was given to Evelyn Hooker.

In 1979 the NGHC initiated and organized the first formal dialogue of LGBT health professionals with the surgeon general of the USPHS. This was one of the several specialized activities supplementing the huge October 1979 March on Washington for Lesbian and Gay Rights. A major recommendation of NGHC's delegation was for the USPHS "to establish a commission to prepare in a year or two a comprehensive report on the special health needs and other health concerns of the nation's sexual minorities" (Cotton, 1993, p. 2611). The NGHC's eight other recommendations for LGBT-relevant services and research are summarized in Table 2.2.

The success of the National Gay Health Conferences made it clear that the educational interests of the LGBT health movement would be greatly furthered by a formal, funded organization. So in 1980, the NGHC and its constituent groups established the National Gay Health Education Foundation; its name was changed in 1985 to the National Lesbian/Gay Health Foundation. In addition to sponsoring the annual national conferences, the Foundation compiled and published *The Sourcebook on Lesbian/Gay Health Care,* a groundbreaking educational contribution about LGBT health issues (Deyton & Lear, 1988).

Several professional organizations now have subunits that review research and recommend policy for LGBT issues in their specific disciplines. For example, the Society for Public Health Education adopted a major policy paper in 2001 on outreach to and education of LGBT people, as well as the need to recruit LGBT individuals to enrich and diversify the organization (Society for Public Health Education, 2002). Also, the Society of Les-

TABLE 2.2. National Gay Health Coalition Recommendations to the U.S. Public Health Service for Expansion of Programs and Services and Contributions to Theory and Practice for Gay and Lesbian People

Goals	Recommendations
Improvement and expansion of services	Financial assistance on a continuing basis from principal Public Health Service funding streams of [sic] lesbian and gay-sponsored health services and women's health clinics
	Updating the definition of sexually transmitted diseases in the PHS venereal disease program to include viral hepatitis and intestinal infections, diseases that, although originally seen largely in gay male populations, will undoubtedly become widespread among all sexually active individuals
	Financial assistance for audio-visual educational materials for health care providers, trained and in-training, particularly nursing and medical students, on the special heath concerns of sexual minorities
	Financial assistance for specially designed and delivered education of the lesbian and gay male communities about physical and mental health
Strengthening theory and practice	Expansion of clinical research on the gynecological and other special health problems of women who do not engage in heterosexual sexual activity
	Expansion of immunological and behavioral research on the prevention of sexually transmitted diseases
	Expansion of behavioral research on homophobia
	Expansion of epidemiological research on alcoholism and other substance abuse among lesbians and gay men

Source: Recommendations taken from a letter to Dr. Julius Richmond, assistant secretary for health, Department of Health & Human Services, and surgeon general, U.S. Public Health Service, from the NGHC, written July 9, 1980. Writing for the NGHC was Walter J. Lear, MD, Convenor of the NGHC. (Letter archived at the Institute of Social Medicine and Community Health, Philadelphia, PA.) Reprinted with permission from the Institute of Social Medicine and Community Health, Philadelphia, Pennsylvania.

bian and Gay Anthropologists of the American Anthropological Association reviews the cultural implications for health in LGBT populations in various countries as well as establishing ethics for researchers in the field. Another LGBT public health highlight deserving note is the appointment in 2003 of the first open lesbian as the dean of a school of public health—Marla Gold at Drexel University in Philadelphia.

The *American Journal of Public Health* had LGBT health as the theme for its June 2001, volume 91, number 6 issue. The demand for copies of this issue was so great it was sold out—the first time this ever happened. As a result, the APHA requested Anthony J. Silvestre, a former Caucus chair, to compile a book of selections from the *AJPH* for publication.

The LGBT health movement has a strong holistic, health-promoting, and kinship character. This is derived in large part from its roots both in public health and in the LGBT community. From the former comes an emphasis on health education, preventive services, and recognition of the total person and continuity of care. From the latter comes a caring and loving identification that transcends the customary distance and division between those providing health services and those receiving them. These roots nourish the understanding of and efforts to oppose the trends to complete medicalization, industrialization, and corporatization of the health care system. The LGBT health movement has demonstrated a remarkable capacity for self-help: to do for itself what the mainstream should do but is unwilling to do or incapable of doing properly and what the mainstream has defined as not being a health service, notably assistance and support for social and emotional needs, which consequently is provided by community members as volunteers.

The LGBT health movement also has an outstanding track record of health activism, a model of participatory democracy in terms of skill, persistence, and magnitude. Such activism has been carried out at the level of health services by LGBT providers and users of these services and the level of city, state, and national health affairs by politically oriented advocacy organizations, some exclusively health focused and others with the broader LGBT agenda. One principal target of this advocacy deserves special note, namely, discrimination against LGBT individuals as both users and providers of health services. As a result, the elimination and reduction of such discrimination is substantial, although far from universal.

[Note: This subsection is largely derived from the following citations (Deyton & Lear, 1988; Lear & Deyton, 1986, 1993; Lesbian, Gay, Bisexual Caucus of Public Health Workers, 1991).]

THE HIV PANDEMIC CHALLENGES
THE LGBT HEALTH MOVEMENT AND PUBLIC HEALTH

The HIV (human immunodeficiency virus) pandemic was first noticed in the United States in 1981 by local clinicians and local health department statisticians (CDC, 1981). What they first saw was the occurrence of several diverse and uncommon diseases in otherwise healthy young men. Within months it became clear that the common element underlying this phenomenon was impairment of the immune systems of these men. A second common element in these first cases was that these men were all identified as gay. As the number of cases increased, the association with homosexual

sexual behavior was reinforced—it became known as "the gay plague," later reworded as GRID, the gay-related immunodeficiency disease. This assumed sociocultural view bore with it society's homophobia, and so government public health agencies were intimidated from immediately taking those public health measures appropriate for a new life-threatening and rapidly spreading disease.

But the LGBT health movement, building on its extensive, well-developed, and multidimensional experience, responded promptly, skillfully, and energetically to the shocking and tragic onset of the pandemic. New and relevantly modified LGBT health services sprang up across the county. Thousands of lesbians volunteered in these services. Self-help and political advocacy reached unprecedented heights. Providing volunteer "buddies" for sick gay men was undertaken with much sophistication and unwavering dedication, despite the large number needed and the volunteers' frequent burnout. The dramatic street demonstrations of AIDS Coalition to Unleash Power (ACT UP) forced a reluctant society to abandon its homophobic-inspired neglect of its mandated responsibility to protect the health of all. ACT UP held its first demonstration in March 1987 to protest the profiteering of pharmaceutical companies. At its height it had thousands of members in more than seventy chapters throughout the country.

The NGTF and the National Gay Health Coalition/National Gay Health Education Foundation convened the first national meeting on acquired immune deficiency on August 15, 1982. This was held in Dallas in conjunction with the NGTF annual leadership conference and was attended by over sixty physicians, public health specialists, health service organizers, political activists, media specialists, and leaders of LGBT organizations. At the plenary session a full report of the then-known epidemiology was presented by James W. Curran, MD, coordinator of the special task force of the CDC, USPHS. Because of the confusion resulting from the use of several names for the disease, the meeting unanimously agreed, with the full concurrence of Curran, that henceforth its name would be acquired immune deficiency syndrome (AIDS). Other decisions were to undertake a campaign for immediate congressional appropriations for AIDS research, to set up an AIDS information exchange center, and to organize another national meeting in conjunction with the next (fifth) National Gay Health Conference in Denver. The meeting also prepared and adopted a guideline for AIDS risk reduction and appointed committees and persons to implement the approved follow-up tasks.

In the United States, little if any recognition was given during the pandemic's first decade to the fact that AIDS was also occurring among nongay men, women, and children. These occurrences were often due to use of unclean needles by drug abusers, contaminated blood transfusions (initially), and infants having HIV-positive mothers. The international public health community knew HIV seropositivity was an equal-opportunity pandemic in almost all nations. It took more than a decade of hard work by the AIDS services community to convince policymakers and societal leaders, funders of health care and medical research, and the general public that all women, men, and children could be at risk of HIV infection. Therefore, broad public health measures had to be implemented to control the AIDS pandemic.

An original and continuing obstacle to public health programs essential for blocking the spread of HIV is the discomfort of the major faith traditions of the Western world with the subject of sexuality, particularly their condemnation of sex that is not for procreation as immoral. For LGBT persons this condemnation is compounded by the view that homosexual sexual activity is especially heinous. Faith activists with such views have engaged in unrelenting and intense, at times even virulent, attacks on tax-supported outreach, education, and services for LGBT people (Miner & Connoley, 2002). Moreover, "polite" society does not like to pay attention to unprotected sex and injection drug use, the principal behaviors that spread the disease. As a result, a number of influential politicians have used their control over public health appropriations, program officials, and appointment of members of professional review and advisory bodies to eliminate or subvert essential public health programs, much to the detriment of the health of millions—particularly those most vulnerable because of poverty, inadequate education, racial discrimination, age, and so-called immoral lifestyles (Lear, 1977).

A number of accomplishments of the AIDS work by LGBT people have influenced the mainstream health field. Notable are the changes made by the Food and Drug Administration in the way it reviews new drugs and the changes by the federal science research agencies in the way they carry out their responsibilities, particularly the addition for the first time of laypeople to research program and grant review committees. As one AIDS activist quipped, the specimens were now looking up the microscope at the researchers!

The AIDS pandemic also produced incontrovertible and publicly visible evidence of the many and serious weaknesses of the U.S. health care system—its inability to plan in response to needs, to assure quality of care, to eliminate unscientific discrimination and indignities, and to control costs. Although the situations involved persons with AIDS, the weaknesses are applicable across the board and confirm that the U.S. health care system is primarily responsive to the profit-oriented controlling interests and not to the people (Fee & Krieger, 1993).

COMMUNITY HEALTH PROGRAMS AND SERVICES

The LGBT community has continued to initiate and maintain public health programs and medical services for LGBT people in a number of cities across the country, either as independent agencies or in partnership with community organizations, hospitals, universities, and local health departments. As was the case with the first such services in the 1970s, these services fill a need that the community at large is still not willing or able to provide because of ignorance, lack of concern, or public hostility derived from the stigma of homosexuality and AIDS.

With increasing administrative sophistication and relentless persistence, the leaders of these programs and services have obtained both recognition for meeting (even surpassing at times) applicable professional standards and financial adequacy with reimbursements from health insurance and government funding programs, grants from foundations, fund-raising in the LGBT community, and fees for services. Although the priorities have been specific LGBT health problems, many such agencies have increased their scope to include general medical care, with a few even providing fertility services, mental health services, and dental services.

This LGBT community achievement, which it can be very proud of, is well represented by the following examples. Programs that offer primary care and related services to the LGBT community include Fenway Community Health in Boston, Howard Brown Health Center in Chicago, Los Angeles LGBT Community Services Center, Lyon-Martin Women's Health Services in San Francisco, Mazzoni Center (formerly Community Health Alternatives) in Philadelphia, and Whitman-Walker Clinic in Washington, DC (Mayer et al., 2001). The Mautner Project in Washington, DC, is an educational, counseling, and support program for lesbians diagnosed with cancer and their partners and families. For men with STDs and AIDS, support is provided by the Chicken Soup Brigade in Seattle (now Lifelong AIDS Alliance), an AIDS nutrition and support program, and the Gay Men's Health Crisis in New York City, perhaps the country's largest educational and service agency of this kind. Other initiatives include the Hetrick-Martin Institute of New York City, a pioneering supplement to mental and physical health care of LGBT youth, Alternatives, Inc., providing LGBT substance abuse and mental health services for over thirty years, and Stonewall Recovery Services in Seattle, offering substance misuse treatment programs. These examples, in addition to benefiting thousands of people with a wide range of major and everyday health care needs, have also been a model for community-based interventions by other subpopulations (Shilts, 1987; Revenson & Schiaffino, 2000).

In contrast to LGBT health agencies, very few government health departments have a clinic, program, or component that is named and publicized as being for LGBT people. Not surprisingly, both New York City and San Francisco health departments have formal offices for LGBT health matters. A number of other local health departments have taken steps to make their services gay friendly and relate to LGBT health needs. The usual steps of this kind are educational materials customized for LGBT people and the employment of physicians, physician assistants, health educators, outreach workers, and other staff who are LGBT and out. This has occurred most often with STD clinics and AIDS programs. Another special health care resource for LGBT people in many cities are out physicians and psychotherapists in private solo or group practices, some of whom advertise in LGBT newspapers.

In addition, specific programs of LGBT professionals have come together to draft statements related to standards of practice for health care provisions for the LGBT community (Clark, Landers, Linde, & Sperber, 2001). These standards address the need for employees to be able to work in clinics that are inclusive and nondiscriminatory and that provide equal benefits and compensation for LGBT employees. Clients in LGBT clinics should expect nondiscrimination and comprehensive, client-friendly procedures, as well as a process to file complaints and have concerns resolved in a fair and equitable manner. Intake and assessment forms should be LGBT friendly (i.e., include provision for a partner or significant other, recognize that there may be children in the family, include partner notification in emergencies, and so on). Policies should be in place to ensure that all agency staff are familiar with LGBT issues as they relate to services and that providers are competent to identify and address specific health problems and treatment issues, as well as providing appropriate treatment and referral when necessary. The provider agency should ensure confidentiality of patient data, including information about sexual orientation and gender identity issues. Clients should be informed about data collection that includes references to sexual orientation and/or gender identity, including how and when such information might be disclosed. Any service should provide safe, appropriate, and confidential treatment to LGBT minors, including informing clients of their legal rights and the possible consequences of any mandatory reporting requirements. In addition, when an agency or program develops community programs, LGBT people should be included in outreach and health-promotion efforts and have representation on agency boards of directors and other institutional bodies (Clark et al., 2001).

THE U.S. PUBLIC HEALTH SERVICE

Public health responsibilities and functions of the federal government come under the jurisdiction of the Department of Health and Human Services (DHHS). The DHHS has a myriad of programs, but most are identified as belonging to one of the eight agencies under HHS. These include such programs as the human service and clinical care programs of the Health Resources and Services Administration and the Indian Health Service; the research programs of the National Institutes of Health; the regulatory supervision of the Food and Drug Administration; and the surveillance and community support of the Centers for Disease Control and Prevention (CDC). These component agencies used to be a part of the U.S. Public Health Service, but in reorganizations in the late 1990s and early 2000s, the USPHS was essentially disbanded and became known as the Office of Public Health Science in the office of the Assistant Secretary for Health. All that remains of the once proud traditions of the PHS are the history and presence of members of the Commissioned Corps of the USPHS. The headquarters of the HHS is in Washington, DC, while the NIH is located on a collegiate-type campus in Bethesda, Maryland. Other HHS programs are headquartered in Rockville, while the CDC and the Agency for Toxic Substances and Disease Registry (ATSDR) are located in Atlanta, Georgia. Serving with distinction in all these agencies are gay and lesbian scientists, administrators, clinicians, and researchers.

The secretary of HHS showed a rare instance of formal interest in LGBT health affairs in an April 1993 meeting called by Secretary Donna Shalala (a Clinton appointee). The hour-long meeting was scheduled to coincide with the third National March on Washington for Lesbian and Gay Equal Rights. The secretary called to this meeting the senior department officials, including the assistant secretary of health Philip Lee. The LGBT delegation of over fifteen were leaders of LGBT health organizations (including the National Gay and Lesbian Health Foundation and several local service agencies) and the National Gay and Lesbian Task Force (AAPHR, 1993). A broad range of issues were addressed. Kate O'Hanlon, president-elect of the gay and lesbian physicians' association the American Association of Physicians for Human Rights (AAPHR), commented afterward: "It was clear that the Secretary's interest in our issues is genuine and heartfelt. Our presentations were greeted by thoughtful questions from both Dr. Shalala and her staff. We're particularly pleased that the Secretary committed HHS to follow-up meetings on the issues raised during our discussion" (Cotton, 1993, p. 2611).

LGBT HEALTH OBJECTIVES FOR THE NATION

Beginning in 1979, DHHS began issuing a document setting health objectives for the nation (Fox, 2002). This is a decennial undertaking, and in each decade the health objectives have been refined and made more specific for various subpopulations within the nation. This is in recognition that morbidity and mortality rates differ from population to population, thus requiring different health objectives for each population.

The 2010 health objectives originally included twenty-nine LGBT-specific objectives (Fox, 2002). When it was learned that these objectives would not be included, LGBT community and individual health providers petitioned HHS to include them. However, the final 2010 health objectives deliberately omitted, probably due to political pressure, any mention of LGBT health.

Believing that LGBT citizens deserved recognition for their health needs and that LGBT populations had differing needs than other minority populations, the Gay and Lesbian Medical Association (GLMA), with partial support from HHS, undertook to develop a companion document to the 2000 health objectives (Gay and Lesbian Medical Association and LGBT Health Experts, 2001; Safford, 2002). The final document *(Healthy People 2010 Companion Document for Lesbian, Gay, Bisexual, and Transgender Health)* paralleled the HHS document in format and focus, but pulled together what research was available on LGBT health and set objectives for LGBT populations. Major portions of this document are available online from GLMA (www.glma.org) and have been published in two special issues of *Clinical Research and Regulatory Affairs* (vol. 19, issues 2 and 3, 2002, and vol. 20, issue 2, 2003).

FUTURE DIRECTIONS AND RESEARCH NEEDS

Since the mid-1970s LGBT health practitioners, programs, and organizations have pioneered and significantly advanced much-needed attention to the health status and health care needs of LGBT people. Nonetheless, influential political forces in this country continue to advocate denial to LGBT people of their basic rights to equality promulgated by the U.S. Constitution, including nondiscrimination in the health field.

Perhaps the most understudied and least-known area in LGBT health is that of transgender people. Aside from the medical and psychological effects of transition, virtually no information is available regarding the special health issues of transgender people or about attaining and maintaining wellness once the transition is accomplished.

Also, research is needed regarding the mental health issues of LGBT people and their families, especially the high suicide rate among LGBT adolescents. Undoubtedly the latter is related to the bullying and abuse of children perceived to be LGBT or those having LGBT parents, compounded by the inexcusable ignorance, indifference, and/or homophobia of school health personnel, teachers, and administrators. Little information is available on the effects of LGBT discrimination in general and in the spiritual sphere (called "Bible abuse" by Rembert Truluck, 2000). A fruitful (but perhaps hazardous) subject for psychological research is the causation of virulent faith-based homophobia.

Studies are needed about the quality, availability, and accessibility of what is being done to address the health issues of LGBT populations, including care and support of medical crises, chronic illness, and everyday health problems as well as recommended preventive care and health-promotion efforts. Improvements and expansion of this spectrum of LGBT health care are, of course, dependent on more and more effective advocacy of LGBT-friendly policies and funding.

Although television in recent years has begun to feature a few LGBT people positively, there is a paucity of information for the general public or the health field about the contributions LGBT people make to their communities, to their professions and vocations, and to the nation's basic democratic and humanitarian values. In this respect, scientifically aggregated and analyzed information about LGBT relationships and families would be of special significance.

Apparent from this discussion of LGBT service and research issues is the essentiality of continuous, customized, and scientifically sound education of all health service providers and administrators, health science school faculties and researchers, social workers, counselors and clergy, social justice advocates, and health policymakers. Awareness with realistic information is the first important step to good public health for LGBT people; next is unqualified respect for the human rights of all—including mainstream acceptance of the diversity of human sexual orientations and gender identifications.

Despite the fact that the American Psychiatric Association determined thirty years ago that homosexuality was not a pathological condition, unscientifically based fear and hostility toward LGBT people, as well as outright discrimination and at times even violence, still persist in most sectors of society, including the health field. Progress has been made, but public health has much more to do to assure that

1. LGBT individuals are included without discrimination as providers and recipients of all medical and public health services;
2. both health professionals and the general public are educated about the science and culture of homosexuality;
3. the health disparities faced by LGBT people and the best methods for addressing these disparities are explored; and
4. that all LGBT people have opportunities equal to those of others for achieving and maintaining optimal health.

REFERENCES

AAPHR. (1993). G & L health leaders hold historic meeting with Shalala. American Association of Physicians for Human Rights. AAPHR *Reporter, 1,* 14.

Aaron, D.J., Markovic, N., Danielson, M.E., Honnold, J.A., Janosky, J.E., & Schmidt, N.J. (2001). Behavioral risk factors for disease and preventive health practices among lesbians. In *Lesbian, gay, bi-sexual, and transgender health issues—Selections from the American Journal of Public Health* (pp. 43-46). Washington, DC: American Public Health Association.

American Public Health Association (1978). *Gay Health Reports, 3*(2).

Bayer, R. (1981). *Homosexuality and American psychiatry: The politics of diagnosis.* New York: Basic Books.

Brown, H.J. (1976). *Familiar faces, hidden lives: The story of homosexual men in America today.* New York: Harcourt Trade Publishers.

Caucus of Gay Public Health Workers. (1977). *Heterosexuality: Can it be cured?* Philadelphia, PA: Author.

Centers for Disease Control (CDC). (1981). Pneumocystis pneumonia—Los Angeles. *Morbidity and Mortality Weekly Report, 30,* 250-252.

Clark, M.E., Landers, S., Linde, R., & Sperber, J. (2001). The GLBT health access project: A state-funded effort to improve access to care. In *Lesbian, gay, bi-sexual, and transgender health issues—Selections from the American Journal of Public Health* (p. 25). Washington, DC: American Public Health Association.

Committee for the Study of Public Health. Institute of Medicine. (1988). *The Future of public health.* Washington, DC: National Academy Press.

Cotton, P. (1993). Gay, lesbian physicians meet, march, tell Shalala bigotry is health hazard. *Journal of the American Medical Association, 269*(20), 2611.

Deyton, B., & Lear, W.J. (1988). A brief history of the gay/lesbian health movement in the U.S.A. In M. Shernoff & W.A. Scott (Eds.), *The sourcebook on lesbian/gay health care.* Washington, DC: National Lesbian and Gay Health Foundation.

Fee, E., & Krieger, N. (1993). Understanding AIDS: Historical interpretations and the limits of biomedical individualism. *American Journal of Public Health, 53*(10), 1477-1486.

Finnegan, D.G., & McNally, E.B. (2002). *Counseling lesbian, gay, bisexual, and transgender substance abusers: Dual identities.* Binghamton, NY: The Haworth Press, Inc.

Fox, C.E. (2002). Difficult challenge for healthy people 2010: Putting policy into practice. *Clinical Research and Regulatory Affairs, 19*(2&3), 119-123.

Fox, K.K., Del Rio, C., Holmen, K.K., Hook, E.W., Judson, F.N., Knapp, J.S., Procop, G.W., Wang, S.A., Whittington, W.L.H., & Levine, W.C. (2001). Gonorrhea in the HIV era: A reversal in trends among men who have sex with men. In *Lesbian, gay, bi-sexual, and transgender health issues—Selections from the American Journal of Public Health* (pp. 29-33). Washington, DC: American Public Health Association.

Gay and Lesbian Medical Association & LGBT health experts. (2001). *Healthy people 2010 companion document of lesbian, gay, bisexual and transgender (LGBT) health.* San Francisco, CA: Gay and Lesbian Medical Association.

Gruskin, E.P., Hart, S., Gordon, N., & Ackerson, L. (2001). Patterns of cigarette smoking and alcohol use among lesbians and bisexual women enrolled in a large health maintenance organization. In *Lesbian, gay, bi-sexual, and transgender health issues—Selections from the American Journal of Public Health* (pp. 167-170). Washington, DC: American Public Health Association.

Last, J.M. (Ed.). (1995). *A dictionary of epidemiology* (3rd ed.). New York: Oxford University Press.

Lear, W.J. (1977). Venereal disease and gay men: Opening remarks. *Sexually Transmitted Disease, 4*(2), 49. [Reprinted in the *American Journal of Public Health, 91*(6), 901-902, June 2001.]

Lear, W.J. (1980). Letter to Dr. Julius Richmond on behalf of NGHC. [Archived.] Philadelphia, PA: Institute of Social Medicine and Community Health.

Lear, W.J., & Deyton, B. (1986). A decade of gay health care: Objectives realized and still to be realized. Paper presented at annual conference of the American Public Health Association, Las Vegas, Nevada, September 28-October 2.

Lear, W.J., & Deyton, B. (1993). The gay and lesbian fight for health care continues. Paper presented at annual conference of the American Public Health Association. San Francisco, California, November 15-19.

Lesbian, Gay, Bisexual Caucus of Public Health Workers. (1991). GLPHWC roots. *LGB Caucus Newsletter,* Winter.

MacKellar, D.A., Valleroy, L.A., Secura, G.M., MacFarland, W., Shehan, D., Ford, W., LaLota, M., Celetano, D.D., Koblin, B.A., Torian, L.V., Thiede, H., & Janssen, R.S. (2001). Two decades after vaccine license: Hepatitis B immunization and infection among men who have sex with men. In *Lesbian, gay, bi-sexual, and transgender health issues—Selections from the American Journal of Public Health* (pp. 35-41). Washington, DC: American Public Health Association.

Marrazzo, J.M., Koutsky, L.A., Kiviat, N.B., Kuypers, J.M., & Stine, K. (2001). Papanicolaou test screening and prevalence of genital papillomavirus among women who have sex with women. In *Lesbian, gay, bi-sexual, and transgender health issues—Selections from the American Journal of Public Health* (pp. 79-84). Washington, DC: American Public Health Association.

Mayer, K., Appelbaum, J., Rogers, T., Lo, W., Bradford, J., & Boswell, S. (2001). The evolution of the Fenway Community Health Model. In *Lesbian, gay, bi-sexual, and transgender health issues—Selections from the American Journal of*

Public Health (pp. 21-23). Washington, DC: American Public Health Association.

Miner, L., & Connoley, J.T. (2002). *The children are free: Reexamining the biblical evidence on same-sex relationships.* Indianapolis, IN: Jesus Metropolitan Community Church.

Revenson, T.A., & Schiaffino, K.M. (2000). Community-based health interventions. In J. Rappaport & E. Seidman (Eds.), *Handbook of community psychology.* (pp. 471-493). New York: Kluwer Academic/Plenum Press.

Rubinstein, G. (1995). The decision to remove homosexuality from the DSM: Twenty years later. *American Journal of Psychotherapy, 49*(3), 416-427.

Safford, L. (2002). Building the pillars of diversity in the U.S. health system: Addressing disparities of sexual orientation and gender identity. *Clinical Research and Regulatory Affairs, 19*(2 & 3), 125-152.

Shilts, R. (1987). *And the band played on: Politics, people and the AIDS epidemic.* New York: St. Martin's Press.

Society for Public Health Education (2002). Resolution on eliminating health disparities based on sexual orientation. Available online at http://www.sophe.org/about/resolutions/sexres.html, accessed January 4, 2004.

Truluck, R. (2000). *Steps to recovery from Bible abuse.* Gaithersburg, MD: Chi Rho Press.

Chapter 3

Lesbian, Gay, Bisexual, and Transgender Public Health Research

Randall L. Sell
Vincent M. B. Silenzio

"Per scientiam ad justitiam"
(Through science to justice)

Magnus Hirschfeld and the Scientific-Humanitarian Committee, 1897;
translation in Steakley, 1997

INTRODUCTION

Lesbian, gay, bisexual, and transgender (LGBT) public health is a relatively new focus of investigation in which even the most important concerns remain largely unexplored. Because the field is so young, researchers are only now identifying what constitutes LGBT public health research. That is, researchers are now thinking more seriously than ever about what "sexual orientation" and "gender" are and why these are important constructs for understanding and improving health. Researchers are also discussing what specific topics need to be or should be explored and, given the nature of the populations, what methods work best for investigating these topics (Gay and Lesbian Medical Association and LGBT Health Experts, 2001; Solarz, 1999; Meyer, 2001).

This chapter explores these issues by examining the importance of defining the populations and terms used, by examining how sexual orientation and gender are measured and categorized in research studies, by providing a theoretical framework for thinking about how and why sexual orientation and gender should be of concern to public health researchers, and by discussing the strengths and limitations of research methods commonly used to study these sometimes hidden populations. First, we put this discussion into context by beginning with a brief history of LGBT public health research.

BACKGROUND

The serious scientific investigation of LGBT public health concerns is relatively new. Although some very notable quasi-public health research published in book form preceded it, including works by Havelock Ellis and John Addington Symonds (1897), Magnus Hirschfeld (1914), Katherine Bement Davis (1929), and George Henry (1948, 1955), the field arguably came into being in 1957 with the publication of Evelyn Hooker's study, funded by the National Institutes of Mental Health, of the social adjustment of a nonclinical sample of gay men. Hooker demonstrated that expert clinical judges could not distinguish the projective test protocols of nonclinical homosexual men from a comparison group of heterosexual men; nor were there differences in adjustment ratings (Hooker, 1957).

The field of LGBT public health then slowly advanced through the 1960s and 1970s, focusing primarily on investigating the spread of sexually transmitted diseases (particularly between men) (Rowan & Gillette, 1978). Arguably, the field really took root with the discovery of HIV/AIDS in the 1980s (Peterkin & Risdon, 2003). However, HIV/AIDS research largely focused on men (usually gay or bisexual) and much less on women (and very rarely lesbians) or transgender people. Although HIV/AIDS may be the single most important topic of research, as determined by its impact upon morbidity and mortality in gay and bisexual men, LGBT public health is much more than any single health concern (as is evidenced by this book).

A significant barrier to conducting public health research had always been the lack of researchers focused on the topic (Solarz, 1999). Only in the 1990s did major research and academic institutions begin to consciously (if not conscientiously) educate students to become investigators with the necessary skills and sensitivity to conduct LGBT public health research. Only then did major research journals begin to publish LGBT-specific public health research articles in any serious way. Unfortunately, funding for LGBT-specific research still is relatively scarce. However, with highly trained researchers becoming interested in the field, in increasing numbers with publications willing to review articles on the topic, and with a few streams of money available to investigate the major causes of morbidity and mortality in these populations, the field is finally coming into its own.

Perhaps the field got its most important recognition and legitimization from the inclusion of sexual orientation in *Healthy People 2010* (HP2010). HP2010 states that its second goal "is to eliminate health disparities among segments of the population, including differences that occur by gender, race or ethnicity, education or income, disability, geographic location, or sexual orientation" (U.S. Department of Health and Human Services, 2000, p. 11). This gave important credence to the notion that sexual orientation should be considered a demographic variable in public health research studies joining such other variables as gender, race or ethnicity, or socioeconomic status. Further, it gave credence to the notion that important health concerns needed to be investigated because they were associated with one sexual orientation more than another. Specifically, sexual orientation was included in twenty-nine of HP's 2010 objectives. These objectives span ten focus areas, including access to care, educational and community-based programs, family planning, HIV, immunization and infectious disease, injury and violence prevention, mental health and mental disorders, sexually transmitted diseases, substance abuse, and tobacco use (Sell & Becker, 2001b).

The National Institute of Mental Health, National Institute on Drug Abuse, and National Institute of Child Health and Human Development (joined by Office of Behavioral and Social Sciences Research, and Office of Research on Women's Health) soon followed HP2010 with the first program announcement (PA-01-96) encouraging scientific investigation into sexual-orientation-associated health disparities. The *American Journal of Public Health*, at about the same time, became the first mainstream health publication to publish a special issue dedicated to LGBT public health (Meyer, 2001).

More than anything else, these events encouraged researchers to think more seriously about how public health concerns may be significantly related to sexual orientations and gender; to write proposals with the belief that they have some chance of getting funding; to analyze data and write papers on these topics, knowing that they have a chance of getting them published in journals recognized by their peers and the public; and just possibly allowed them to believe that all of this work may one day reduce morbidity and mortality and increase quality of life in these populations.

WHAT IS "SEXUAL ORIENTATION" AND "GENDER" AND WHY ARE DEFINITIONS IMPORTANT?

In his book *All the Sexes*, Henry recognized, fifty years ago, that "unless the word homosexual is clearly defined, objective discussion regarding it is futile, and misunderstanding and erroneous conclusions are inevitable" (Henry, 1955, p. 70). To this day, despite Henry's warning, the construct of the "homosexual" or the more encompassing constructs of "sexual orientation" and "gender" have eluded clear definition despite, or perhaps because of, attempts by many to do so (Sell, 1997).

Numerous constructs used in public health research are not well-defined, including demographic variables other than sexual orientation and gender, such as race or ethnicity and socioeconomic status (Krieger, 2000b). It is therefore not surprising that the constructs of most relevance to LGBT public health, sexual orientation and gender, are likewise not well-defined. Although the lack of a clear definition is not essential to conducting research (as is evidenced by the volumes of public health research examining race and ethnicity) and should not prevent the initiation of new research, it is important, especially for a new field of research focusing on types or categories of people, to at least try to define these categories (Sudman, 1976).

If for no other reason, logical conceptualizations of the constructs are necessary in order to develop valid and reliable measures of sexual orientation and gender from which associations with health can be identified in research and consequently addressed through public health practice. Addressing these issues is also fundamental to defining the field of LGBT public health, because such definitions conceptually delineate the topic of investigation. Practically, the issues must be examined because the definitions ultimately determine who is included in studies of LGBT health (as well as who is included as heterosexual controls or as nontransgender controls) and who is consequently the target of health interventions and policy that may result from the research.

The literature debating how the constructs of race and ethnicity should be defined and measured for use in public health research demonstrates the importance and difficulty of defining populations and categories of people for research and public health purposes. Particularly relevant to this discussion are the extensive deliberations that occurred concerning the impact and utility of new measures of race and ethnicity introduced with the 2000 U.S. Census (Krieger, 2000a; Wallman, Evinger, & Schechter, 2000; Sondik, Lucas, Madans, & Smith, 2000; Fullilove, 1998). Efforts to study and provide health care to LGBT people would be well informed by a close review of this literature. Like discussions about the definition and measurement of race and ethnicity, discussions about the definition and measurement of sexual orientation and gender are not and may never produce definitive conclusions, but they are necessary for the field to advance and be taken seriously. Assessing where we are in being able to answer the question of what is a gay or a bisexual man, a lesbian or bisexual woman, a transgender person, or, more broadly, what is sexual orientation and gender, and how these constructs might have meaningful associations with health is of course a central proposition of this book.

Having just argued strongly for the importance of developing definitions of sexual orientation and gender, it may be surprising that no definitions will be presented here. This is because definitions remain extremely elusive, and a full discussion is beyond the scope of this chapter. In articles published elsewhere, attempts have been made to show the tremendous variability in definitions and the meanings implicit in these definitions (Sell, 1997). One review of actual research studies found that definitions are rarely discussed and often can only be inferred from publications with difficulty (Sell & Petrulio, 1996). Rather than recommending specific definitions here, we call upon researchers in future publications to explicitly state the definitions of the constructs underlying or implicit in their research design. Further, we call upon researchers to remember these definitions as they interpret their findings and incorporate them in any presentation of their results.

However, having pointed out that no single, clear definition for either sexual orientation or gender has been developed is not to say that there are not any major trends in definitions of these constructs. For example, definitions of sexual orientation usually contain one (or some combination) of three additional constructs, which we will refer to here as "dimensions of sexual orientation": (1) sexual orientation identity, (2) sexual behavior, or (3) sexual attraction (Sell, 1997). Yet, no clear trends have been noted regarding which of these dimensions is most commonly mentioned, nor is there much consistency in how they are described. Without clear definitions of the central theoretical constructs, how can we measure them in public health research in order to identify subjects for research studies?

HOW ARE LGBT PEOPLE IDENTIFIED FOR PUBLIC HEALTH RESEARCH?

Measures of sexual orientation and gender that are capable of identifying specific sexual orientations and people who are transgender are of course necessary in order to conduct LGBT public health research studies. The current state of sexual orientation measurement as well as some suggested measures of sexual orientation are discussed here.

When assessed, the sexual orientation of a research subject is generally measured by the selection (either by the researcher or the subject) of a single category from a list of a few discrete categories provided as responses to a single question about either (1) the sex of people to which the respondent has been sexually attracted, (2) the sex of people the respondent has had sexual contact with, or (3) how the respondent identifies his or her sexual orientation (sexual orientation identity) (Sell & Petrulio, 1996). Not surprisingly, these correspond with the list of the three most common constructs/dimensions mentioned in definitions of the sexual orientation construct.

Although it would be convenient if measures of each of these dimensions identified the same population, they do not. The National Health and Social Life Survey, which is one of the best surveys to have collected sexual orientation data in the United States, demonstrates that sexual attraction, sexual behavior, and sexual orientation identity measures of sexual orientation identify different (albeit overlapping) populations. Laumann, Gagnon, Michael, & Michaels (1994) found that of the 8.6 percent of women reporting some same-gender sexuality, 88 percent reported same-gender sexual desire, 41 percent reported some same-gender sexual behavior, and 16 percent reported a lesbian or gay identity. Of 10.1 percent of men reporting some same-gender sexuality, 75 percent reported same-gender sexual desire, 52 percent reported some same-gender sexual behavior, and 27 percent reported a gay identity. Other surveys have had similar results (Sell, Wells, & Wypij, 1995; Russell, Franz, & Driscoll, 2001).

Examples of questions that can be used to assess each of these three dimensions are provided in the second column of Table 3.1. The questions are presented here only as examples of questions that can be utilized to assess each of the dimensions of sexual orientation. The identity and behavior questions, with slight modification, are taken from the Massachusetts Youth Risk Behavior Survey (MYRBS) (Massachusetts Department of Education, 2002). MYRBS researchers have examined the properties of these questions fairly extensively and have modified them based upon their experience over five administrations of the survey, beginning in 1993. The sexual attraction question was newly created for this chapter and crafted to mirror the sexual behavior question. A summary of questions used in additional research studies is available elsewhere (Sell & Becker, 2001b).

No matter what question is chosen to assess sexual orientation, the validity and reliability of the measure should be investigated. Few if any measures of sexual orientation or gender have ever undergone the level of serious examination that, for example, questions used to assess race and ethnicity have undergone (Miller, 2002). Elsewhere Sell and Becker (2001b) have recommended that research on sexual orientation measures investigate how the questions are interpreted in diverse populations, and how the mode of data collection, question wording, and nonresponse impact validity and reliability. Further, they recommend that studies also examine the best methods of analyzing and tabulating sexual orientation data and the skills and training mecessary for researchers responsible for collecting and maintaining sexual orientation data.

The questions in Table 3.1 are practical for researchers and health care practitioners who want to assess sexual orientation quickly and without

TABLE 3.1. A Framework for Gay and Bisexual Men's Health Research and Practice

Dimensions of Sexual Orientation	Example of Assessment	Associated Health Concerns
Sexual orientation identity	Which of the following best describes you? a) Heterosexual (straight) b) Gay c) Lesbian d) Bisexual e) Not sure	• Access to care • Tobacco use • Cancers (e.g., lung, stomach) • Alcohol use • Drug use • Violence victimization • Teen suicide attempts • Eating disorders/nutrition • Parenting/marriage • Aging
Sexual behavior	During the past year, the person(s) with whom you have had sexual contact is (are): a) I have not had sexual contact with anyone b) Female(s) c) Male(s) d) Female(s) and male(s)	• Sexually transmitted diseases (e.g., herpes, hepatitis, syphilis, human papillomavirus, chlamydia, gonorrhea) • HIV/AIDS • Cancers (e.g., anorectal, Kaposi's sarcoma, breast, endometrial, ovarian)
Sexual attraction	During the past year, the person(s) to whom you have been sexually attracted is (are)? a) I have not been sexually attracted to anyone b) Female(s) c) Male(s) d) Female(s) and male(s)	• Mental health concerns related to "coming out" • Prevention interventions
Cross-cutting		• Violence • Access to care (e.g., health insurance, sexual orientation history) • Sexual health • Public health education/media

complication. The questions, with little or no modification, may be utilized in many different types of research or health care delivery settings, and may be administered in many different formats, including face-to-face interviews or self-completed questionnaires. However, others have recognized the limitations of these single-item measures, believing that they may oversimplify the assessment of a complex construct. The three chief complaints with these types of sexual orientation measures are that (1) they do not recognize sexual orientation as a complex continuum between heterosexuality and homosexuality, (2) they may inappropriately combine the constructs of heterosexuality and homosexuality, which would be better measured independently, and (3) such measures may not adequately reflect the cultural differences in the interpretation or expression of same-sex sexuality (Sell, 1997; Silenzio, 1997).

Addressing the first concern, Kinsey, Pomeroy, and Martin (1948) noted that

> It is a fundamental of taxonomy that nature rarely deals with discrete categories. Only the human mind invents categories and tries to force facts into separated pigeonholes. The living world is a continuum in each and every one of its aspects. The sooner we learn this concerning human sexual behavior the sooner we shall reach a sound understanding of the realities of sex. (p. 639)

Based upon these views, Kinsey developed the Kinsey Scale, which rates sexual orientations on a seven-point continuum from 0 (exclusively heterosexual) to 6 (exclusively homosexual), with 3 being the midpoint (equally heterosexual and homosexual) (Kinsey et al., 1948).

The second concern is more complicated and requires a more complex solution. Shively and DeCecco, who first put forth the idea that heterosexuality and homosexuality should be thought of as discrete constructs and measured independently, proposed a solution in a five-point scale on which heterosexuality and homosexuality would be independently assessed (Shively & DeCecco, 1977). Their scale, however, has largely been forgotten, and its validity and reliability remain untested.

The third concern recognizes that current biomedical and sociological frameworks addressing same-sex sexual expression have been heavily influenced by the cultural milieu from which these frameworks have emerged (Herdt, 1998). However, a multiplicity of competing frameworks exist, often simultaneously, within varied social and cultural settings. Beyond our current categorical framework of heterosexual, homosexual, and related concepts, other frameworks have existed historically and persist to the present day. These can be broadly situated within at least three additional conceptual categories defined by age, gender, or profession.

In *age-defined* frameworks such as that of classical Greece, sexual expression between members of the same sex occurs as part of normal maturation from childhood to adulthood. Such relations, typically between older and younger individuals, may or may not be considered essential to normal development, depending on the culture. *Gender-defined* frameworks provide for same-sex sexual expression in the context of individuals who assume the gender of the opposite sex, or who possess a combined or "third" gender. Examples include the *activo-pasivo* distinction made within several societies in or influenced by the Mediterranean basin cultural area (such as Latin America), as well as two-spirit traditions in Native American societies. *Profession-defined* frameworks address same-sex sexual expression that occurs within a professional or occupational context. Examples include male or female impersonators and the shamans of several societies along the Pacific Rim. The significance of these diverse patterns for researchers is in the fundamental influence upon subjects' responses to questions measuring same-sex sexual expression framed within Western cultural terms (Silenzio, 2003).

Recognizing the many concerns that have been raised, even more complex assessments of sexual orientation have been proposed (Sell, 1998; Klein, Sepekoff, & Wolf, 1985; Sambrooks & MacCulloch, 1973; Coleman, 1990; Berkey, Perelman-Hall, & Kurdek, 1990). Unfortunately, for the most part, the complexity of these assessments makes them impractical for most research purposes and, like the Shively and DeCecco scale, their validity and reliability remain unexamined. The development and testing of sexual orientation measures is in its infancy. Arguably, the measurement of gender is even further behind in development and testing (Israel & Tarver, 1997).

Yet without consensus concerning how the constructs of sexual orientation and gender should be measured, researchers have proceeded to examine associations between sexual orientation and health and the health of transgender people. In fact, there may never be consensus concerning how to best measure these constructs, or arguments over measurement standards may never be conclusively settled (as in the case with race and ethnicity). However, researchers presenting their results should explicitly outline and discuss how they assessed sexual orientation, and what they believe to be the limitations of the methods they chose. The next section outlines a framework for investigating public health research based upon the discussion thus far and continues the discussion of limitations of the measurement of sexual orientation and gender.

A FRAMEWORK FOR THE INVESTIGATION
OF LGBT PUBLIC HEALTH

The dimensions of sexual orientation that are most commonly included in definitions and measures of sexual orientation as described in the previous two sections (sexual orientation identity, sexual behavior, and sexual attraction) are presented in the first column of Table 3.1 as part of a theoretical framework that can be used to illustrate the scope of LGBT public health research. Although it would be efficient to define and measure sexual orientation by assessing only one of the three dimensions, there may be reasons why each of them might have importance for understanding associations between sexual orientation and health. An attempt to relate the definitions and measures to actual public health concerns will be made here and is intended as a guide for conducting research.

It should be noted at this point that this framework focuses on lesbian, gay, and bisexual health; a similar framework can hopefully be identified for understanding transgender health. That is, it is hoped that a framework could be developed to illustrate how definitions and measures of gender can be theoretically and in practice linked to specific health concerns. Likewise, such a framework could be used to direct and interpret public health research related to transgender health (Israel & Tarver, 1997).

The framework relating dimensions and measures of sexual orientation to health in Table 3.1 is fairly straightforward. The third column of Table 3.1 provides a summary of health concerns that we believe might be more closely associated with one dimension of sexual orientation than another. Researchers may want to consider how the selection of a sample based upon this dimension of sexual orientation may be more relevant to their research than selection based upon another dimension.

For example, it is not surprising that when researching and discussing HIV/AIDS and sexually transmitted diseases among sexual minority men, the label for the at-risk population most commonly used is "men who have sex with men" (Catania et al., 2001; Fox et al., 2001). Focusing on sexual behaviors not only provides a more targeted focus for understanding the spread of HIV/AIDS, but also has a strong public health rationale. This is not to say that the other dimensions of sexual orientation do not have value in understanding HIV/AIDS issues. For example, men who are sexually attracted to other men but who have not had sexual contact with other men may be the targets of HIV/AIDS prevention efforts. Likewise, prevention efforts may be very different depending upon whether they target men who have sex with other men who identify as gay or bisexual or men who do not identify as gay or bisexual.

The health concerns associated with the different dimensions of sexual orientation presented in Table 3.1 are meant only to provide insight into and provoke discussion of possible relationships between sexual orientations and health. Further, the list is not meant to be exhaustive, and although hopefully logical, little empirical evidence supports the arrangement of some of the concerns into these categories. Some of the most interesting evidence, however, comes from Youth Risk Behavior Survey (YRBS) data. Since the Centers for Disease Control, which sponsors the YRBS, does not mandate the collection of sexual orientation data in the survey, the collection of these data has not been standardized across the states that have independently decided to collect the information. States and cities have consequently added an array of sexual orientation identity, sexual behavior, and sexual attraction questions to their otherwise standardized survey instruments (Sell & Becker, 2001b).

YRBS data from the localities assessing sexual orientation have shown, regardless of which dimension of sexual orientation they assess (including even perceived sexual orientation), that lesbian, gay, and bisexual youth have higher rates of suicidal thoughts and attempts, victimization by school violence, drug and alcohol abuse, early onset of sexual behavior, and eating disorders (Russell et al., 2001; Faulkner & Cranston, 1998; Garofalo, Wolf, Kessel, Palfrey, & DuRant, 1998; Garofalo, Wolf, Wissow, Woods, & Goodman, 1999; Vermont Department of Health, 1999; DuRant, Krowchuk, & Sinal, 1998; French, Story, Remafedi, Resnick, & Blum, 1996; Oregon Health Division, 1997; Reis & Saewyc, 1999; Remafedi, French, Story, Resnick, & Blum, 1998). However, as suggested in Table 3.1, some dimensions of sexual orientation have been shown to be more highly correlated with specific outcomes. For example, reporting suicide attempts in the previous year were 5 percent of male youth with same-sex attractions or relationships, 28 percent of male youth with same-sex behavior, and 35 percent of youth who identified as gay, lesbian, or bisexual (data on boys and girls were not presented separately, but the percentage for males would have exceeded 35 percent) (Faulkner & Cranston, 1998; Garofalo et al., 1998; Russell & Joyner, 2001).

In another example of the framework, sexual behaviors (or the lack of heterosexual sexual behavior) can put lesbian and bisexual women at increased risk for certain cancers. Although lesbian and bisexual women can and do have children, they may have fewer children than heterosexual women. Because nulliparity is believed to be a risk factor for breast, endometrial, and ovarian cancer, lesbian and bisexual women may be at increased risk for these cancers. Further, oral contraceptives, which may be prescribed to homosexual women less often than to heterosexual women, may provide some protection from ovarian cancer (but may possibly increase the risk of breast cancer). Finally, homosexual men may be at increased risk for anorectal cancer as a result of their increased risk of contracting human papillomavirus through sexual behavior (Gay and Lesbian Medical Association and LGBT Health Experts, 2001).

Further, the development of a lesbian, gay, or bisexual identity may be associated with participation in these communities, and these communities may consequently promote certain safe and unsafe behaviors that result in either positive or negative health outcomes. For example, a common meeting place for lesbians, gays, and bisexuals has traditionally been bars (D'Emilio, 1984). Because of the availability of alcohol, tobacco, and other drugs at bars and the use of these substances by peers and potential sexual partners, lesbians, gays, and bisexuals may be at increased risk of using or abusing these substances. This participation in bar settings could also, in theory, put them at increased risk of developing lung cancer in localities in which smoking is still permitted in these settings. Further, the abuse of these substances could put them at increased risk of participating in "unsafe sex" (Semple, Patterson, & Grant, 2003).

Other chapters of this book will discuss the current state of knowledge concerning the health of lesbians, gays, and bisexuals. Therefore, the inclusion and placement of each of the health concerns listed in Table 3.1 will not be fully justified in this chapter. However, in other chapters in this book it may be helpful for public health researchers to think about how specific health concerns may relate to this framework.

Finally, a number of health concerns do not easily fit into the three dimensions of sexual orientation, consequently showing some the limitations to this framework (see the final row of Table 3.1). For example, access to health care spans all three of the dimensions of sexual orientation. Access to health care is of concern for two reasons. First, lesbians, gays, and bisexuals may not provide a full or accurate account of their sexual orientation to their health care provider when it is requested, and health care providers may not be trained to ask the appropriate questions to assess sexual orientations. When the health care provider does not know the sexual orientation of the patient, the patient does not have true access to the health care system because the special health problems discussed in this book may not be thoroughly investigated, and other health concerns (such as oral contraceptives for lesbians not sexually active with men) may be inappropriately addressed (Klitzman & Greenberg, 2002; Gay and Lesbian Medical Association and LGBT Health Experts, 2001).

Second, health insurance, or the lack thereof, prevents access to health care. Gay and bisexual men may have difficulties obtaining or retaining insurance due to their HIV status or their perceived risk of contracting HIV. Lesbian and bisexual women may have trouble obtaining insurance because women are more likely than men to be employed in settings that do not provide health insurance. Also, women's incomes are lower on average than men's, allowing them less disposable income to purchase insurance. Further, most lesbian, gay, and bisexual men and women are not able to obtain health insurance through the workplace of their same-sex "significant others," as heterosexual couples are often permitted to do (Gay and Lesbian Medical Association and LGBT Health Experts, 2001).

Further, the health of lesbians, gays, and bisexuals can be affected by the fear or sometimes hatred of homosexuality and bisexuality that permeates society. In particular, as a result of homophobia, homosexuals and bisexuals are at a higher risk of being victimized through "hate crimes." When a lesbian, gay, or bisexual person is physically or verbally harassed, the perpetrator may not be acting based upon the person's actual sexual orientation identity, their actual sexual behaviors, or because of their actual same-sex sexual attractions, but rather based upon what they perceive these to be in their victim. In fact, it may be gender-atypical behavior more than their sexual orientation that puts the person at risk for violence (Willis, 2004).

Finally, it is important to mention that researchers should not necessarily focus solely upon looking for and researching the existence and causes of health inequalities related to sexual orientations and gender. Although these might be an essential aspect of research into LGBT public health and may be fundamental to the framework presented here, researchers should also investigate qualitative differences in health based upon sexual orientation and gender. For example, even if it is found that LGBT people are the victims of violence at rates equal to (as opposed to greater or less than) other populations, the experience of this violence may be very different in ways that are not easily quantifiable.

LIMITATIONS OF RESEARCH METHODS FOR INVESTIGATING LGBT HEALTH

The complexity of issues in LGBT health requires researchers to draw upon the full range of available methods. Relatively speaking, sexual minority populations remain rare and hidden. Although geographic concentration within large conurbations has been appreciated for some time, data from the 2000 U.S. Census have underscored that sexual minority populations are found in every area of the nation (Sell et al., 1995; Laumann et al., 1994; Associated Press, 2001).

Much controversy has surrounded the so-called essentialist-constructionist debate surrounding same-sex sexuality (Padgug, 1992). Simply stated, the debate regards whether same-sex sexuality is an essential feature of human nature or whether it is a phenomenon produced by social structures. Fortunately, the steam has run out of the engines of those holding the most extreme theoretical positions in this debate. Most researchers have arrived at a middle ground, recognizing the truth behind both of these viewpoints and the conceptual utility of both (Crompton, 2003).

Anthropological and sociological studies of sexuality have advanced our current understanding of sexual identity development, social factors influencing sexual behavioral patterns, and the myriad interpretive frameworks for sexual expression that exist within any given social structure. Moreover, in conjunction with historical research these issues can be understood as exhibiting dynamic change over time. What guided the sexual expression of men and women of classical Greece, Victorian England, and American society at the turn of the millennium shares many features, but differs profoundly in others. More recently, anthropological research has pointed to the differences among LGBT subgroups based on geographic setting, racial or ethnic background, social class, and so on, further underscoring the need for sophisticated research methods in studying this highly diverse population (Crompton, 2003).

How, then, does one appropriately address the issues of difficulty in accessing significant numbers of LGBT people for research? Provided it is adequately measured, sexual orientation should be considered a core variable in all data collection systems and instruments (Sell & Becker, 2001a). With the wide geographic dispersion, social diversity, and social stigmatization of sexual minority populations, quantitative social science studies of the relationships among health, sexual orientations, and transgender identity must overcome the barriers in obtaining sufficient sample sizes for study. Relatively rare populations can present certain methodological and financial challenges when constructing representative samples (Sell et al., 1995; Martin & Dean, 1990; Sudman, Sirken, & Cowan, 1988; Sudman, 1976). To a larger extent, unlike in the areas of defining and measuring the populations as discussed previously, research outside the field of sexual orientations and gender can be examined, modified, and applied to the construction of research samples (Lee, 1993; Renzetti & Lee, 1993).

Although the analytical and interpretive issues related to sample size and representativeness of the population under study differ between quantitative and qualitative research approaches, these concerns remain central to both lines of inquiry. A multiplicity of qualitative approaches exist to address these concerns (Bernard, 1998, 2000). One illustrative example of qualitative sample generation involves a systematic development of contacts over time (Silenzio, 2003) (see Table 3.2). This represents a basic ethnographic approach to gaining entry into a social group, with an emphasis on rapid assessment. Nonetheless, ethnographic approaches provide detailed, qualitative information about the population under study, suggesting interpretations that may be transferable to other populations and in other periods of time (Crabtree & Miller, 1999).

The approach in Table 3.2 displays much in common with the methods that have been most often used to construct samples of LGBT populations in quantitative studies. In the case of LGBT populations, these sampling approaches include the following:

- *List Sampling*—Sample populations are derived from a list, such as members of an LGBT organization. This may include the entire list or a selection of members from the list.
- *Multipurpose Sampling*—Samples initially constructed for a separate purpose are drawn upon to study issues related to LGBT health. For example, a study to examine women and suicide, by stratifying the sample by sexual orientation, can be expanded to examine the relative risks of various factors by sexual orientation.
- *Screening Sampling*—A larger, general population sample is screened using a question or set of questions to identify LGBT people for inclusion into the research study.
- *Network or Snowball Sampling*—In this approach, the researcher builds from a core sample of the population of interest. Members of this core then identify other members of the target population who are consequently contacted and included in the study. These additional individuals can then be used to build the overall study sample through subsequent recruitment waves (referred to as the so-called snowballing effect), which can continue until the desired sample size is obtained.
- *Outcropping Sampling*—This approach identifies individuals of rare populations at venues frequented by the populations. For example, lesbian and gay pride events, lesbian and gay neighborhoods, and online venues such as a gay- or lesbian-themed chat room serve as "outcroppings" of individuals from which to draw study samples.
- *Advertising Sampling*—This approach uses commercial advertisements to recruit subjects. Advertisements are usually placed in media outlets catering to the population of interest or posted in venues frequented by the population.
- *Servicing Sampling*—Services can be offered to a study subject as an inducement to participate in a study. Examples would include transsexuals recruited through an offer of free hormone-replacement counseling or gay men recruited through free or reduced-price hepatitis vaccinations.

TABLE 3.2. Rapid Ethnographic Assessment for LGBT and Other Sexual Minority Populations

Action Step	Objective
Define the target or at-risk populations	Development of preliminary working definitions of the population(s) of interest
Search for information and gaps in knowledge about the target population	Conduct a thorough search of the literature and other documentary evidence to identifying gaps in knowledge about the target population
Survey internal staff members who have knowledge of the target community	Identifying internal staff members and others with knowledge of the target population and collecting data through semistructured interviews or surveys
Survey external systems staff and volunteers with knowledge of the target communities	Move beyond immediate staff and contacts to gather additional information from other formal agencies or professionals familiar with the target community
Survey "interactors"	Interactors are defined as individuals who have informal contact with the target community, but are not themselves part of the target community
Reduce and integrate information from the internal and external interviews	This involves close examination and integration of the data generated and provides the foundation for subsequent steps
Define and prioritize sectors and subgroupings of the target population	The taxonomies developed initially are revised in light of the data that emerge. The sectors and subgroupings developed are prioritized for study based upon issues such as accessibility, levels of risk, and relative size of the population
Obtain access through "gatekeepers" and other means to conduct observations	Gatekeepers are individuals who can control access to the target population for participant or nonparticipant observation
Interview key participants or members of the target community	In-depth, semistructured, or structured interviews to gather "insider" views of the sectors and subgroupings of interest
Interpret data from all the previous steps	Formal data reduction, analysis, and interpretation
Conduct focus groups with members of the target communities	Formal use of focus groups to provide critiques of individual interview data and to conduct "member checking" of findings, interpretations, and conclusions

Source: Adapted from Silenzio, 2003, and Higgins et al., 1996.

Although systematic biases are introduced through each of these approaches, one or more of these methods can be and often are used simultaneously to construct samples. Although they are beyond the scope of the present discussion, these biases must be addressed in analyzing and interpreting study findings. Nonetheless, these sampling approaches are frequently used because they are relatively convenient and feasible with limited available resources (Meyer & Colten, 1999).

One further challenge to studies of LGBT health is that of sampling and studying "sensitive" topics. Sensitive research areas are defined by Sieber and Stanley (1988) as "studies in which there are potential consequences or implications, either directly for the participants in the research or for the class of individuals represented by the research" (p. 50). For individuals whose sexuality may not be public knowledge, study subjects may face risks of social stigmatization, victimization, violence, discrimination, and other concerns due to participation in research. Revealing sexual orientation or transgender identity can be difficult because of cultural taboos or because some subjects may have unresolved concerns relating to these issues (Ryan & Futterman, 1998; Sell et al., 1995). Without protection of confidentiality, subjects can place themselves at risk for violence and discrimination through participation (Lee, 1993). Although the legal scene regarding same-sex behavior is rapidly changing, study participants may reveal or imply the conduct of certain sexual behaviors classified as criminal in some jurisdictions (Hunter, Michaelson, & Stoddard, 1992). Our available approaches to studies of LGBT health and other sensitive topics must therefore be examined in the context of such concerns that are not frequently relevant to other areas of health research (Lee, 1993; Renzetti & Lee, 1993). The sensitive nature of LGBT health research affects the entire research process, including the formulation of research questions, study design and conduct, and dissemination of research results. LGBT health researchers must be able to competently address a range of methodological, ethical, political, and legal challenges.

Several approaches have been developed to successfully assist researchers addressing sensitive topics. In terms of the development of survey questions, the following techniques have been widely used:

- *Loading questions*—This refers to the process of biasing a question to influence a participant's comfort with providing a response. For example, a question can be phrased to imply that a certain behavior is common or socially acceptable. Questions can also be worded to assume that a respondent has participated in specific behaviors, forcing the subject to respond in the negative if they have not (Lee, 1993).
- *Familiar words*—Questions that include wording commonly used by the subject or the population to describe the sensitive topic being ex-

plored have been shown to improve the subject's understanding and increase comfort with responding to questions (Bradburn, 1983).

- *Long questions*—For most purposes, short questions are almost always preferable to long questions; however, long questions can sometimes provide memory clues to the respondent or give the respondent more time to recall past experiences on sensitive topics (Bradburn, 1983).
- *Embedded questions*—Questions that are sensitive can be purposefully embedded throughout the questionnaire to decrease the level of threat or discomfort they may pose. For example, questions regarding same-sex sexual behavior are less threatening in a general survey of sexual behavior. Questions regarding past behavior or practice tend to be perceived as less threatening than current behavior or practice, and are therefore frequently asked first. Questions concerning the present can then be asked to follow up whenever a respondent reports "ever" expressing the behavior (Lee, 1993).

Researchers can address other aspects of the research process to better examine sensitive topics. These can include some of the following techniques, described in detail in the references cited: randomized response, nominative techniques, and microaggregation techniques (Lee, 1993; Duffy & Waterton, 1984; Bradburn, 1983; Boruch & Cecil, 1979). Finally, when studying sensitive topics, assuring confidentiality can improve response rates and the validity of research subjects' responses. Assuring confidentiality can be a complex process; however, every researcher studying LGBT health should be aware of procedures to do so and must be able to competently implement these procedures (Boruch & Cecil, 1979).

DISCUSSION

LGBT public health research is at an exciting phase of development and an important crossroad in history. A few academic institutions are at last purposely training researchers who can critically and intelligently explore the essential issues. Funders are beginning to put money toward the research of these issues, and peer-reviewed public health publications are increasingly willing to issue articles on the topic. However, LGBT public health research has a number of fundamental issues that must be explored before the field can be truly realized. As discussed in this chapter, different definitions and measures of sexual orientation and gender will identify different populations, and the epidemiology of health will differ between these populations. The implication of this obvious statement for LGBT public health has not been adequately examined. This chapter has attempted to explore this concern by suggesting a framework to assist in the discovery and interpretation of associations between sexual orientation and health.

Clearly, much can be learned from similar work and analyses examining relationships between race and ethnicity and health. Perhaps the most important of these lessons is the value of standardization in population measures. Although the measures of race and ethnicity included in the 2000 U.S. Census may not be perfect and satisfy all constituencies, they have become at least temporary standards to which those looking for associations between race and ethnicity and health can adhere. The results of one study can therefore be compared with the results of another study, and the racial and ethnic distributions found in a sample can be compared to distributions in the general population. At present, comparable standards for measuring sexual orientation and gender (i.e., capable of identifying transgender people) do not exist, and no obvious sources or authorities exist for producing such measures. Perhaps measures from the YRBS as presented in Table 3.1 or from work being conducted at the National Center for Health Statistics can serve as foundations for future work related to the measurement of sexual orientation. These issues need to be more clearly examined and generally acceptable solutions found, particularly as they relate to gender, if the field is to advance.

Finally, methods need to be developed and tested across all public health subdisciplines (such as epidemiology, sociology, anthropology, political science, etc.) that can be used to study LGBT public health. Because the populations are relatively rare and can sometimes be hidden, they often pose particular challenges to researchers. However, despite the challenges of defining, measuring, and sampling sexual orientation and gender discussed in this chapter, researchers are forging ahead with studies that provide important information concerning the links between health, sexual orientation, and gender, as well as providing valuable insights into the conduct of such research.

QUESTIONS TO CONSIDER

1. Does your agency collect lesbian-, gay-, bisexual-, and transgender-specific health data?
2. How can your agency include lesbian, gay, bisexual, and transgender items on research and needs-assessment instruments?

3. How can you advocate for researchers to include lesbian, gay, bisexual, and transgender items in/on current research instruments?
4. What benefits will the collection of lesbian, gay, bisexual, and transgender health data provide to your agency?

REFERENCES

Associated Press. (2001, August 22). Households headed by gays rose in the 90's, data shows. *The New York Times*, p. A17.

Berkey, B. R., Perelman-Hall, T., & Kurdek, L. A. (1990). The multidimensional scale of sexuality. *Journal of Homosexuality, 19*(4), 67-87.

Bernard, H. R. (Ed.). (1998). *Handbook of methods in cultural anthropology*. Walnut Creek, MD: AltaMira Press.

Bernard H. R. (2000). *Social research methods: Qualitative and quantitative approaches*. Thousand Oaks, CA: Sage Publications.

Boruch, R. F., & Cecil, J. S. (1979). *Assuring the confidentiality of social research data*. Philadelphia: University of Pennsylvania Press.

Bradburn, N. M. (1983). Response effects. In P. H. Rossi, J. D. Write, and Andy B. Anderson (Eds.), *Handbook of survey research* (pp. 289-328). New York: Academic Press.

Catania, J. A., Osmond, D., Stall, R. D., Pollack, L., Paul, J. P., Blower, S., Binson, D., Canchola, J. A., Mills, T. C., Fisher, L., Choi, K. H., Porco, T., Turner, C., Blair, J., Henne, J., Bye, L. L., & Coates, T. J. (2001). The continuing HIV epidemic among men who have sex with men. *American Journal of Public Health, 91*(6), 907-914.

Coleman, E. (1990). Toward a synthetic understanding of sexual orientation. In D. P. McWhirter, S. A. Sanders, & J. M. Reinisch (Eds.), *Homosexuality/heterosexuality: Concepts of sexual orientation* (pp. 267-276). New York: Oxford University Press.

Crabtree, B. F., & Miller, W. L. (1999). *Doing qualitative research* (2nd ed.). Thousand Oaks, CA: Sage Publications.

Crompton, L. (2003). *Homosexuality and civilization*. Cambridge, MA: The Belknap Press of Harvard University.

Davis, K. B. (1929). *Factors in the sex life of twenty-two hundred women*. New York: Harper & Brothers Publishers.

D'Emilio, J. (1984). *Sexual politics, sexual communities*. Chicago: University of Chicago Press.

Duffy, J. C., & Waterton, J. J. (1984). Randomized response models for estimating the distribution function of a quantitative character. *International Review, 52*, 165-172.

DuRant, R., Krowchuk, D., & Sinal, S. (1998). Victimization, use of violence, and drug use at school among male adolescents who engage in same-sex sexual behavior. *Journal of Pediatrics, 133*(1), 113-118.

Ellis, H., & Symonds, J. A. (1897). *Sexual inversion*. London: Wilson and Macmillan.

Faulkner, A. H., & Cranston, K. (1998). Correlates of same-sex sexual behavior in a random sample of Massachusetts high school students. *American Journal of Public Health, 88*(2), 262-266.

Fox, K. K., del Rio, C., Holmes, K. K., Hook, E. W., III, Judson, F. N., Knapp, J. S., Procop, G. W., Wang, S. A., Whittington, W. L., & Levine, W. C. (2001). Gonorrhea in the HIV era: A reversal in trends among men who have sex with men. *American Journal of Public Health, 91*(6), 959-64.

French, S. A., Story, M., Remafedi, G., Resnick, M. D., & Blum, R. W. (1996). Sexual orientation and prevalence of body dissatisfaction and eating disordered behaviors: A population-based study of adolescents. *International Journal of Eating Disorders, 19*(2), 119-126.

Fullilove, M. T. (1998). Comment: Abandoning "race" as a variable in public health research—An idea whose time has come. *American Journal of Public Health, 88,* 1297-1298.

Garofalo, R., Wolf, R. C., Kessel, S., Palfrey, J., & DuRant, R. (1998). The association between health risk behaviors and sexual orientation among a school-based sample of adolescents. *Pediatrics, 101*(5), 895-902.

Garofalo, R., Wolf, R. C., Wissow, L. S., Woods, E. R., & Goodman, E. (1999). Sexual orientation and risk of suicide attempts among a representative sample of youth. *Archives of Pediatric Adolescent Medicine, 153,* 487-493.

Gay and Lesbian Medical Association and LGBT Health Experts (2001). *Healthy people 2010 companion document for lesbian, gay, bisexual and transgender (LGBT) health.* San Francisco, CA: Gay and Lesbian Medical Association.

Henry, G. W. (1948). *Sex variants: A study of homosexual patterns.* New York: Paul B. Hoeber.

Henry, G. W. (1955). *All the sexes: A study of masculinity and femininity.* New York: Rinehart and Company, Inc.

Herdt, G. (1998). *Same sex, different cultures: Exploring gay and lesbian lives.* New York: Westview Press.

Higgins, D. L., O'Reilly, K., Tashima, N., Crain, C., Beeker, C., Goldbaum G., Elifson, C. S., Galavotti, C., & Guenther-Grey, C. (1996). Using formative research to lay the foundation for community level HIV prevention efforts: An example from the AIDS Community Demonstration Projects. *Public Health Reports, 111* (Part 1), 28-35.

Hirschfeld, M. (1914). *Die homosexualität des mannes und des wiebes.* Berlin, Germany: Louis Marcus.

Hooker, E. (1957). The adjustment of the male overt homosexual. *Journal of Projective Techniques, 21,*18-31.

Hunter, N. D., Michaelson, S. E., & Stoddard, T. B. (1992). *The rights of lesbians and gay men.* Carbondale and Edwardsville, IL: Southern Illinois University Press.

Israel, G. E., & Tarver, D. E. (1997). *Transgender care.* Philadelphia, PA: Temple University Press.

Kinsey, A. C., Pomeroy, W. B., & Martin, C. E. (1948). *Sexual behavior in the human male.* Philadelphia, PA: W. B. Saunders.

Klein, F., Sepekoff, B., & Wolf, T. J. (1985). Sexual orientation: A multi-variable dynamic process. *Journal of Homosexuality, 11,* 35-49.

Klitzman, R. L., & Greenberg, J. D. (2002). Patterns of communication between gay and lesbian patients and their health care providers. *Journal of Homosexuality, 42*(4), 65-75.

Krieger, N. (2000a). Counting accountably: Implications of the new approaches to classifying race/ethnicity in the 2000 census. *American Journal of Public Health, 90*(11), 1687-1689.

Krieger, N. (2000b). Refiguring "race": Epidemiology, racialized biology, and biological expressions of race relations. *International Journal of Health Services, 30*(1), 211-216.

Laumann, E., Gagnon, J., Michael, R., & Michaels, S. (1994). *The social organization of sexuality: Sexual practices in the United States.* Chicago: University of Chicago Press.

Lee, R. M. (1993). *Doing research on sensitive topics.* London: Sage Publications.

Martin, J. L., & Dean, L. (1990). Developing a community sample of gay men for an epidemiological study of AIDS. *American Behavioral Scientist, 33*(5), 546-561.

Massachusetts Department of Education. (2004). 2003 Youth Risk Behavior Survey results. Retrieved August 31, 2005, from http://www.doe.mass.edu/hssss/yrbs/03/results.pdf.

Meyer, I. (2001). Why lesbian, gay, bisexual, and transgender public health? *American Journal of Public Health, 91*(6), 856-859.

Meyer, I., & Colten, M. E. (1999). Sampling gay men: Random digit dialing versus sources in the gay community. *Journal of Homosexuality, 37*(4), 99-110.

Miller, K. (2002). *Cognitive analysis of sexual identity, attraction, and behavior questions.* Cognitive Methods Staff Working Paper Series, no. 32. Hyattsville, MD: Office of Research and Methodology, National Center for Health Statistics.

Oregon Health Division, Center for Health Statistics and Vital Records. (1997). *Suicidal behavior: A survey of Oregon high school students, 1997.* Retrieved June 22, 2005, from http://www.oregon.gov/DHS/ph/chs/data/hsi/teensuic/teensuic.shtml.

Padgug, R. (1992). Sexual matters: On conceptualizing sexuality in history. In E. Stein (Ed.), *Forms of desire: Sexual orientation and the social constructionist controversy* (pp. 43-67). New York: Routledge.

Peterkin, A., & Risdon, C. (2003). *Caring for lesbian and gay people: A clinical guide.* Toronto: University of Toronto Press.

Reis, B., & Saewyc, E. (1999). *Eighty-three thousand youth: Selected findings from eight population-based studies as they pertain to anti-gay harassment and the safety and well-being of sexual minority students.* Seattle: Safe Schools of Washington Coalition.

Remafedi, G., French, S., Story, M., Resnick, M. D., & Blum, R. (1988). The relationship between suicide risk and sexual orientation: Results of a population-based study. *American Journal of Public Health, 88*(1), 57-60.

Renzetti, C. M., & Lee, R. M. (Eds.). (1993). *Researching sensitive topics.* London: Sage Publications.

Rowan, R. L., & Gillette, P. J. (1978). *The gay health guide: A complete medical reference for homosexually active men and women.* Boston: Little, Brown and Company.

Russell, S. T., Franz, B., & Driscoll, A. K. (2001). Same-sex romantic attraction and violence experiences in adolescence. *American Journal of Public Health, 91*(6), 903-906.

Russell, S. T., & Joyner, K. (2001). Adolescent sexual orientation and suicide risk: Evidence from a national study. *American Journal of Public Health, 91*(8), 1276-1281.

Ryan, C., & Futterman, D. (1998). *Lesbian and gay youth: Care and counseling.* New York: Columbia University Press.

Sambrooks, J. E., & MacCulloch, M. J. (1973). A modification of the sexual orientation method and automated technique for presentation and scoring. *British Journal of Social and Clinical Psychology, 12,* 163-174.

Sell, R. L. (1997). Defining and measuring sexual orientation: A review. *Archives of Sexual Behavior, 26*(6), 643-658.

Sell, R. L. (1998). The Sell assessment of sexual orientation: Background and scoring. *Journal of Gay, Lesbian, and Bisexual Identity, 1*(4), 295-310.

Sell, R. L., & Becker J. B. (2001a). *Sexual orientation data: Inclusion in information systems and databases of the Department of Health and Human Services.* Prepared for the Office of the Assistant Secretary for Planning and Evaluation. 5 March 2001.

Sell, R. L., & Becker, J. B. (2001b). Sexual orientation data: Inclusion in health information systems used to monitor HP2010. *American Journal of Public Health, 91*(6), 876-882.

Sell, R. L., & Petrulio, C. (1996). Sampling homosexuals, bisexuals, gays and lesbians for public health research: A review of the literature from 1990-1992. *Journal of Homosexuality, 30*(4), 31-47.

Sell, R. L., Wells, J. A., & Wypij, D. (1995). The prevalence of homosexual behavior and attraction in the United States, the United Kingdom and France: Results of national population-based samples. *Archives of Sexual Behavior, 24*(3), 235-248.

Semple, S. J., Patterson, T. L., & Grant, I. (2003). HIV-positive gay and bisexual men: Predictors of unsafe sex. *AIDS Care, 15*(1), 3-15.

Shively, M. G., & DeCecco, J. P. (1977). Components of sexual identity. *Journal of Homosexuality, 3,* 41-48.

Sieber, J. E., & Stanley, B. (1988). Ethical and professional dimensions of socially sensitive research. *American Psychologist, 43,* 49-55.

Silenzio, V. M. B. (1997). Lesbian, gay and bisexual health in cross-cultural perspective. *Journal of the Gay and Lesbian Medical Association, 1*(2), 75-86.

Silenzio, V. M. B. (2003). Anthropological assessment for culturally appropriate interventions targeting men who have sex with men. *American Journal of Public Health, 93*(6), 867-871.

Solarz, A. L. (Ed.). (1999). *Lesbian health: Current assessment and directions for the future.* Washington, DC: Institute of Medicine, National Academy Press.

Sondik, E. J., Lucas, J. W., Madans, J. H., & Smith, S. S. (2000). Race/ethnicity and the 2000 census: Implications for public health. *American Journal of Public Health, 90*(11), 1709-1713.

Steakley, J. D. (1997). Per scientiam ad justitiam: Magnus Hirschfeld and the sexual politics of innate homosexuality. In R. Vernon (Ed.), *Science and homosexualities* (pp. 133-154). New York: Routledge.

Sudman, S. (1976). *Applied sampling.* New York: Academic Press.

Sudman, S., Sirken, M. G., & Cowan, C. D. (1988). Sampling rare and elusive populations. *Science, 240,* 991-996.

U.S. Department of Health and Human Services. (2000). *Healthy People 2010: Understanding and improving health* (2nd ed.). Washington, DC: U.S. Government Printing Office.

Vermont Department of Health, Office of Alcohol and Drug Abuse Programs. (1999). *1999 Vermont youth risk behavior survey statewide report.* Retrieved September 1, 2005, from http://www.state.vt.us/adap/1999YRBS/YRBSST991.htm.

Wallman, K. K., Evinger, S., & Schechter, S. (2000). Measuring our nation's diversity: Developing a common language for data on race/ethnicity. *American Journal of Public Health, 90*(11), 1704-1708.

Willis, D. G. (2004). Hate crimes against gay males: An overview. *Issues in Mental Health Nursing, 25*(2), 115-132.

PART II:
ACADEMIA

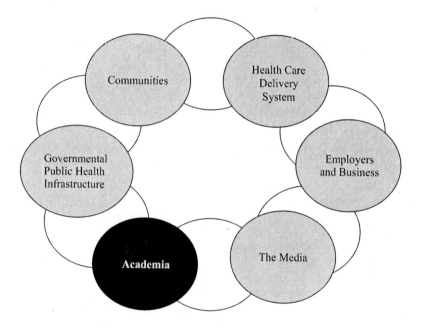

Chapter 4

Lesbian, Gay, Bisexual, and Transgender Cultural Competency for Public Health Practitioners

Katherine L. Turner
Wayne L. Wilson
M. Kate Shirah

INTRODUCTION AND BACKGROUND

Public health services rendered to LGBT people are negatively impacted by practitioners' lack of knowledge about or sensitivity to sexual or gender orientation, ignorance about specific health concerns, and real or perceived homophobia and heterosexism. Ignorance, fear, and aversion by both practitioners and LGBT clients can lead to suboptimal care or a lack of provisions of public health services (Gay and Lesbian Medical Association and LGBT Health Experts, 2001; Lee, 2000). LGBT cultural competency training can help practitioners overcome these barriers, resulting in improved public health services for LGBT people.

Beyond the individual practitioner level exists a growing body of work designed to create a public health environment that is more accessible and services that are appropriate for LGBT individuals. To achieve this, LGBT individuals should be included in public health research, interventions, and policy development. Public health practice standards and guidelines on culturally appropriate health care services for LGBT people are also needed at the national, state, and local level.

The authors wish to acknowledge the following for their support and guidance: Sandra Crouse Quinn, Eugenia Eng, Karen Strazza Moore, students in the UNC–Chapel Hill Department of Health Behavior and Health Education who helped plan and facilitate LGBT competency workshops, Lesbian Resource Center, and Triangle Community Works.

In the absence of national or state policy standards and a coordinated effort to implement them, individual organizations have developed guidelines, training curricula, and materials to prepare public health practitioners in LGBT cultural competency. These could serve as a foundation for the development of future standards. In Massachusetts, the Gay, Lesbian, Bisexual, and Transgender Health Access Project created a set of community standards of practice and indicators for the provision of quality health care for LGBT clients (see Exhibit 4.1.) (GLBT Health Access Project, 1999).

The Society for Public Health Education (SOPHE) passed a resolution, based on the United States Department of Health and Human Services document for Healthy People 2010, that measures should be taken to eliminate health disparities based on sexual orientation.

The Society for Public Health Education (SOPHE) is an independent, international professional association organized to promote healthy behaviors, healthy communities, and healthy environments through its membership, its network of local chapters, and its numerous partnerships with other organizations. With its primary focus on public health education, SOPHE provides leadership through a code of ethics, standards for professional preparation, research, and practice; professional development; and public outreach.

Among other actions, this resolution calls for professional training to increase LGBT cultural competency of public health and health care professionals (SOPHE, 2001). Likewise, the American Public Health Association (APHA) has passed two resolutions that, respectively, supported increased inclusion of LGBT people in research efforts (APHA, 1998) and specifically acknowledged transgendered individuals in research and clinical practice (APHA, 1999). A milestone in LGBT health care guidance was achieved with the coordinated effort of the Gay and Lesbian Medical Association and LGBT health researchers to develop the *Healthy People 2010 Companion Document for Lesbian, Gay, Bisexual, and Transgender Health* (Gay and Lesbian Medical Association and LGBT Health Experts, 2001).

LGBT competency is one of many aspects of cultural competency. To date, much of the work and literature on cultural competency has focused on racial and ethnic minorities. The U.S. Office of Minority Health (OMH) has created guidelines and culturally and linguistically appropriate standards for cultural, racial, and ethnic competency in health care (OMH, 2003). Many individuals belong to multiple cultures; for example, they may be racial/ethnic minorities as well as LGBT. Care must be taken when developing cultural competency standards not to infuse biases, such as a heterosexual bias in racial/ethnic competency standards or a white bias in LGBT competency standards. Although some similarities exist regarding

**EXHIBIT 4.1. Massachusetts GLBT Health Project
Standards Example**

The community standards of practice and quality indicators identified were designed to guide and assist providers in achieving specific goals of eliminating bias and prejudice while supporting a safe health care environment for LGBT people.

The standards address both agency administrative practices and service delivery components, including the following areas:

Personnel
Client's Rights
Intake and Assessment
Service Planning and Delivery
Confidentiality
Community Outreach and Health Promotion

Following is an example of a standard and indicators in the area of service planning and delivery:

Standard: All agency staff shall have a basic familiarity with gay, lesbian, bisexual, and transgender issues as they pertain to services provided by the agency.

Indicator: Development and implementation or revision of agency training and programs on diversity, harassment, and antidiscrimination to assure explicit inclusion of gay, lesbian, bisexual, and transgender issues.

Indicator: Development and implementation of training for all intake, assessment, supervisory, human resource, case management, and direct care staff on basic gay, lesbian, bisexual, and transgender issues.

how to approach cultural competence in racial/ethnic and LGBT populations, each community's characteristics and histories of stigma and discrimination require that specific competency standards be established to address their unique concerns. Advocating for one type of cultural competency does not diminish the importance or need for other types.

The goal of this chapter is to provide a framework for understanding, assessing, and developing training to enable public health practitioners to provide competent and sensitive services to LGBT people. The LGBT Cultural Competency Framework for Public Health Practitioners introduced in this chapter, organized by topic areas and including specific objectives, covers each progressive stage leading to cultural competency. The framework is designed to aid the development of LGBT cultural competency training for public health practitioners and, ultimately, lead to consistently equitable and high-quality public health services for LGBT people.

CONTEXT FOR TERMINOLOGY AND DEFINITIONS

In discussions on LGBT cultural competency, consistent and common terminology is needed, including the terms culture, cultural competency, awareness, sensitivity, competency, and mastery. *Culture* can be defined as a specific set of social, educational, religious, or professional behaviors, practices, and values that individuals learn and adhere to while participating in or out of groups with which they usually interact (DiversityRX, 1997). Cultural competency has been extensively discussed and defined in the literature (DiversityRX, 1997; Goldsmith, 2000; Messina, 1994; OMH, 2003; Sullivan, 1995). For the purposes of this chapter, *cultural competency* will be discussed as an evolution through a series of stages, from awareness of the culture, to sensitivity to cultural issues, to competent practice within the culture, and ultimately, to mastery as a trainer of cultural competence. *Cultural awareness* is understood as knowledge about a particular group and about oneself in relation to that group. Awareness is gained primarily through reading, studying, observing, or training. *Cultural sensitivity* is defined as having a deeper understanding, appropriate attitudes, and a commitment to addressing disparities in a particular group in relation to other groups (Messina, 1994). *Cultural competency* is defined as a set of knowledge, attitudes, and skills that can be demonstrated by an individual under specific conditions and evaluated on predetermined standards based on the premise of respect for individuals and differences and the implementation of a trust-promoting method of practice (DiversityRX, 1997; Sullivan, 1995) (see Figure 4.1). Usually, a tandem process of personal and professional transformation occurs during the journey toward cultural competency and mastery. Even when one has attained mastery, learning and evolving one's cultural skills should be an ongoing process.

RATIONALE

LGBT individuals deserve health care services that are appropriately and competently provided at the same level of access and quality as they are to all other members of the larger society. Practitioners need to realize that LGBT individuals are accessing services as well as working as their peers

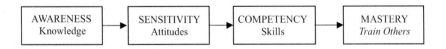

FIGURE 4.1. Stages of Cultural Competency

and colleagues. Two of the biggest barriers to culturally competent care are practitioners' lack of awareness that LGBT individuals have specific health service needs and, even if they are aware of specific needs, their inability to provide services competently. Once practitioners are sensitized to LGBT needs, they can begin developing appropriate attitudes and skills to attain LGBT cultural competence.

"When I asked if they had seen any other gay people, she said, 'We treat all our patients the same,' and my first thought was, 'Uh-oh . . . warning sign.' " — Gay man (Turner, Wilson, & Shirah, 2003)

Because of ignorance about the diversity within the LGBT community, a lesbian, gay, bisexual, or transgender person who does not fit a stereotype may not be recognized or identified as LGBT. For example, if practitioners only recognize effeminate, white, gay men as LGBT, the needs of the remaining members of the LGBT community are ignored or inadequately served. This limited view of LGBT individuals continues to perpetuate service and health disparities among LGBT people.

In some instances, LGBT people may face similar barriers to health care access as in the general population, for example, because of low income or lack of health insurance. However, certain barriers are unique to LGBT people. Transgender people have in some instances been refused service specifically because of their gender orientation or appearance. Lesbians and bisexual women on average may have reduced means to afford services because of lower earnings than their male counterparts (Perry & O'Hanlan, 1997). Inequitable quality of care for LGBT people has been documented (Bowen, 2001; Perry & O'Hanlan, 1997); specific examples include

- Overt prejudice, discrimination, disdain, or denial within health systems that leads to LGBT people feeling unsafe or uncomfortable with disclosure of sexual or gender orientation and intimate relationships and can result in avoidance of care;
- Overt homophobia, subtler heterosexism, or denial of LGBT-specific norms and needs that impairs practitioners' interactions with clients and decreases effectiveness of service delivery;
- Ignorance regarding issues of sexual and gender orientation and the health needs of LGBT people by practitioners;
- Assumption of risk factors based on sexual or gender orientation rather than individual behaviors and health history, resulting in inappropriate services;

- Inadequate protection of individual and same-gendered couples' rights in health policies and a lack of recognition of LGBT people's intimate relationships and families; and
- Inadequate research on LGBT health issues, exclusion of LGBT people or means of identifying them in general research, and general reluctance of LGBT participants to participate or disclose their identity in research.

"It's kind of Russian roulette because you don't know how a doctor is going to react when you come out to them and there have definitely been times when I haven't because already from the doctor's manner or things he or she has said, I just feel like it's not safe." — Lesbian (Shirah, 2002)

Many public health practitioners do not recognize how their assumptions and biases affect their interactions with LGBT peers and clients as well as the quality of services they deliver, even when those biases are unconscious or communicated nonverbally (Cranton & King, 2003; Duffy, 2001). For example, practitioners may avoid eye contact, maintain more distance, place a physical barrier such as a desk between themselves and their clients, or put on more physical barriers (such as two pairs of latex gloves) before making contact with clients. Practitioners can also convey assumptions or discomfort through spoken language, such as using words or asking questions that assume heterosexuality, ignoring or not responding to clients' comments about their sexual or gender orientation, or even using blunt or abrasive language with LGBT clients (Dean et al., 2000; Matthews, Peterman, Delaney, Menard, & Brandenburg, 2002; Shirah, 2002). Nonverbal and verbal communication speaks volumes to clients about the practitioners' receptivity to them and, in turn, clients may be less likely to seek or return for health care services or provide adequate information for the practitioner to provide quality services (Clark, Landers, Linde, & Sperber, 2001).

"Even when they're nice, I don't like seeing doctors. It's like going to a judge or priest: They're authorities, they always know and you don't. My sexual choices are suspect and I'm supposed to believe them." — Bisexual man (Turner, Wilson, & Shirah, 2003)

Some specific examples of how anti-LGBT bias can negatively impact health services include defining gay men's health needs only in the context of HIV and ignoring broader health needs; missing the importance of cervical cancer or sexually transmitted infection screening in sexually active lesbian clients; or failing to understand why a female-to-male transgender person who still has breasts would need a clinical breast exam, even if he does not relate comfortably to his female body parts.

LGBT individuals often make rational assumptions about health services and practitioners due to the social stigma they have faced in their broader life experiences. Fear or hatred (homophobia or transphobia) and denial (heterosexism or strict gender roles) of LGBT people in our society creates an environment in which LGBT people may rightly be wary when accessing new health services or seeing a practitioner for the first time. Health systems and practitioners have often perpetuated discrimination and homophobia with LGBT clients. Some health practitioners continue to maintain biases against LGBT people, fail to recognize LGBT health concerns, or make heterosexist assumptions (Perry & O'Hanlan, 1997; Ryan, Brotman, & Rowe, 2000). Service and organizational polices need to address potential presumptions by LGBT people that they may need to hide their sexual or gender orientation in order to receive adequate and equitable care. Taking steps to reduce biases and create an environment that is supportive to appropriate self-disclosure can increase service quality.

"He [the doctor] said, 'You're an aberration. You should expect this kind of treatment.' There have been others, but that stands out particularly in my mind . . . he did absolutely nothing to make me want to stay on this plane of existence." — Male-to-female transgender (Turner, Wilson, & Shirah, 2003)

That the previously mentioned biases continue to be experienced and documented indicates a need to establish standards for LGBT cultural competency for all public health practitioners that can be implemented in all health services. Establishing standards for working with LGBT communities provides a structure for public health practitioners and institutions to follow. As part of their evolution from awareness to sensitivity, practitioners need to learn about the characteristics of LGBT cultures. As with every culture, unique norms of behavior and communication impact the quality of interactions. The diversity within the LGBT community creates unique variations in language that need to be explored and understood. Once an initial awareness and sensitivity toward LGBT culture and needs are addressed for individuals, the process can then move to the service-delivery level to create a more welcoming environment for LGBT people. This progression would include institutionalizing policies to address LGBT competency and making commitments to provide training in core preservice educational curricula as well as in-service training for established public health practitioners.

Practitioners may be concerned that providing culturally competent care for LGBT people might be unacceptable to their non-LGBT clients and that they could be perceived as promoting homosexuality and transgenderism. It is helpful to understand the difference between affirming LGBT communities and promoting homosexuality. To "affirm" LGBT communities is to communicate positively about their existence and value; to "promote" LGBT communities would be to advance or put LGBT people in a higher position than another group (Hedgepeth, 2000). A practitioner would be promoting homosexuality and transgenderism if the messages stated they are preferable to or better than being heterosexual or nontransgendered. Affirming the LGBT community in health services builds on the awareness that LGBT people exist and deserve fair treatment and that LGBT people represent a valuable part of the community as a whole.

Every public health practitioner has an ethical and professional responsibility to provide the best care and services possible to every person who needs them. Public health practitioners may have difficulty reconciling professional standards while remaining true to personal values. Because some of their clients will be LGBT, practitioners may need to assess their attitudes and beliefs and then explore how they impact individual practice and the health services environment as a whole. Support and training for providers through LGBT cultural competency curricula would provide them with the opportunity for this necessary reflection and evolution.

Public health institutions and individual practitioners must take the initiative to assess the state of their intentions and readiness to provide LGBT-positive health services to diverse LGBT individuals and communities. Given the persistent biases keeping individuals from providing competent care, there is a clear need to create standards and training curricula that support LGBT competency. In doing so, these standards and training curricula will help to eliminate systemic, institutional, and individual barriers to appropriate and sensitive services and create culturally competent public health environments for LGBT individuals.

AN LGBT CULTURAL COMPETENCY FRAMEWORK

Based on rationales already outlined in this chapter, public health institutions of higher learning and professional organizations must effectively prepare public health practitioners to address LGBT health disparities and thus institutionalize LGBT cultural competency training into the core curriculum and ongoing certification requirements. To date, no widely accepted LGBT cultural competency framework for training public health practitioners has been developed. However, identifying and defining the core public health competencies needed for practitioners to effectively conduct research, deliver services in a practice, and advocate for policies concerning LGBT individuals and communities is a crucial step in developing such a framework.

The LGBT Cultural Competency Framework for Public Health Practitioners is outlined in Table 4.1. This framework identifies topic areas necessary to achieving LGBT cultural competency with related learning objec-

TABLE 4.1. LGBT Cultural Competency Framework for Public Health Practitioners

Topic Area	Objectives by Stage		
	Awareness	Sensitivity	Competency
Inclusion	Recognize the presence of LGBT people in every community and culture, encountered in both personal and professional lives	Demonstrate understanding of the importance of designing and delivering health services inclusive of LGBT people	Provide services that are inclusive of LGBT people
Sex and gender	Differentiate between sexual and gender orientation and identity	Demonstrate sensitivity toward the diversity of sexual and gender orientations and identities	Deliver services that are appropriate to people's self-identification of gender and sexual orientation
Terminology	Define key terminology and concepts used by LGBT individuals and communities	Demonstrate understanding of the importance of terminology to LGBT identity and community	Use LGBT terminology appropriately in practice
Roles and family structures	Identify partnership and family structures and individuals' roles within them	Respect individual roles and partnership and family structures	Provide services that respect individual roles and appropriately include LGBT people's partners and families
Diversity	Recognize the diversity within LGBT communities	Appreciate the diversity within LGBT communities	Design and provide services that meet LGBT people's diverse health needs
Stigma	Describe heterosexism, homophobia, and transphobia, their institutionalization in the public health systems, and impact on LGBT people's health	Accept responsibility for addressing stigma at the individual and organizational level	Institute policies and practice norms that create a safe and welcoming environment for LGBT practitioners and clients within public health organizations and services

TABLE 4.1 *(continued)*

	Objectives by Stage		
Topic Area	Awareness	Sensitivity	Competency
Sociopolitical factors	Discuss sociopolitical factors that impact the health and quality of life of LGBT individuals	Demonstrate concern about the social and political environment for LGBT individuals	Advocate for legal and civil policies and laws that promote LGBT health and quality of life
Health status	Describe current demographics and health status of LGBT populations	Demonstrate concern for LGBT people's health status and means of improving it	Design and provide public health services that improve LGBT people's health
Access to care	Identify unique factors affecting LGBT individuals' access to health care	Accept responsibility for reducing barriers to health care access for LGBT individuals	Proactively reach out to LGBT clients and implement strategies to facilitate access to services
Quality of care	Identify factors affecting quality of health services provided to LGBT individuals	Demonstrate commitment to improving health services for LGBT individuals	Design and deliver consistently high-quality public health services for LGBT people
Personal values	Recognize personal beliefs and biases related to LGBT individuals and communities	Accept responsibility for personal beliefs and biases related to LGBT individuals and communities and how they impact service delivery	Practice effective, respectful, and trust-building interaction and communication with LGBT people

tives for each topic area. Each topic area's learning objectives are listed as a progression through the cultural competency stages identified earlier in this chapter: awareness, sensitivity, and competency. (The mastery stage mentioned previously will not be addressed here, as it lies beyond the scope of this chapter.)

The framework serves as a basis for achieving general LGBT cultural competency and can be used as a guide for developing LGBT cultural competency training materials and curricula. For individual public health and related disciplines, additional topic areas or more specific learning objectives may need to be developed to address particular practice areas and guidelines (e.g., gynecological screening standards for transgender patients).

The first topic area addressed, inclusion, illustrates the first step in achieving LGBT cultural competency: acknowledgement of the presence of LGBT people in the world and, hence, the need to provide services that are inclusive of LGBT people. The next topic areas—sex and gender, terminology, roles and family structures, and diversity—consist of internal factors of LGBT (and heterosexual) communities and individuals. The existence of external factors that affect LGBT communities shapes the next two topic areas: stigma and sociopolitical factors. Stigma refers to heterosexism, homophobia, and transphobia on an individual and organizational level. Sociopolitical factors include laws, policies, and social structures that affect, intentionally and unintentionally, the lives of LGBT people.

Health status, access to care, and quality of care describe the health of LGBT individuals as well as what and how internal and external factors affect LGBT individuals' health status, access to care, and the quality of care they receive. For public health practitioners, these topic areas illustrate the particular health needs of LGBT people and what factors may help or hinder the ability to address those needs. The last topic area, personal values, focuses on the individual public health practitioner's own beliefs and biases related to LGBT communities and individuals.

Awareness

Basic awareness (Figure 4.2) begins through the acknowledgement that LGBT people exist in every family, organization, community, and culture whether these individuals are recognized or identify as LGBT or not. Differentiating sex and gender, both sexual and gender orientation, as well as sexual and gender identities, shapes the understanding of continuums of sex, gender, and sexual orientation identification. Learning essential terminology and concepts that are used to describe LGBT subcommunities, family structures, and other defining characteristics provides a context for understanding the beliefs and practices of LGBT people.

Multiple factors affect access to quality health care and general quality of life issues for LGBT individuals and communities. Perhaps the most significant of these is stigma, both actual and perceived, which plays out in not only the individual lives of LGBT people but also in the social and political environment in which individuals function (Dean et al., 2000). Therefore, practitioners should be able to identify forms of stigma, sociopolitical factors

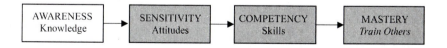

FIGURE 4.2. Stages of Cultural Competency: Awareness

that perpetuate prejudice and discrimination, and other factors that influence health status, access to care, and quality of care.

One of the more difficult steps in achieving cultural competency is becoming aware of one's own personal biases and stereotypes (Dedier, Penson, Williams, & Lynch, 1999). In order to effectively work with LGBT individuals and communities, public health practitioners must acknowledge the assumptions and stereotypes that color their interactions with clients (Welch, 2002).

Sensitivity

Although public health practitioners may have an awareness of the issues surrounding professional interactions with LGBT individuals and communities, they must also become sensitive (Figure 4.3) to the norms that shape their clients' lives. Resnicow, Baranowski, Ahluwalia, and Braithwaite (1999) suggest that culturally competent practice begins with the ability to incorporate awareness of experiences, beliefs, and practices within a historical, social, and political context. The sensitivity stage, therefore, should guide practitioners to distance themselves from a heteronormative perspective, in which the existence of LGBT people, clients, and peers is not recognized or valued, through developing respect and appreciation for the culture of LGBT communities and individuals.

With movement toward cultural sensitivity, public health practitioners should foster appreciation for and validation of diversity in sex and gender orientations and identities; respect for family structures, functions, and roles within LGBT culture; and appreciation of the diversity within and among LGBT communities and individuals. They must also begin to understand and acknowledge the relationship between the social environment and the lives of LGBT individuals (e.g., how lack of same-sex marriage rights prevents automatic visitation privileges and health care decision making of same-sex partners).

Public health practitioners can become more culturally flexible and sensitive by identifying crucial sociopolitical factors and particular cultural beliefs and practices and then incorporating and validating these factors in their practice (Welch, 2002). Similarly, it is important for practitioners to

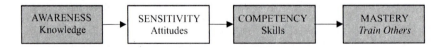

FIGURE 4.3. Stages of Cultural Competency: Sensitivity

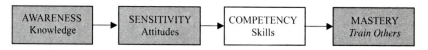

FIGURE 4.4. Stages of Cultural Competency: Competency

accept responsibility for their personal beliefs and biases, and respect when others' beliefs and practices may be different from their own.

Competency

Achieving cultural competency (Figure 4.4) among all public health practitioners should be the goal of both preservice and in-service curricula. Although achieving LGBT cultural awareness and sensitivity learning objectives signifies good intentions, competency combines both the desire and ability to effectively serve the public health needs of LGBT individuals and communities (Welch, 2002). Cultural competency entails modifying one's own practice as well as working to create a supportive organizational and sociopolitical environment in partnership with LGBT individuals and the community (OMH, 2001; GLMA & LGBT Health Experts, 2001).

Culturally competent practitioners are able to effectively assess and provide services in an inclusive and respectful manner. They are able to advocate for policies and practice norms within their organizations and communities that create a safe and welcoming environment for LGBT people. Further, public health practitioners should be able to design and implement health services and programs that are inclusive and respectful of LGBT individuals, as well as attempt to overcome the barriers that prevent LGBT individuals from accessing those services. This can be achieved by practicing trust building and effective interaction and communication skills, as well as suspending personal beliefs and practices in order to maintain a perspective of LGBT individuals' beliefs and practices.

LGBT AWARENESS, SENSITIVITY, AND COMPETENCY TRAINING

This section will address both preservice and in-service training for public health students and current practitioners on the continuum from awareness to sensitivity to competency. Students and in-service trainees will be described as participants, while faculty and facilitators conducting the training will be referred to as instructors.

LGBT and allied faculty, students, staff, and practitioners may be the individuals to initially advocate with school and organization administrators for the inclusion of LGBT competency training in the core curriculum and ongoing certification requirements or staff development (see Exhibit 4.2 for tips on advocating). However, it is important that the burden does not fall on only LGBT people to ensure LGBT competency training. It has been the authors' experience that if LGBT issues are only or mostly addressed when certain people raise them, this can lead to LGBT training becoming inconsistent and sporadic, with varying levels of quality.

LGBT training cannot be a one-time occurrence. It takes time and experience under varied circumstances to attain sensitivity and competency. Rather than only offering one discrete course, LGBT training is more effective when it is interwoven in all public health courses (Garcia, Wright, & Corey, 1991; Stephenson, Peloquin, Richmond, Hinman, & Christiansen, 2002). Courses can include case studies, essay questions, field practicums, and other learning exercises that include diverse scenarios of LGBT people and their health concerns. LGBT and allied faculty, students, staff, alumni, practitioners, and community groups can be excellent resources to schools and organizations that need assistance in developing appropriate training policies and materials.

Practitioners are raised, as all people are, with a wide range of beliefs about sex, gender, and human sexuality. The ultimate goal of LGBT competency training is to build upon the range of experiences and support the participants' personal transformation and attainment of professional skills. Public health practitioners cannot be blamed for not having been exposed to LGBT cultural competency training when standards and policies are not

EXHIBIT 4.2. Advocating for LGBT Cultural Competency in Training Curricula

- Identify public health curricula, courses, professional conferences, and other preservice or continuing education events that present an opportunity for introducing LGBT competency training.
- Identify the decision makers who have the authority to include LGBT competency training, such as faculty, administrators, instructors, conference organizers, and panel moderators.
- Identify key stakeholders who will actively support efforts to include LGBT competency training, such as faculty, alumni, administrators, professional organization officers, and LGBT advocates and leaders.
- Mobilize key stakeholders to gather support and precedence, advocate for inclusion, and work with decision makers to implement proposed policy or curriculum changes.
- Work with faculty, instructors, organizers, and LGBT advocates to develop or adapt appropriate training curricula and activities.

widely recognized, accepted, and instituted. However, once offered the opportunity, public health practitioners must be willing to work toward developing LGBT awareness, sensitivity, and competency to be able to provide competent care for everyone. Ultimately, if they are unwilling to work toward LGBT cultural competency, then they are not fulfilling the roles and responsibilities of a public health practitioner (Pew Health Professions Commission, 1995; Stephenson et al., 2002).

Creating a Productive Learning Environment

For effective public health training on LGBT awareness, sensitivity, and competency, the instructor creates a learning space that is both safe and challenging (Hutchinson, 2003; Newell, 1999). Instructors need to have participants create, agree upon, and remain aware of group guidelines, as well as ensuring enforcement when they are being violated. Group guidelines help establish safe parameters within which participants can take risks and still remain supported in their learning (Porter, 1984; Wegs, Turner, & Randall-David, 2003).

Perhaps because many are motivated by service to people, public health students and practitioners can be hesitant to explore or reveal their biases in front of their peers. Instructors may need to work diligently to create a nonjudgmental and supportive learning space that allows for open exploration and discussion without negative repercussions for those who express unpopular or minority opinions. Instructors can remind participants that a variety of viewpoints is common in every group and ask participants to take risks and voice their ideas or opinions, even if they are challenging for others. As long as participants are voicing their sincere opinions and are not intending to hurt anyone's feelings, instructors should continue to maintain an open space for a diversity of ideas and viewpoints. Instructors need to refrain from becoming defensive or taking comments personally when people voice opposing opinions. These differences of opinion can be channeled into important learning opportunities when instructors handle them effectively.

Awareness Training

LGBT Existence

LGBT awareness training can begin with a presentation that informs participants of the existence of LGBT people in every family, organization, community, and culture. This can be accomplished through the introduction of a trigger, or presentation, designed to stimulate thoughtful discussion, followed by a progression of questions and facilitated discussion. The trigger could be a quote, image, skit, panel of LGBT people, or clip from a mainstream television show or film that deals with the invisibility of an LGBT character's sexual or gender orientation. Instructors can then split the participants up into pairs or small groups to discuss questions about their own experiences with LGBT people, relative LGBT invisibility in a heterosexist society, and reasons for this invisibility.

LGBT Terminology

Other important components of LGBT awareness training are desensitization to LGBT terms and images and the development of a common vocabulary to ensure clear communication throughout the training. This includes airing terms and images that are considered pejorative by some, neutral by others, and that may have been co-opted as positive language by some members of the LGBT community.

During a desensitization and vocabulary-building activity, instructors may ask participants to fill in the blanks for each of the following statements: "A lesbian is . . ." "A transgender person is . . ." Continue with "gay man," "bisexual woman," "bisexual man," "heterosexual woman," and "heterosexual man." Instructors can help participants overcome their hesitations to use words or images that may be considered stereotypical or demeaning by saying them first, thus demonstrating that this language is acceptable in that learning space. Instructors can encourage participants to call out their responses in a "stream of consciousness" manner without censoring their thoughts. The idea is to explore the words, images, and assumptions that first come to mind when people hear the words, "gay man," "lesbian," and so on and to become more comfortable using the terminology. Instructors can have participants brainstorm as many words and images as come to mind for each term, one at a time. Participants are then asked a series of discussion questions to provoke a deeper understanding of where these associations come from and what effects they may have on interactions with LGBT people.

These discussion questions could include the following:

- What are some ways you can overcome assumptions about LGBT and heterosexual people?
- What did you learn about the words and images you associate with LGBT and heterosexual people?
- What assumptions did you make?
- As public health practitioners, how might these associations and assumptions affect your interactions with LGBT and heterosexual co-workers and clients?

This exercise requires attentive facilitation and a healthy dose of humor to encourage a free-flowing group brainstorm and exploration without crossing the line to becoming a socially acceptable group bashing of LGBT or heterosexual people.

Awareness of One's Own Biases

Public health practitioners must learn how their assumptions and biases affect the quality of their interactions with LGBT clients and peers and, ultimately, the quality of the services provided. Instructors can have participants reflect on situations they have experienced personally. For example, a time when the participants knew without being told that someone else was making an assumption about them, or a time when someone held a bias against a participant because of a characteristic that was out of their control. For example, a participant may share her experiences with people assuming she was dumb because she was blonde and attractive. Some may have experienced bias because of their appearance or accent. Instructors can then ask participants how being the recipient of bias made them feel about themselves and about that person, and how the bias affected their interaction with and trust of the person. This type of reflection may help participants gain a better understanding of how assumptions and biases can have profound negative effects on people's interactions and the outcomes of those interactions (Cranton & King, 2003).

Sensitivity Training

Values Clarification

A necessary element of LGBT sensitivity training is the opportunity for participants to reflect on their values and attitudes in such a way that leads to personal and professional transformation. Most people, including many LGBT people, are unaware of the extent of their own homophobia and heterosexism. Personal relationships with LGBT people are key to this process. It can be helpful for instructors to have participants reflect on LGBT people in their lives or characters on television or in film to whom they can relate. Then the instructor can facilitate a process in which participants experience an LGBT person's pain and see themselves as part of the source of that pain. Again, this can be accomplished through the presentation of a trigger followed by a series of discussion questions that elicit participants' learned heterosexism and homophobia in order to make them more conscious of the ways they may unwittingly feed into those biases and assist them in identifying the ways they can alleviate the suffering they cause.

Values clarification is an important element in sensitivity training. It helps participants become more aware of their values and attitudes, gain a deeper understanding of others, question their personal beliefs, and gain empathy for LGBT people by demonstrating the stigma that they face. One extremely effective values clarification activity is "Four Corners." In advance, the instructor posts a sign in each of the four courners of the room that reads "strongly agree," "agree," "disagree," or "strongly disagree." The instructor distributes worksheets to participants, who anonymously indicate their responses (strongly agree, agree, disagree, or strongly disagree) to a series of statements about LGBT people, policies, and civil rights. The instructor collects and redistributes the worksheets so every participant has one that is most likely not their own. The instructor then reads one of the statements and asks participants to go to the corner of the room with the sign that corresponds with the response on their worksheet. A group is now in each of the four corners. All four groups are given a few minutes to develop the strongest arguments they can think of in support of the response on their worksheet, regardless of whether it aligns with their own beliefs. A reporter for each group then presents their group's arguments to the other three groups. This is repeated two to three times using different statements on the worksheet. Participants then sit back down and debrief the activity. By having to construct arguments for opinions they may or may not hold, this activity serves to help participants clarify their values and gain empathy for others. Participants will identify their own attitudes about LGBT issues and have the opportunity to better understand other people's opinions, hear additional or different arguments about their own opinions, and hear discussion and questions about their beliefs.

Empathy Development

Another important process in sensitivity training is empathy development. A variety of empathy exercises help participants better understand life as an LGBT person, the unique challenges and stigmas they face, and what actions could make life less stressful and more enjoyable for LGBT people. A visualization activity is often very effective in accomplishing this process by having people imagine what their everyday lives would be like if they were members of a sexual or gender minority in an intolerant world. Participants close their eyes and the instructor leads them through a number of scenarios in which they imagine their lives as part of a sexual or gender minority. This is usually a sobering experience for people who have taken their sexual and gender orientation, and the privileges they are accorded because of them, for granted. One example of an experiential empathy activity is the LGBT homework assignment. Participants are given a list of activities and asked to do at least one of them in the two weeks following the LGBT sensitivity training. They are paired with a buddy, with whom they will debrief their action once they have completed the assignment. Examples of empathy-building activities include trying to keep their romantic relationship closeted for a week; raising LGBT issues or concerns to a group of peers; or buying, carrying, and reading an LGBT publication in public.

Competency Training

Building upon the attainment of awareness and sensitivity, participants need to acquire and apply skills in both simulated and actual settings in order to reach competency. Competency training needs to be skill based and provide opportunities for participants to practice their skills with LGBT people. The skills practiced by participants need to be relevant and applicable to their work as public health practitioners. The instructor also needs to provide opportunities for participants to anticipate barriers they will face in advocating for LGBT inclusion and how they will overcome those challenges. The goal of competency training is for participants to practice and get feedback on addressing LGBT competency issues with their standard public health skills until they have reached an acceptable established standard.

Critical Analysis

Skill activities may include practice with critical analysis on public health case scenarios to determine the potential implications for LGBT people. Participants read case studies and answer questions about how the particular scenario could potentially impact LGBT people and their health.

Development of LGBT-Inclusive Interventions

Another skill activity is for participants to develop public health programs, research, and policies that are LGBT inclusive. Small groups can work on designing LGBT-inclusive health education or health-promotion materials and programs, research designs and measures, and public health policies. In addition to identifying the language, images, outreach, promotion strategies, and definitions they would employ, groups would identify potential barriers they could face in advocating for LGBT inclusion and methods for overcoming them (see Exhibits 4.3 and 4.4).

**EXHIBIT 4.3. Case Example Preservice Training:
Introduction to LGBT Competency Workshop
for Public Health Education Master's Students**

At the UNC–Chapel Hill School of Public Health, public health education master's students and alumni advocated for the inclusion of LGBT training for all first-year master's-level students. One faculty member was supportive and set aside a class for this training.

The faculty member allowed the instructors autonomy with workshop design and facilitation and had well-defined participation in the workshop. The instructors designed and conducted a needs assessment with the students to determine their levels of experience with LGBT issues, attitudes about working with LGBT people, and potential training needs. Evaluations from a previously conducted antiracism workshop the students had participated in were also analyzed. The instructors formed a committee with students to help plan and prepare for the workshop. They tailored the agenda and activities to the unique needs, experiences, group dynamics, and range of experiences with LGBT people and topics. Based on the needs assessment and other workshop evaluations, instructors knew the workshop needed to be relevant, practical, and skills focused. Due to the relatively short time allotted for the workshop, instructors also maximized group learning time by assigning independent readings and LGBT-awareness homework assignments before and after the workshop and then a follow-up LGBT homework assignment with a planned debriefing in pairs. Despite this level of planning, instructors remained flexible to make changes throughout the workshop if the planned activities or discussions weren't having the desired effect or students expressed other expectations of the workshop. They conducted an evaluation to determine if students' needs were met and facilitate planning for the next year's workshop.

Note: Due to continued support by subsequent faculty, this workshop is now an annual part of first-year student training.

Recommendations

- LGBT cultural competency needs to be included in national public health standards and guidelines.
- LGBT cultural competency training needs to be integrated into public health and in-service curricula for public health practitioners.
- LGBT training cannot be a one-time occurrence. It is more effective when it is interwoven in all public health courses.
- Every practitioner, whether LGBT or not, needs to raise issues of increasing LGBT competency so the burden does not fall solely on LGBT communities.

- LGBT competencies need to be further developed and tailored for specific public health disciplines.
- Training curricula need to be developed to train practitioners to competency within their public health discipline.
- LGBT and LGBT-allied faculty, students, staff, alumni, practitioners, and community groups can be consulted as resources to schools and organizations that need assistance developing appropriate training policies and materials.

EXHIBIT 4.4. Case Example In-Service Training: Culturally Competent Care Training Curriculum

A preliminary needs assessment conducted by the Lesbian Resource Center (LRC), a nonprofit organization in Durham, North Carolina, highlighted the overwhelming need for additional services to address lesbian health care service delivery needs. In addition to increased national attention on the health issues affecting women who partner with women (WPW), the organization received a vast number of requests for recommendations for friendly and knowledgeable health care providers and detailed information about those providers' qualifications. The organization identified the need to develop a standardized training curriculum for health care providers that would be implemented by volunteer trainers.

Utilizing a cultural competency framework, the development of the curriculum involved three key elements: an extensive review of existing LGBT training guides and manuals; interviews with health care providers to determine the most appropriate format, delivery, and content of a training on the health issues of WPW; and interviews and focus groups with community members to identify particular health care needs of local WPW.

The goal of the training curriculum is to educate clinical health care providers on the health care concerns, issues, and needs of WPW living in the North Carolina Triangle area (Durham, Orange, and Wake Counties). The curriculum covers information, skills, and resources health care providers need to create a WPW-friendly health care practice. Based on providers' identified need for flexibility in training, the core components of the curriculum, two ready-to-go training modules and several mix-and-match modules, allow for variety in training length, design, and setting.

"Culturally Competent Care for Women Who Partner with Women in the North Carolina Triangle Area" serves as an excellent resource for the LRC in offering trainings to Triangle health care providers. In addition, it may be used as a starting point for other individuals and agencies to offer health care provider trainings in their own communities (Shirah, 2002). More information on the curriculum can be found at www.trianglelrc.org.

CONCLUSION

LGBT people are in every family, community, workplace, and client population and are deserving of the same high-quality public health services as all other members of society. Health disparities experienced by lesbian, gay, bisexual, and transgender individuals and the LGBT community are sufficiently documented and must be eliminated. This chapter has begun charting LGBT cultural competency objectives, and additional work must be done to complete, standardize, and institutionalize these competencies in public health standards, guidelines, and curricula. It is the duty of public health practitioners to serve the public, and LGBT people are part of that public. Public health practitioners, in order to fulfill their roles and responsibilities, must be trained to competently serve LGBT people.

"I liked that we're all leaving assumptions behind. We need constant reminders. We needed more time to discuss, unpack our stereotypes." — Health education master's student/training participant (Turner, Wilson, & Shirah, 2003)

QUESTIONS TO CONSIDER

1. What are some specific examples of how public health practitioners' biases can affect services provided to LGBT people?
2. How can cultural competency training for public health practitioners improve health services for LGBT people?
3. If differences were to exist, how can health care practitioners reconcile their personal beliefs about LGBT people with their professional responsibility to provide high-quality care to all clients?
4. As they progress through each stage of the LGBT Cultural Competency Framework, what are some examples of the knowledge and skills public health practitioners should possess concerning LGBT people at the
   • Awareness stage?
   • Sensitivity stage?
   • Competency stage?
5. What are some training activities that can help public health practitioners improve their LGBT cultural competency?
6. What are some steps individuals can take to advocate for the inclusion of LGBT cultural competency in preservice or in-service training for public health practitioners?
7. Has your academic institutional review board (IRB) been educated about LGBT cultural competency issues and LGBT health issues?

REFERENCES

American Public Health Association (APHA). (1998). *Policy #9819: The need for public health research on gender identity and sexual orientation.* Retrieved September 1, 2005, from http://www.apha.org/legislative/policy/policysearch/index.cfm?fuseaction=view&id=171.

American Public Health Association (APHA). (1999). *Policy #9933: The need for acknowledging transgendered individuals within research and clinical practice.* Retrieved September 1, 2005, from http://www.apha.org/legislative/policy/policysearch/index.cfm?fuseaction=view&id=204.

Bowen, S. (2001). Access to health services for underserved populations in Canada. In "Certain circumstances": Issues in equity and responsiveness in access to health care in Canada. Retrieved September 1, 2005, from http://www.hc-sc.gc.ca/hppb/healthcare/pdf/circumstances.pdf.

Clark, M.E., Landers, S., Linde, R., & Sperber, J. (2001). The GLBT Health Access Project: A state-funded effort to improve access to care [Electronic version]. *American Journal of Public Health, 91*(6), 895-896.

Cranton, P., & King, K.P. (2003). Transformative learning as a professional development goal [Electronic version]. *New Directions for Adult and Continuing Education, 98,* 31-37.

Dean, L., Meyer, I.H., Robinson, K., Sell, R.L., Sember, R., Silenzio, V.M.B., Bowen, D.J., Bradford, J., Rothblum, E., Scout, White, J., Dunn, P., Lawrence, A., Wolfe, D., & Xavier, J. (2000). Lesbian, gay, bisexual, and transgender health: Findings and concerns. *Journal of the Gay and Lesbian Medical Association, 4*(3), 101-151.

Dedier, J., Penson, R., Williams, W., & Lynch, T., Jr. (1999). Race, ethnicity, and the patient-caregiver relationship. *The Oncologist, 4,* 325-331.

DiversityRX. (1997). *DiversityRX: Glossary.* (August 14). Retrieved September 1, 2005, from http://www.diversityrx.org/HTML/ESGLOS.htm.

Duffy, M.E. (2001). A critique of cultural education in nursing [Electronic version]. *Journal of Advanced Nursing, 36*(4), 487-495.

Garcia, M.H., Wright, J.W., & Corey, G. (1991). A multicultural perspective in an undergraduate human services program [Electronic version]. *Journal of Counseling & Development, 70,* 86-90.

Gay and Lesbian Medical Association (GLMA) and LGBT Health Experts (2001). *Healthy People 2010 companion document for lesbian, gay, bisexual, and transgender (LGBT) health.* San Francisco, CA: Gay and Lesbian Medical Association.

Gay, Lesbian, Bisexual and Transgender Health Access Project. (1999). Community standards of practice for provision of quality health care services for gay, lesbian, bisexual and transgendered clients. Retrieved September 1, 2005, from http://www.glbthealth.org/documents/SOP.pdf.

Goldsmith, O. (2000). Culturally competent health care [Electronic version]. *The Permanente Journal, 4*(2), 53-55.

Hedgepeth, E. (2000). *What does it really mean to "affirm" versus "promote"?* Retrieved September 1, 2005, from http://www.lifespaneducation.com/affirmation-vs-promotion.pdf.

Hutchinson, L. (2003). Educational environment [Electronic version]. *British Medical Journal, 326,* 810-812.

Lee, R. (2000). Health care problems of lesbian, gay, bisexual, and transgender patients. *Western Journal of Medicine, 172*(6), 403-408.

Matthews, A.K., Peterman, A.H., Delaney, P., Menard, L., & Brandenburg, D. (2002). A qualitative exploration of the experiences of lesbian and heterosexual patients with breast cancer [Electronic version]. *Oncology Nursing Forum, 29*(10), 1455-1462.

Messina, S.A. (1994). *A youth leader's guide to building cultural competence.* Retrieved September 1, 2005, from Advocates for Youth Web site http://www.advocatesforyouth.org/publications/guide/.

Newell, W.H. (1999). The promise of integrative learning [Electronic version]. *About Campus, 4*(2), 17-23.

Office of Minority Health, U.S. Department of Health and Human Services. (2001). *Draft—A practical guide for implementing the recommended national standards for culturally and linguistically appropriate services in health care.* Retrieved September 1, 2005, from http://www.omhrc.gov/clas/ guideintro.htm.

Office of Minority Health, U.S. Department of Health and Human Services. (2003). *National standards for culturally and linguistically appropriate services in health care final report.* Retrieved September 1, 2005, from http://www.omhrc.gov/omh/programs/2pgprograms/finalreport.pdf.

Perry, M.J., & O'Hanlan, K.A. (1997). Lesbian health: Barriers to accessing quality care. In E. Blechman (Ed.), *Behavioral medicine for women: A comprehensive handbook* (pp. 843-848). New York: Guilford Publications.

Pew Health Professions Commission. (1995). *Critical challenges: Revitalizing the health professions for the twenty-first century.* Retrieved September 1, 2005, from http://www.futurehealth.ucsf.edu/pdf_files/challenges.pdf.

Porter, L. (1984). Group norms: Some things can't be legislated. In L. Porter & B. Mohr (Eds.), *NTL reading book for human relations training,* Seventh edition (pp. 42-45). Arlington, VA: NTL Institute.

Resnicow, K., Baranowski, T., Ahluwalia, J.S., & Braithwaite, R.L. (1999). Cultural sensitivity in public health: Defined and demystified. *Ethnicity and Disease, 9,* 10-21.

Ryan, B., Brotman, S., & Rowe, B. (2000). *Access to care: Exploring the health and well-being of gay, lesbian, bisexual, and two-spirit people in Canada.* Montreal: McGill Centre for Applied Family Studies.

Shirah, M.K. (2002). Culturally competent care for women who partner with women in the North Carolina triangle area: A training curriculum for health care providers. In "Homophobia in health care is unhealthy": Development of a provider curriculum on the health care needs of women who partner with women in the Triangle Area, NC. Unpublished master's thesis, University of North Carolina, Chapel Hill.

Society for Public Health Education (SOPHE). (2001). *Resolution on eliminating health disparities based on sexual orientation.* Retrieved September 1, 2005, from http://www.sophe.org/about/resolutions/sexres.html.

Stephenson, K.S., Peloquin, S.M., Richmond, S.A., Hinman, M.A., & Christiansen, C.H. (2002). Changing educational paradigms to prepare allied health professionals for the 21st century [Electronic version]. *Education for Health, 15*(1), 37-49.

Sullivan, R.S. (1995). *The competency-based approach to training.* Retrieved September 1, 2005, from http://www.reproline.jhu.edu/english/6read/6training/cbt/sp601web.pdf.

Turner, K.L., Wilson, W.L., & Shirah, K. (2003). Introduction to LGBT competency for public health practitioners. Unpublished training guide.

Wegs, C., Turner, K., & Randall-David, B. (2003). *Effective training in reproductive health: Course design and delivery.* Chapel Hill, NC: Ipas.

Welch, M. (2002). *Concept paper: Culturally competent care.* Report prepared for the Office of Minority Health. Washington, DC: American Institutes for Research.

PART III:
THE COMMUNITY

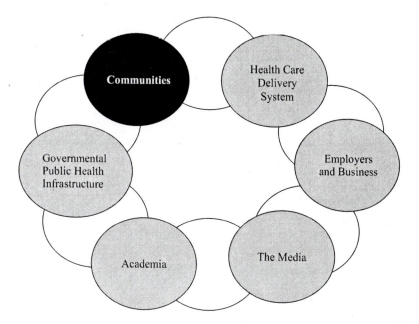

Figure reprinted with permission from *The Future of the Public's Health in the 21st Century.* ©2002 by the National Academy of Sciences, courtesy of the National Academies Press, Washington, DC.

Chapter 5

Lesbian and Bisexual Women's Public Health

Amy Baernstein
Wendy B. Bostwick
Kathleen R. Carrick
Patricia M. Dunn
Kim W. Goodman
Tonda L. Hughes
Nina Markovic
Jeanne M. Marrazzo
Helen A. Smith

INTRODUCTION

During the past decade, the National Institute of Mental Health, Centers for Disease Control and Prevention, American Medical Association, American Public Health Association, and Institute of Medicine have issued reports noting that health care and health care research affecting gay, lesbian, bisexual, and transgender people are inadequate. The Institute of Medicine (IOM) released a report on the current assessment and future directions regarding lesbian health. The first research priority identified in that report was to "better understand the physical and mental health status of lesbians and to determine whether there are health problems for which lesbians are at higher risk as well as conditions for which protective factors operate to reduce their risk" (IOM, 1999, p. 10). This recommendation followed a review of the current body of knowledge regarding the health of lesbians, which was determined to be inadequate, and supported the need for additional data to determine if there is an increased risk of certain diseases among lesbian women.

The factor that separates lesbian women from heterosexual women is "lesbianism." Health issues that concern lesbian women are thought to be largely similar to those that concern heterosexual women. The uniqueness of "lesbianism" is characterized by self-identity, sexual partnering behaviors, and/or by affectional preference, and lesbians may be classified as such by any one or a combination of these factors (IOM, 1999). The contributors to this chapter discuss the relevance of lesbianism and the method of classifying women as lesbians in their review of specific health-related topics.

It is important to note that although this chapter is about lesbians and bisexual women, few health-related studies have actually focused on bisexual women as a separate category for analysis; rather, most combine lesbians and bisexual women, reflecting an untested assumption that they are more similar than different (for exceptions, see Diamant, Wold, Spritzer, & Gelberg, 2000; Diamant & Wold, 2003; Jorm, Korten, Rodgers, Jacomb, & Christensen, 2002; Koh, 2000). Although some of the findings related to health status and health behaviors discussed here are likely relevant to bisexual women, particularly in terms of risk related to sexual behaviors, the extent to which these two sexual minority groups share common risk factors is unclear. Therefore, results discussed here should be cautiously interpreted to reflect bisexual women's health. The authors recognize the acute need for more research focusing specifically on self-identified bisexual women.

From a public health perspective, the number of individuals in a target population is relevant in allocation of resources to address concerns. The number of lesbians in the United States is not well documented, and it will vary depending upon the definition of "lesbian" and whether bisexual women are included in the planning of programmatic activities. Accurate and reliable estimates of the population are problematic; however, estimates range from a low of 1.3 percent to as high as 8.6 percent of the total U.S. population. Public health and demographic researchers are beginning to more accurately enumerate the population, which is important as it will allow for better programming to address the public health impact of specific behaviors/diseases in the population.

Many authors contributed their individual expertise to this chapter. The overall intent of this chapter was to address some of the conditions that may disproportionately affect lesbians and conditions that may affect lesbian women differently than heterosexual women. Notably, compared to heterosexual women, sexually transmitted infections may differ in the lesbian population related to sexual partner contacts; alcohol and tobacco use may differ in the lesbian population related to current perceived social norms in the population; and risk for chronic diseases may also differ among lesbians, as detailed in the section using cardiovascular disease as the example. Finally, intimate partner violence may differ in appearance and reaction by officials as it presents in the lesbian population.

SEXUALLY TRANSMITTED DISEASES AND INFECTIONS

The chance of transmission of specific bacteria and viruses during female-female sexual activity is for the most part unknown. What is known about transmission of sexually transmitted infections between women is summarized here to help guide those who provide health care to lesbian and bisexual women and for those who promote public health for these populations. In this section we use the term "lesbian" to refer to women who have sex with other women, rather than to describe sexual identity.

The data regarding sexually transmitted infections and lesbians come from three sources. First, researchers may review records from sexually transmitted infection clinics. In studies like this, women who report sexual contact with other women are identified and the results of their laboratory testing are compiled. These studies have the advantage of studying well-defined diagnoses. However, they focus on a biased sample of women who, while reporting same-sex behavior, are likely not representative of lesbians as a whole. A second type of study recruits self-identified lesbians and surveys them regarding sexually transmitted infections they have had. This type of study may capture a more representative sample of lesbians but suffers from the imprecision inherent in using self-report of sexually transmitted infections rather than confirmed laboratory testing. Further, such studies may be biased by the fact that both providers and lesbians themselves may view risk for sexually transmitted infections as low, and therefore they may be undertested and underdiagnosed (Bauer & Welles, 2001; Ferris, Batish, Wright, Cushing, & Scott, 1996). Finally, a study may recruit lesbians in various ways and then test them for the infections of interest. Studies of this type are few.

To evaluate the risk of sexually transmitted infections in lesbians, providers should ask clients their number of recent and lifetime sexual partners, both male and female. Assuming that a self-identified lesbian is not previously or currently sexually active with men is usually incorrect. In one study, 74 percent of self-identified lesbians had had male partners in the past, and of self-identified bisexual women, 98 percent had prior or current male partners (Bauer & Welles, 2001). Of lesbians recruited for studies in Seattle, 80 to 86 percent reported prior sex with men, 23 to 28 percent had had sex with a man in the past year, and the median number of male and female lifetime partners was the same (Marrazzo, Koutsky, Kiviat, Kuypers, & Stine, 2001; Marrazzo et al., 1998; Marrazzo, Stine, & Wald, 2003). In a sample of women seen at a clinic for sexually transmitted infections in London, 69 percent of those identifying as lesbian had had prior male partners (Evans, Kell, Bond, & MacRae, 1998), and at another London clinic specializing in the sexual health of lesbians, 91 percent had had prior male partners (Skinner, Stokes, Kirlew, Kavanagh, & Forster, 1996). Heterosexual intercourse transmits the full range of sexually transmitted infections, some of which may be undetected for years.

Women who have sex with both men and women appear to have more sexual partners over their lifetimes than women who have sex exclusively with either men or women. Scheer et al. (2002) found in a population-based survey in low-income neighborhoods that women who had sex with only men reported a mean of 16 lifetime partners, whereas women reporting sex with men and women reported a mean of 307 lifetime partners (number reflects responses from sex workers). Similarly, in clients attending a sexually transmitted infection clinic in Seattle, women with only female partners in the previous two months had 3.4 partners in the past year, women with only male partners had 5.3 partners in the past year, and women with male and female partners had 16.5 partners in the past year (Marrazzo, Koutsky, & Handsfield, 2001). Women who report sex with both men and women are likely to be at highest risk for sexually transmitted infections.

Lesbian and bisexual women may have male partners who are at higher risk for HIV and sexually transmitted infections than the partners of women who have sex with men only. In one sexually transmitted infection clinic study, 10 percent of women who had sex with only women in the previous two months had had a prior male partner who was gay or bisexual, compared to 6 percent of women reporting sex with men only. Of women reporting sex with both men and women in the prior two months, 29 percent had had a prior gay or bisexual male partner. Women who reported sex with both men and women in the previous two months were also more likely than women who had sex with only men or only women to have had more than four male sexual partners in a year, more likely to exchange sex for money or drugs, and more likely to have used intravenous drugs themselves (Marrazzo, Koutsky, & Handsfield, 2001). In summary, lesbian and bisexual women may have past or current sex partners at high risk for HIV and other sexually transmitted infections.

Women may transmit infections to one another during sex (including oral, genital, anal, and digital contact) and through use of sex toys. The specific infections that may be transmitted this way are discussed in the following sections.

Human Immunodeficiency Virus (HIV)

Case reports of HIV transmission between women exist (Kwakwa & Ghobrial, 2003; Rich, Buck, Tuomala, & Kazanjian, 1993). Oral-genital contact, mucosa-to-mucosa genital contact, contact with genital herpes lesions, and vigorous use of sex toys are the theorized mechanisms for transmitting the virus. However, reports of female-female transmission are rare. Decisions about screening lesbian and bisexual women for HIV should be based on other risk factors such as unprotected sex with men, particularly bisexual men, and intravenous drug use. A study that reviewed HIV testing in New York State from 1993 to 1994 found that women reporting sex with both men and women had a higher rate of HIV (4.8 percent) than women who had sex with women only (3.0 percent) or men only (2.9 percent). Intravenous drug use was the most common risk factor in HIV-infected women who had sex with women (Shotsky, 1996). A targeted sampling study in San Francisco in 1993 had similar results, finding that women who reported sex with both men and women or who characterized themselves as bisexual had a greater risk of HIV infection than other women did. Most of the HIV-infected women in this study reported intravenous drug use (Lemp et al., 1995). Similarly, a population-based study of residents of low-income neighborhoods in California from 1996 to 1998 found that women who had sex with both men and women were much more likely than exclusively heterosexual women to report high-risk behaviors, such as sex with a man known to be HIV infected, sex in exchange for money or drugs, sex with multiple male partners, and intravenous drug use (Scheer et al., 2002). Review of sexually transmitted infection clinic records in Seattle from 1993 to 1997 found no HIV-infected women who reported sex with women only (Marrazzo, Koutsky, & Handsfield, 2001). In summary, transmission of HIV between women during sex is rare, but providers should interview all women about high-risk behaviors regardless of sexual identity.

Genital Herpes

Genital herpes, usually caused by herpes simplex virus-2 (HSV-2) but occasionally caused by herpes simplex virus-1 (HSV-1), can be transmitted by contact of mucous membrane to mucous membrane or vulnerable skin. Therefore, transmission between women is theoretically possible. Most people infected with HSV-2 are not aware of their infection, and transmission may occur when the infected individual is asymptomatic. Genital herpes has been reported in women with no prior sexual contact with men (Carroll, Goldstein, Lo, & Mayer, 1997; Skinner et al., 1996). In a study of lesbians in Seattle from 1998 to 2001, 2.6 percent of women who reported no male partners had antibodies to HSV-2. Likelihood of having HSV-2 antibodies increased with increasing lifetime number of male sex partners. The authors concluded that HSV-2 can be transmitted between women, though less efficiently than between men and women. Likelihood of having antibodies to HSV-1, which typically causes oral herpes, increased with increasing number of lifetime female partners (Marrazzo et al., 2003), suggesting a role for orogenital sex in facilitating transmission in this population.

Human Papillomavirus (HPV)

Evidence exists that HPV, a family of viruses that cause anogenital warts and cervical cancer, may be transmissible between women by skin-to-skin contact, digital-genital contact, and use of sex toys. Women who report never having sexual contact with men were found to have vulvar warts and abnormal pap smears (Edwards & Thin, 1990), cervical neoplasia associated with HPV (Ferris et al., 1996; O'Hanlon & Crum, 1996), or HPV DNA by genetic probe (Marrazzo, Koutsky, Kiviat, et al., 2001; Marrazzo et al., 1998). In one sample, 19 percent of women with no prior sexual contact with men had HPV DNA detected by genetic probe and 14 percent had cervical dysplasia (Marrazzo et al., 1998). Anogenital warts and/or abnormal pap smears were also self-reported by women with no prior sexual contact with men (Bauer & Welles, 2001; Carroll et al., 1997). In studies using genetic probes to detect HPV, women who had sex with both men and women in the previous year were more than twice as likely to have HPV than women who had sex with only women in the previous year (Marrazzo, Koutsky, Kiviat, et al., 2001; Marrazzo et al., 1998).

The finding that HPV is present in women whose sexual contact with men is either remote or nonexistent has important implications regarding pap screening for these women. Such women may consider themselves at low risk for cervical cancer, and their health care providers may assume the same (Marrazzo, Stine, & Koutsky, 2000). For example, of 248 women who have sex with women interviewed by Marrazzo and colleagues in Seattle from 1998 to 2000, 36 percent had not had a pap smear in the previous two years and 9 percent said they were told by a physician that they did not need pap screening (Marrazzo, Koutsky, Kiviat, et al., 2001). Thus, routine screening for cervical dysplasia may be neglected in these women (Ferris et al., 1996; Marrazzo et al., 2000). Women who have sex with women should receive pap screening for cervical dysplasia according to the same guidelines as other sexually active women.

Trichomoniasis

Trichomoniasis was self-reported by women with no prior sex with men in studies by Bauer and Welles (2001) and Carroll et al. (1997). Trichomoniasis was reported in both members of a lesbian couple by Skinner et al. (1996) and Kellock and O'Mahony (1996). Kellock and O'Mahony's report documents a metronidazole-resistant strain of trichomonas in both partners, furthering the suspicion that it was transmitted from one to the other by transmission of infected vaginal fluid, probably through digital-vaginal sex.

Bacterial Vaginosis

Bacterial vaginosis is commonly self-reported by lesbians (Carroll et al., 1997). It is the most common diagnosis in lesbians evaluated at sexually transmitted infection clinics and is more common than in heterosexual women at those clinics (Edwards & Thin, 1990; Skinner et al., 1996). This may reflect the fact that the symptoms of bacterial vaginosis mimic other sexually transmitted infections and therefore bring lesbians to sexually transmitted infection clinics. Marrazzo et al. (2002) found that in a community-based sample of women who have sex with women, 35 percent had bacterial vaginosis, and 58 percent of those were symptomatic. A greater number of lifetime female sex partners was associated with increased likelihood of bacterial vaginosis, though a greater number of lifetime male sex partners was not. Furthermore, lesbian couples were very likely to be concordant for bacterial vaginosis. Of specific sexual practices, use of a shared, vaginally inserted sex toy and receptive oral-anal sex were the most strongly associated with bacterial vaginosis (Marrazzo et al., 2002). The exact cause of bacterial vaginosis is unknown, but these data suggest that some factor that promotes bacterial vaginosis may be transmissible between women during sexual activity. Whether female partners of women diagnosed with bacterial vaginosis should be routinely tested and treated is not known.

Other Sexually Transmitted Infections

Chlamydia and pelvic inflammatory disease were self-reported by women with no prior sex with men (Bauer & Welles, 2001), but no cases were confirmed in case series except in women with previous male partners. Campos-Outcalt and Hurwitz (2002) reported one case of a woman contracting syphilis via receptive oral sex with her female partner. No cases of gonorrhea transmission between women have been documented.

In summary, human papillomavirus, which causes genital warts and cervical dysplasia, and herpes simplex viruses are probably the sexually transmitted infections most commonly transmitted between women. Bacterial vaginosis may eventually be defined as a sexually transmitted infection between women, but the exact etiology of the condition remains unknown.

Pap screening should be performed for lesbians following current national guidelines that apply to heterosexual women. In assessing a lesbian or bisexual woman's risk of sexually transmitted infection, clinicians should consider the patient's risk behaviors, not her sexual identity.

ALCOHOL USE AND ABUSE

As discussed in Chapter 9, although earlier claims of widespread alcohol abuse among lesbians (and gay men) have been revised, more recent research findings *do* suggest that lesbian and bisexual women differ from heterosexual counterparts in their patterns of drinking and drinking-related problems. Lesbians are less likely than heterosexual women to abstain from drinking alcoholic beverages, less likely to decrease their drinking with age, and more likely to report drinking-related problems. To design more effective interventions, greater understanding of these differences is needed. Researchers and clinicians need to ask not only "Do lesbians drink more?" but also examine reasons *why* lesbians may be at heightened risk.

Following is a brief discussion of some of the factors believed to influence lesbians' patterns of drinking and drinking-related problems.

Risk Factors

Few studies have focused on bisexual women as a separate category for analysis; most combine lesbians and bisexual women, reflecting an untested assumption that they are more similar than different. Although some of the findings related to risk and protective factors for drinking among lesbians are likely relevant to bisexual women, the extent to which these two sexual minority groups share common risk factors is unclear. Therefore, this discussion relates primarily to lesbians. Further, although the term "risk factor" is used to suggest a potential causal relationship, no longitudinal studies of lesbians' drinking have been completed.

The risk factors for lesbians' (and gay men's) heavy drinking and drinking-related problems most commonly mentioned in the literature are reliance on "gay" bars for socialization and the stress associated with being part of a stigmatized and marginalized population group. Although important, these risks are generally offered without further explanation or discussion of underlying processes.

Drinking behaviors are governed to a large extent by social structures (rules, role expectations, norms, and values) of the individual's cultural group and by the drinking behavior of peers. For example, lower rates of drinking and drinking-related problems among black women in the general population are believed to result from drinking norms that are less permissive than those of white women (Herd, 1993). Although drinking norms appear to be changing, more permissive drinking norms in lesbian communities (compared with norms for women in general) likely contributes to higher prevalence of drinking. Peer influence also likely plays an important role in lesbians' drinking. A recent longitudinal study of young married couples found that having a heavy-drinking peer network was strongly related to heavier drinking in both men and women, and this relationship was independent of the partner's drinking (Leonard & Mudar, 2000). Similarly, Weinberg (1994) found evidence for both partner and peer influence on gay men's drinking. Alcohol consumption was higher and alcohol-related problems greater among men whose partners were heavy drinkers. Weinberg also found that gay men whose social lives revolved around bar settings were likely to have friends who were heavier drinkers. Socializing in bars was associated with both availability of alcohol and peer pressure to drink. Similarly, McKirnan and Peterson (1989) and Bloomfield (1993) found that regularly visiting bars was associated with heavier drinking and drinking-related problems in lesbians.

Social roles, such as marriage and parenting, are believed to be protective against drinking problems among heterosexual women. Reasons include social support gained from family, increased responsibilities, and greater social monitoring and feedback, all of which may discourage excessive drinking (Wilsnack, 1995). At present, lesbians are less likely than heterosexual women to bear or raise children (Patterson, 1998). Until recently, lesbians have been unable to legally marry their same-gender partners, and even same-gender partners in stable, long-term relationships receive less sanction and support for their relationships than do unmarried heterosexual cohabiting couples. However, several studies have documented that compared with heterosexual relationships, same-gender relationships tend to be more equitable in terms of household and family responsibilities (Caldwell & Peplau, 1984; Schneider, 1986). Further, in comparing relationship satisfaction of lesbian and heterosexual couples, one finds few, if any, differences (Kurdek & Schmitt, 1986; Peplau, Cochran, & Mays, 1997; Zak & McDonald, 1997). These factors are important buffers against stress and may reduce the risk of heavy or problematic drinking.

Other factors, such as childhood sexual abuse (CSA) and depression, suggested by some studies to be more prevalent among lesbians than heterosexual women, have only recently been discussed in the literature on lesbian health. Although there is ample evidence of an association between higher levels of alcohol use and abuse and CSA and depression among women in the general population, the extent to which these experiences are more prevalent, or whether their association with alcohol use differs for lesbians, is unclear.

It is possible that higher rates of CSA and depression in studies of lesbians can be explained, at least in part, by self-selection bias. Lesbians who participate in research are predominately Caucasian, well-educated, and more often than not live in or near large cities. By definition, women who volunteer to participate in lesbian-health studies are willing to disclose their sexual orientation. It seems reasonable that these women may also be willing to disclose other experiences, such as CSA or psychiatric disorders, which also tend to be stigmatized (Hughes & Wilsnack, 1997). In addition, studies suggest that lesbians are substantially more likely than heterosexual women to seek mental health counseling (Bradford & Ryan, 1988; Hughes, Haas, Razzano, Cassidy, & Matthews, 2000; Morgan, 1992; Sorenson & Roberts, 1997), which may serve as an important coping resource and protective factor against heavy drinking. Further, whether the reasons for seeking help relate to self-improvement or emotional distress stemming from problems related to sexual orientation, women who participate in therapy may be more likely to recall, label, and report experiences of CSA and depression. Nevertheless, given current limitations in research, findings of higher rates of CSA, depression, and other mental health problems must be interpreted cautiously (Hughes, Wilsnack, & Johnson, 2005; Hughes & Eliason, 2002; Meyer, 2003).

Among women who have experienced CSA or depression, the relative risk for alcohol problems may differ by sexual orientation. For example, lesbians must learn to manage stigma and cope in a world that is hostile toward them. Some lesbians may find that this experience helps them to cope more effectively and protects them to various degrees when faced with negative life experiences. Conversely, other lesbians may be at relatively higher risk (than heterosexual women) for negative coping because of the effect of chronic stresses related to their minority status.

The previous discussion of risk factors is clearly abbreviated; alcohol abuse is a complex problem that results from the interaction of numerous risk factors. It is important that we continue to move beyond questions of prevalence to more theoretical questions related to the underlying processes of risk. In addition, it is imperative to remember that even in the presence of multiple risk factors, the majority of lesbians do *not* drink excessively or experience alcohol-related problems. This suggests that many lesbians have developed adaptive coping skills and resiliency that serve to protect them from heavy drinking. Understanding how resiliency develops in members of sexual minority groups would greatly enhance the development of effective prevention, early intervention, and treatment strategies.

TOBACCO USE

Data on smoking among lesbian and bisexual women are limited. A recent review by Ryan, Wortley, Easton, Pederson, & Greenwood (2001) identified eight adult studies from 1987 to 2000 that included questions on tobacco use. Of these eight studies, six included lesbian and bisexual women. All six determined sexual orientation through self-identification. Current smoking was not defined in three of the six studies, and two of the remaining three used definitions different from the standard definition for adults. Of these six studies, two combined lesbians and bisexual women into one category, two included lesbian women only, and two categorized lesbians and bisexual women separately. The majority of studies were based on nonprobability (convenience) samples, with only one study using probability-based sampling. Overall, respondents tended to be white, in their thirties, and college educated. Estimated smoking rates ranged from 11 percent to 50 percent.

Among more recent studies, Gruskin, Hart, Gordon, & Ackerson (2001) looked at patterns of cigarette smoking and alcohol use among lesbians and bisexual women enrolled in a large health maintenance organization. In this study, lesbians and bisexual women (25.4 percent) were significantly more likely than heterosexual women (12.6 percent) to be current smokers. A recent review by Hughes, Matthews, Razzano, & Aranda (2003) focused specifically on sexual orientation and women's smoking. In addition to reviewing smoking prevalence, risk factors for smoking among lesbians were presented, including negative affect and depression, body image and weight, marketing and advertising, personal characteristics and gender roles, other substance abuse, and smoking behavior of significant others.

Although smoking prevalence data in the published literature are limited, available data consistently show that smoking rates among lesbian and bisexual women are higher than those seen in the general population. Additional research is needed to better understand the reasons lesbian and bisexual women smoke more than the general population and the barriers to quitting—both those unique to sexual minority women and those shared with all women and the general population. Barriers to quitting likely include limited access to quality health care and culturally appropriate and sensitive tobacco cessation programs and materials. Most employers do not provide health insurance coverage to gay and lesbian partners of employees, and any employees who do receive health coverage for their gay or lesbian partners must pay federal income taxes on the value of the insurance.

Also, lesbians are less likely to obtain medical care, meaning they may receive less tobacco-cessation education and counseling.

> Many lesbians avoid seeking health care because of past negative expe-
> riences with homophobic practitioners. These experiences have been
> well-documented within the medical literature and may include patron-
> izing treatment, intimidation, attempts to change the patient's sexual
> orientation, hostility toward the patient or her partner(s), breach of con-
> fidentiality; invasive and inappropriate personal questioning, neglect,
> denial of care, undue roughness in the physical exam, and sexual as-
> sault. (O'Hanlan, Dibble, Hagan, & Davids, 2004, p. 229)

Lesbians and bisexual women may be more likely to smoke due to a variety of unique factors and less frequently receive or respond to prevention
messages. For example, lesbians are believed to face a disproportionate
amount of daily stress due to homophobia and discrimination, and smoking
has been found to be more prevalent among groups experiencing high levels
of stress. Because of the increased stress and other reasons, behavior associated with smoking, such as alcohol and drug use, may be higher among lesbians and bisexual women than among their heterosexual counterparts.
Places where smoking is prevalent—such as bars—historically have been
an important social focus for lesbians and bisexual women, possibly because of a history of exclusion from or discrimination in other social settings. Moreover, since the early 1990s, the tobacco industry has targeted the
gay market through direct advertisement, sponsorship, and promotional
events.

These risk factors and access problems are exacerbated for lesbians and
bisexual women who also have low incomes, have low education levels, are
racial or ethnic minorities, live in nonurban areas, and/or are young. Research suggests that young lesbians and young bisexual and questioning
women are more likely to be depressed, lonely, isolated, discriminated
against, physically or verbally victimized, or to attempt suicide than their
heterosexual counterparts. All of these factors likely contribute to increased
substance use, including smoking.

The public health system has begun developing responses addressing the
elevated rates of smoking, the barriers to quitting, and the unique needs relevant to lesbians and bisexual women. Most strategies are grounded in the
early work and grassroots programs started within LGBT communities.
Two LGBT cessation models developed in the 1990s were the "Out and
Free" program by the Sexual Minorities Tobacco Coalition in Seattle and
The Last Drag Program in San Francisco.

Other major national LGBT-focused activities initiated during the past
decade have included the Gay American Smoke Out, modeled after the
Great American Smoke Out; the Centers for Disease Control and Prevention–funded Lesbian, Gay, Bisexual, and Transgender Tobacco Prevention

and Control Project, coordinated by the National Association of LGBT Community Centers; and counteradvertising campaigns to promote health-positive messages targeted to LGBT people. As of August 2005, approximately nine cessation programs tailored to the LGBT community were listed, one of which is based at the Mautner Project for lesbian health (begun over ten years ago and designed originally to target solely lesbians/women who partner with women [WPW]) and two others specifically targeting lesbians and bisexual women—the Chicago-based Lesbian Community Cancer Project's Bitch to Quit Program, and Gurlz Kick Ash, a program of the Bronx Lesbian and Gay Health Resource Consortium.

Several public-health-based tobacco-cessation approaches that have been utilized for the general population are now being adapted for use in LGBT communities, including phone and Internet quit lines such as the University of California at San Francisco's *iQuit,* an Internet-based cessation program for LGBT smokers; promotion of the U.S. Public Health Service's clinical practice guideline, *Treating Tobacco Use and Dependence* (Fiore et al., 2000), among health care providers who care for LGBT patients; LGBT-focused antitobacco media campaigns to counter tobacco advertising and disseminate LGBT-inclusive messages, including some, such as the Mautner Project's multimedia campaign, that are targeted solely to lesbians/WPW; and production of a CD-ROM on LGBT populations and tobacco by the Tobacco Technical Assistance Consortium at Emory University, which includes information regarding tobacco-industry marketing to LGBT people and strategies to counteract it, and a call to action for tobacco control professionals to work to decrease tobacco-use prevalence among LGBT people (the CD-ROM can now be ordered from the TTAC Web site at www.ttac.org/products/index.html).

CARDIOVASCULAR DISEASE

Cardiovascular disease (CVD) is the leading cause of mortality among women living in the United States. Coronary heart disease and cerebro-vascular disease rank as the first and second causes of death, respectively, regardless of race and ethnicity (Centers for Disease Control and Prevention, 1999). Morbidity data show a similar trend, rating hypertension, diabetes, CVD, and stroke as the four leading chronic diseases among American women (Centers for Disease Control and Prevention, 1994). According to the American Heart Association, in 2002, 52.3 percent of all deaths from cardiovascular diseases occurred in women (American Heart Association, 2005). The National Heart, Lung, and Blood Institute reports that one in ten women from ages forty-five to sixty-four years of age has some form of heart disease, a figure that increases to one in four women over sixty-five years of age (National Institutes of Health, 1998).

Previous research has identified certain risk and protective factors for cardiovascular disease in women. It has been suggested that prevalence rates for these factors may systematically vary between lesbians and heterosexual women. Compared to their heterosexual counterparts, some evidence suggests that lesbians may have higher rates of cigarette smoking, alcohol abuse, and obesity, thus increasing their risk for CVD. In contrast, lesbians may be more physically active and may have higher educational attainment compared to heterosexual women, thus imparting a reduced risk of CVD.

Self-reported behaviors and health status among self-identified lesbians were compared to a probability sample of women from the general population, providing evidence that there may be differences between lesbian and heterosexual women on several of the documented modifiable risk factors for CVD (Aaron et al., 2001). However, these differences in health behavior have not been confirmed in a large investigation utilizing an age- and education-matched control group of heterosexual women, and there is a paucity of information on potential differences between lesbian and heterosexual women regarding physiological factors known to increase the risk of CVD (e.g., lipids, blood pressure, etc.).

The major risk factors for CVD have been well established (Willet, Green, & Stampfer, 1987) and include smoking (Willet et al., 1987), high blood pressure (Whelton, He, & Appel, 1996; Saltzberg, Stroh, & Frishman, 1988), high blood cholesterol (Sempos, Cleeman, & Carroll, 1993; Manolio, Pearson, & Wenger, 1992), excess body weight (Manson, Stampfer, & Colditz, 1990; Wing, Kuller, & Bunker, 1989), physical inactivity (Paffenbarger & Lee, 1996; Owens, Matthew, Wing, & Kuller, 1990), and diabetes (Manson & Spelsbert, 1996; Geiss, Herman, & Smith, 1995). In addition, factors such as personality attributes and excess alcohol intake have been associated with an increased risk of CVD in women (National Institutes of Health, 1998). Many of these factors are indicative of an overall unhealthy lifestyle and may occur in combination. Due to the behavioral construct of smoking, excess body weight, physical inactivity, and alcohol use, they are considered modifiable risk factors. These behavioral risk factors also contribute to the development of other conditions known to increase the risk for CVD, namely high blood pressure, high blood cholesterol, and diabetes. Tobacco use, physical activity patterns, and alcohol abuse have been reported as the top three causes of death in the United States (McGinnis & Foege, 1993). Specific to cardiovascular disease deaths, 17 to 30 percent of CVD deaths can be attributed to tobacco use, and 22 to 30 percent can be attributed to activity patterns. Clearly, modifiable behavioral risk factors have a tremendous impact on CVD morbidity and mortality.

Cigarette Smoking

Most published prevalence rates of current cigarette smoking among lesbian women report estimates of 20 to 30 percent (Denenberg, 1995; Moran, 1996; Rankow & Tessaro, 1998; Bradford & Ryan, 1987). One study has reported very low current smoking rates among lesbians (11 percent), which was lower than a heterosexual comparison group (23 percent). Current cigarette use among lesbian women in the ESTHER (Epidemiological Study of Health Risk in Lesbians) study was 5 to 10 percent higher than the reported prevalence from the Behavioral Risk Factor Surveillance System (BRFSS) (Aaron et al., 2001). Data from the Women's Health Initiative (WHI), a study of older, postmenopausal women, indicate that lesbian women may have a higher lifetime exposure to tobacco. Among heterosexual women, 43 percent were past smokers and 7 percent were current smokers; among lesbians, 54 percent were past smokers and 12 percent were current smokers (Valanis et al., 2000).

Excess Body Weight

The limited data available indicate that lesbian women may have higher body mass index (BMI) and thus higher rates of overweightness compared to the general population of women. In a study of college students, lesbians had an average BMI of 24.7 kg/m^2 compared to an average BMI of 22.0 kg/m^2 for heterosexual women (Siever, 1994). Likewise, in a sample of middle-aged women, lesbians had a significantly higher BMI when compared to a sample of middle-aged heterosexual women (Roberts, Dibble, & Scanlon, 1998). The rate of overweight/obesity of lesbian women in the ESTHER study was 7 percent higher than that reported from the BRFSS. Rates of overweight/obesity of the lesbian women in WHI were 5.4 percent higher than the rates in heterosexual women (Valanis et al., 2000).

Physical Activity Patterns

A paucity of data exists pertaining to dietary and physical activity patterns among lesbian women. Some evidence suggests that lesbian women may be more physically active than heterosexual women. Patton, Millard, and Kessenich (1998), in a study of risk factors for osteoporosis, reported that 71 percent of the women in the lesbian sample exercised regularly compared to 58 percent of heterosexuals. Data indicate that not only are lesbian women less likely than heterosexual women to be sedentary, but they are more likely to engage in vigorous physical activity (Aaron, Markovic, Danielson, Janosky, & Schmidt, 2000). The WHI data revealed little difference in physical activity between lesbian and heterosexual women in this older group of women (Valanis et al., 2000).

Alcohol Use

In contrast to the other behavioral factors discussed previously, extensive research has been conducted regarding the association between sexual orientation and alcohol use/abuse. Much of the earlier research has been criticized due to the methodology used to recruit subjects (Bux, 1996; Hughes & Wilsnack, 1994, 1997). Historically, one of the primary social outlets for lesbians was bars and clubs (Bradford & Ryan, 1988). As such, many early studies recruited subjects in these establishments and, not surprisingly, reported higher rates of alcohol use and abuse than reported in heterosexual women. Recent studies have utilized more rigorous sampling techniques to limit the selection bias, and reported rates of current drinking have ranged from 52 percent to 83 percent (McKirnan & Peterson, 1989; Bloomfield, 1993; Hughes, Haas, & Avery, 1997). The primary difference in alcohol use between lesbian and heterosexual women has been in the rates of abstinence, with more heterosexual women reporting abstinence (McKirnan & Peterson, 1989; Hughes et al., 1997). Among the lesbian women in a preliminary study, 65 percent were classified as current drinkers compared to 41 percent of women in the BRFSS. Data from the WHI indicate that lesbians were more likely to use alcohol and to use more of it compared to heterosexual women (Valanis et al., 2000).

Based on this evidence, it appears that lesbian and heterosexual women may differ markedly in their health behaviors. The apparent higher prevalence of cigarette smoking and excess body weight may impart an increased risk of CVD. However, the limited data indicate that lesbian women may be more physically active and engage in more vigorous physical activity, which would act as a protective factor related to the risk of CVD. Data from the Cooper Clinic strongly support the hypothesis that increased cardiorespiratory fitness, which is achieved by participating in vigorous physical activity, is one of the primary factors related to reducing all causes of mortality and CVD mortality, even in the presence of increased body weight (Lee, Blair, & Jackson, 1999; Wei, Kampert, & Barlow, 1999). Nonabstinence from alcohol may also be protective, as moderate consumption (one to two drinks per day) may impart some protection against CVD.

REPRODUCTIVE CANCERS

Although no known biological differences exist between lesbians and heterosexual women that put lesbians at greater risk for chronic diseases (Aaron et al., 2001), studies indicate that lesbians may have a greater combination of concerns that could lead to certain diseases, such as reproductive cancers (Aaron et al., 2001; Carroll, 1999; Dibble & Roberts, 2003; Gruskin et al., 2001; Matthews, Brandenburgh, Johnson, & Hughes, 2004). Barriers to health care and specific risk factors are two important informational pieces to consider when it comes to decreasing lesbians' chances of being diagnosed with gynecological or breast cancer.

Findings suggest that the constellation of risk factors could possibly place lesbians at greater risk of developing reproductive cancers than heterosexual women. Avoidance of gynecological and breast screenings (for early detection), absence of childbirth and oral contraceptive use, alcohol consumption and smoking, and obesity are risk factors for developing reproductive cancers. Although these indicators are present in the general population of women, to have them all concentrated in the lesbian population may be unique.

Gynecological and Breast Screenings

Studies show that since lesbians are unlikely to receive routine gynecological tests for birth control and prenatal care, they are screened less for breast and cervical cancer (Matthews et al., 2004). When screening intervals are lengthened, such as receiving a gynecological exam with a pap smear every third or fourth year, early detection and treatment can be delayed. All women need regular pap smears starting at the age of eighteen or first sexual encounter (Dibble & Roberts, 2003).

Pregnancy and Oral Contraceptives

Research reveals lesbians are less likely to have ever used oral contraceptives and have a likelihood of nulliparity or first pregnancies past the age of thirty. Bearing a child before thirty, breast-feeding, and oral contraceptive use have been identified as contributing to lower risk of reproductive cancers (Carroll, 1999; Cochran et al., 2001).

Alcohol Consumption and Smoking

Research indicates that lesbians and bisexual women under fifty are more likely than heterosexuals to engage in cigarette smoking and heavy drinking (Aaron et al., 2001; Gruskin et al., 2001; Cochran et al., 2001; Dibble & Roberts, 2002). Lesbians have been identified as heavier smokers compared with heterosexual women.

Obesity/Body Mass Index

BMI is an objective scientific measure that is used to predict health status primarily as related to obesity. BMI uses height and weight measurements to estimate body fat, and the result predicts one's chances of morbidity and mortality. Studies find that lesbians have a greater BMI than heterosexual women, which means that lesbians are more likely to be overweight or obese (Carroll, 1999; Aaron et al., 2001; Cochran et al., 2001).

Aside from differing rates of risk factors related to reproductive cancers, studies also indicate that lesbians face other concerns when it comes to getting needed health care. Discrimination, misinformation, and finances pose as three health care barriers related to access to medical care among lesbian women.

Discrimination

Research documents that lesbians do not utilize health care services as often as medically recommended nor as often as heterosexual women. Some lesbians report they do not partake in regular gynecological and breast exams because of previous negative experiences with health care providers. For example, some feel they have received substandard care, were refused health care, and heard derogatory comments by health care providers because of sexual identity and/or behavior. Dibble & Roberts note that the "hostility, fear, and discomfort experienced by lesbians in healthcare system should not be underestimated" (Dibble & Roberts, 2003, p. 77).

Misinformation

Some physicians and health care providers make the inaccurate assumption that lesbians do not have or have never had sex with men. Because of this misassumption, discussions regarding oral contraceptives and safer sex practices do not take place between lesbian patients and their health care providers. In addition, some physicians still do not recognize the need for routine physicals and gynecological exams, including pap smears, as often as for heterosexual women. Further, many lesbians do not receive the education they need because informational packets and screening programs are designed for heterosexual audiences (Dibble & Roberts, 2003).

Finances

Lesbians are less likely to have health care coverage through a spouse/partner than heterosexual women. In addition, lesbians' household incomes are lower than heterosexual household incomes, which may impact health-care-seeking behaviors (Aaron et al., 2001).

Distinctive patterns of risk factors and barriers to care may converge in the lesbian population, negatively altering the risk of reproductive cancers compared to heterosexual women. It is notable that bisexual women may share some of the same experiences as lesbians when it comes to risk factors and barriers to care. Further research might elucidate the fine differences and similarities between lesbians, bisexual women, and heterosexual women and risk for cancers of the female reproductive system.

INTIMATE PARTNER VIOLENCE AND LESBIANS

The inadequacies of using a heterosexual framework of domestic violence to assist lesbian couples were outlined in an early paper by Lobel (1986). Despite continued calls for lesbian-specific interventions in cases of domestic violence, it appears that little has changed in the ways that lesbian battering is addressed by service providers (Hammond, 1989; Leventhal & Lundy, 1999; Giorgio, 2002). Heterosexual bias can be defined as "conceptualizing human experience in strictly heterosexual terms and consequently ignoring, invalidating, or derogating homosexual behaviors and sexual orientation, and lesbian, gay male, and bisexual relationships and lifestyles" (Herek, Kimmel, Amaro, & Melton, 1991, p. 957). Society's failure to recognize gay and lesbian relationships has contributed to the lack of services available to address lesbian partner violence (National Coalition of Anti-Violence Programs, 1998).

Violence in lesbian relationships raises broader theoretical questions about gender and heterosexual assumptions regarding the causes of violence (Hart, 1986; Renzetti, 1988). Conventional and feminist notions of domestic violence that suggest violence is solely the province of men disrupt basic notions about the causes of battering as well as meanings of "efficient" interventions. Considering the causes of lesbian battering means explanations of abusive behaviors cannot be reduced to male socialization or male privilege (Renzetti, 1988). It also means we can no longer view women as simply passive victims in need of protection.

Socially sanctioned "masculine" or "feminine" roles and heterosexual bias influence how a lesbian might be perceived as either "batterer" or "victim." If a lesbian batterer is perceived as being more "masculine" and the victim is perceived as being more "feminine," it fits within our current heterosexually influenced understanding of domestic violence. However, at the same time, it sets up a conceptual barrier to viewing battering behaviors without a gender-defined context (Prentice & Carranza, 2002). Normative gender definitions that inform the coordinated community response model do not account for the case of a "masculine" lesbian who is battered, nor does it help identify a "feminine" batterer.

Shelters, services, training, and interventions have all been engineered on a model that presupposes that heterosexuality is the norm when responding to domestic violence (Walker, 2000). If most domestic violence shelters assume that a battered woman is heterosexual, for example, shelter staff members and hotline volunteers respond with "What's his name?" when a woman calls a shelter to inquire about services. Individuals in shelters are often required to participate in group counseling. Lesbians could be concerned that if they reveal their partner was female they will encounter homophobia from shelter residents and staff. Often lesbians will switch pronouns from a "she" to "he" in telling their stories in a mixed group in order to be accepted by the goup.

CVC programs are very clear in providing services based on legal "family" definitions. Because of a lack of legal status for their relationships, lesbians are not often eligible for compensation. The situation is often quite complicated. If a lesbian is seeking services as an individual, then she is eligible. But, for example, if a lesbian is a partner seeking services (such as counseling to cope with the stalking of her female partner by an ex-husband) then they are not eligible for services under CVC program guidelines.

Prioritizing information specific to lesbian couples, including issues of outing and community reluctance as well as institutionalized barriers, will provide the empirical basis for adapting the coordinated community response model to the specific needs of lesbians.

Nonetheless, professional domestic violence organizations' funding remains tied to reported prevalence rates of violence within their community (National Coalition Against Domestic Violence, 2002).

However, what shelters and hotlines "count" are actually *reported* incidents of *heterosexual* intimate partner violence based upon help-seeking behaviors. Reliance on prevalence rates continues to reinforce implicit gender assumptions that perpetrators of violence are exclusively male and that battered women are exclusively heterosexual, and thus it fails to account for abuse within gay and lesbian relationships.

Lesbian Partner Violence

Silence about lesbian battering among professionals, police (Younglove, Kerr, & Vitello, 2002), courts (Hammond,1989), therapists (Ristock, 2001), researchers (Leventhal & Lundy, 1999), theorists, and activists (Beckett & Macey, 2001), as well as dynamics within the lesbian community have contributed to the "invisibility" of the issue of same-sex domestic violence (Greene & Herek, 1994; McLauglin & Rozee, 2001). In fact, even lesbians will identify and associate domestic violence with heterosexual relationships (Ristock, 2001). Once revealed, however, lesbian partner violence poses unique challenges to heteronormative assumptions and gender-role expectations regarding women and domestic violence.

Degrees of "being out" are specific factors that pose unique opportunities for points of control or leverage in a lesbian relationship and can increase risk for abuse and violence (Ocamb, 2000). Lesbians who report that they fear disclosure of their sexual orientation by being "outed" are more likely to self-report anxiety, isolation, lower self-esteem, and less social support (Jordan & Deluty, 1998). Lesbians who batter their intimate partners may choose to take advantage of their partners' fear of being "outed" to control their partners' behaviors and limit their choices. Abusive lesbians may use this fear as leverage to blackmail their partners to remain in the relationship.

LBGT communities may be reluctant to respond to cases of domestic violence due to fear of exacerbating the larger society's negative attitudes about gays and lesbians (Niolan, 2000). Alexander (2002) asserts that by not asking questions about violence when interacting with members of the LBGT community, we not only miss the opportunity for intervention but also contribute to further isolation within the community.

Institutional Barriers and Lesbian Partner Violence

Walker (2000) found that heterosexual victims of domestic violence often do not report domestic violence for fear of retaliation from the abusive partner. Battered lesbians also fear retaliation; however, reluctance to report lesbian partner violence is more strongly associated with a fear of confronting homophobia in the process of reporting the abuse (Island & Letellier, 1991). Lesbians who are battered face inconsistent reception and treatment from hospital, emergency personnel, and traditional domestic violence shelters. They may also be reluctant to involve police and judicial personnel in their "personal" affairs, since historically such institutions have codified and responded to homosexuality as a "crime." A history of police raids in gay and lesbian bars and antisodomy laws contribute to the persistent fear that the legal system will not treat lesbians fairly (e.g., *Bowers v. Hardwick,* 1986; *Lawrence & Garner v. Texas,* 2003).

Many states in the United States have legislated mandatory arrest policies to help address victim's fear in prosecuting. Mandatory arrest takes the burden of prosecution off the victim and increases the likelihood of a more consistent criminal justice intervention in domestic violence cases, ultimately better serving victims. In states that adopt mandatory arrest, law officers are required to arrest the primary aggressor in all domestic violence incidents where there is probable cause. Correct identification of the primary aggressor is a significant challenge in domestic violence calls (Crager, Cousin, & Hardy, 2003). Identification of the primary aggressor becomes even more difficult when both partners are female (Poorman & Seelau, 2001).

The lack of legal recognition of kinship or familial ties for lesbian relationships has important consequences for access to social services. For example, nationally, the Crime Victims Compensation (CVC) programs were created to help remunerate victims for the costs incurred as a result of a crime (Stuehling, 2001). Domestic violence advocates often link (heterosexual) battered women to CVC programs to help reimburse out-of-pocket losses (such as broken eyeglasses, replacement of prescription medication) or services required as a result of injuries (such as hospital bills, physical therapy, or counseling fees). In Pennsylvania Act 139 of 1976 (PA CVC Act), a *family* is defined as anyone related by blood or marriage (within three generations), or residing in the same household with that individual for at least thirty or more days (Stuehling, 2001). Theoretically, then, the PA CVC act should also benefit battered gays and lesbians who cohabitated with their abusive partners. However, eligibility guidelines for counseling in cases resulting in a homicide are limited to legal next of kin by blood or marriage (Stuehling, 2001).

Because lesbian couples are not currently eligible for legal marriage, lesbian domestic violence cases are especially complicated. For example, if a remarried woman in a legal heterosexual marriage is killed by her ex-husband, her widower is eligible for CVC services. However, if a woman in a current lesbian relationship is killed by a former partner (either male or female), her current female partner is not eligible for CVC services; legally, she is not recognized as next of kin by blood or marriage.

Saulnier (2002) found that lesbians seeking physical or mental health services experienced a range of provider reactions that then influenced their decisions for future care. These reactions ranged from homophobia and heterosexism to tolerance, lesbian sensitivity, and lesbian affirmation. Saulnier (2002) concluded that lesbian care decisions and especially compliance with treatment depended on the reactions that lesbians received when they came out to the health care provider. This issue is crucial when we consider existing domestic violence services for battered women. Lesbians will assess staff and agency responses to see if they will be supported during their crisis.

Recommendations for a Lesbian-Inclusive Coordinated Community Response

The successful implementation of the coordinated community model requires basic education, materials, and training about domestic violence. The 2000 National Training Project, Creating a Public Response to Private Violence (Duluth Domestic Abuse Intervention Project, 2000), was a great step forward in providing inclusive training materials. This represented a collaborative effort to provide a template for any community wishing to improve their response to violence. Yet this benchmark manual contains no information, resources, or acknowledgement that violence occurs within same-sex couples. When even basic information about same-sex battering is missing it should be no surprise that services still do not effectively address the needs of battered lesbians. Some have advocated the creation of segregated services specializing in providing domestic violence services to same-sex couples (Community United Against Violence, 2000). However, segregation of services could reinforce a dangerous precedent in which any minority group could be classified as "other" (i.e., in need of specialized services) rather than part and parcel of training for a coordinated community model. Tigert (2001) points out that much of the domestic violence information we have obtained from heterosexual batterers multiplies the barriers to accessing domestic violence services for battered lesbians. Expanding our views about intimate partner violence will make service provision inclusive as well as challenge us to consider why intimate violence is tolerated in any community.

QUESTIONS TO CONSIDER

1. Do you advertise services in targeted lesbian and bisexual women's publications?
2. Do you help to sponsor lesbian and bisexual women's health events?
3. Have you and your staff participated in LGBT diversity training programs?
4. Does your reception area display posters and/or publications with images of lesbian and bisexual women?

5. Do you have brochures on health issues that may disproportionately affect lesbian and bisexual women? Do these publications have images and/or make reference to lesbian and bisexual women?
6. Do your intake forms allow women to indicate a "partner" or "marriage-like relationship" (as opposed to "husband")? Do your intake forms ask about "sex with men, women, or both" (as opposed to assuming sex with men only)?
7. Do you have "living wills" and "power of attorney" forms available for women to complete, and do you routinely ask *all* women if they have completed these items?
8. Do you maintain a list of competent referral sources for lesbian and bisexual women who may require care outside of your service(s)?
9. Do you know the name, address, and telephone number of one (or more) local gay, lesbian, bisexual, and transgender individual support centers or organizations?

REFERENCES

Aaron, D.J., Markovic, N., Danielson, M.E., Honnold, J.A., Janosky, J.E., & Schmidt, N.J. (2001). Behavioral risk factors for disease and preventive health practices among lesbians. *American Journal of Public Health, 91*(6), 972-975.

Aaron, D.J., Markovic, N., Danielson, M.E., Janosky, J.E., & Schmidt, N.J. (2000). Physical activity of lesbian women and associations with other health behaviors. *Medicine and Science in Sports and Exercise, 2,* S167.

Alexander, C. (2002). Violence in gay and lesbian relationships. *Journal of Gay and Lesbian Social Services, 14* (1), 95-98.

American Heart Association. (2005). *2005 heart and stroke statistical update.* Dallas, TX: American Heart Association.

Bauer, G.R., & Welles, S.L. (2001). Beyond assumptions of negligible risk: Sexually transmitted diseases and women who have sex with women. *American Journal of Public Health, 91*(8), 1282-1286.

Beckett, C., & Macey, M. (2001). Race, gender and sexuality: The oppression of multiculturalism. *Women's Studies International Forum, 24*(3/4), 309-319.

Bloomfield, K.A. (1993). A comparison of alcohol consumption between lesbians and heterosexual women in an urban population. *Drug and Alcohol Dependence, 33,* 257-269.

Bradford, J., & Ryan, C. (1988). *The national lesbian health care survey.* Washington, DC: National Lesbian and Gay Health Foundation.

Bux, D.A. (1996). The epidemiology of problem drinking in gay men and lesbians: A critical review. *Clinical Psychology Review, 16,* 277-298.

Caldwell, M.A., & Peplau, L.A. (1984). The balance of power in lesbian relationships. *Sex Roles, 10,* 587-599.

Campos-Outcalt, D., & Hurwitz, S. (2002). Female-to-female transmission of syphilis: A case report. *Sexually Transmitted Diseases, 23,* 119-120.

Carroll, N.M. (1999). Optimal gynecologic and obstetric care for lesbians. *Obstetrics & Gynecology, 93*(4), 611-613.

Carroll, N.M., Goldstein, R.S., Lo, W., & Mayer, K. (1997). Gynecological infections and sexual practices of Massachusetts lesbian and bisexual women. *Journal of the Gay and Lesbian Medical Association, 1*(1), 15-23.

Centers for Disease Control and Prevention. (1994). *Chronic disease in minority populations.* Atlanta, GA: Centers for Disease Control and Prevention.

Centers for Disease Control and Prevention. (1999). Deaths: Final data for 1997. *National Vital Statistics Reports, 47*(19), 1-104.

Cochran, S., Mays, V.M., Bowen, D., Gage, S., Bybee, D., Roberts, S., Goldstein, R.S., Robison, A., Rankow, E.J., & White, J. (2001). Cancer-related risk indicators and preventive screening behaviors among lesbians and bisexual women. *American Journal of Public Health, 91*(4), 591-597.

Community United Against Violence. (2000). From our lives, for our lives: Culturally appropriate responses to relationship violence in lesbian, bisexual, and transgender women of color communities. Workshop packet handed out at the National Coalition Against Domestic Violence Conference, San Francisco, California.

Crager, M., Cousin, M., & Hardy, T. (2003). Victim-defendants: An emerging challenge in responding to domestic violence in Seattle and the King County region. Retrieved January 18, 2004, from http://www.mincava.edu.

Denenberg, R. (1995). Report on lesbian health. *Women's Health Journal, 5,* 1-11.

Diamant, A.L., & Wold, C. (2003). Sexual orientation and variation in physical and mental health status among women. *Journal of Women's Health, 12*(3), 41-49.

Diamant, A.L., Wold, C., Spritzer, K., & Gelberg, L. (2000). Health behaviors, health status, and access to and use of health care. *Archive of Family Medicine, 9,* 1043-1051.

Dibble, S.L., & Roberts, S.A. (2002). A comparison of breast cancer diagnosis and treatment between lesbian and heterosexual women. *Journal of the Gay and Lesbian Medical Association, 6*(1), 9-17.

Dibble, S.L., & Roberts, S.A. (2003). Improving cancer screening among lesbians over 50: Results of a pilot study. *Oncology Nursing Forum, 30*(4), 569.

Duluth Domestic Abuse Intervention Project. (2000). Creating a Public Response to Private Violence. Duluth, MN: National Training Project.

Edwards, A., & Thin, R.N. (1990). Sexually transmitted diseases in lesbians. *International Journal of STD & AIDS, 1,* 178-181.

Evans, B.A., Kell, P.D., Bond, R.A., & MacRae, K.D. (1998). Racial origin, sexual lifestyle, and genital infection among women attending a genitourinary medicine clinic in London. *Sexually Transmitted Infections, 74*(1), 45-49.

Ferris, D.G., Batish, S., Wright, T.C., Cushing, C., & Scott, E.H. (1996). A neglected lesbian health concern: Cervical neoplasia. *Journal of Family Practice, 43*(6), 581-584.

Fiore, M.C., Bailey, W.C., Cohen, S.J., Dorfman, S.F., Goldstein, M.G., Gritz, E.R., Heyman, R.B., Jaen, C.R., Kottke, T.E., Lando, H.A., et al. (2000). *Treating to-*

bacco use and dependence. Quick Reference Guide for Clinicians. Rockville, MD: U.S. Department of Health and Human Services, Public Health Service.

Geiss, L.S., Herman, W.H., & Smith, P.J. (1995). *Mortality in non-insulin-dependent diabetes.* In M.I. Harris, C.C. Cowie, M.P. Stern, E.J. Boyko, G.E. Reiber, & P.H. Bennett (Eds.), *Diabetes in America* (pp. 233-258). Bethesda, MD: National Institutes of Health, National Institute of Diabetes and Digestive and Kidney Disease.

Giorgio, G. (2000). Speaking silence: Definitional dialogues in abusive lesbian relationships. *Violence Against Women, 8*(10), 1233-1259.

Greene, B., & Herek, G.M. (Eds.). (1994). *Lesbian and gay psychology: Theory, research, and clinical applications.* Thousand Oaks, CA: Sage Publications.

Gruskin, E., Hart, S., Gordon, N., & Ackerson, L. (2001). Patterns of cigarette smoking and alcohol use among lesbians and bisexual women enrolled in a large health maintenance organization. *American Journal of Public Health, 91*(6), 976-979.

Hammond, N. (1989). Lesbian victims of relationship violence. *Women & Therapy, 8*(1/2), 89-105.

Hart, B. (1986). Lesbian battering: An examination. In K. Lobel (Ed.), *Naming the violence: Speaking out about lesbian battering.* Seattle, WA: Seal Press.

Herd, D. (1993). An analysis of alcohol-related problems in black and white women drinkers. *Addiction Research, 1*(3), 181-198.

Herek, G., Kimmel, D.C., Amaro, H., & Melton, G.B. (1991). Avoiding heterosexist bias in psychological research. *American Psychologist, 46*(9), 957-963.

Hughes, T.L. (2005). Alcohol use and alcohol-related problems among lesbians and gay men. *Annual Review of Nursing Research, 23,* 283-325.

Hughes, T.L., & Eliason, M. (2002). Substance use and abuse in lesbian, gay, bisexual, and transgender populations. *The Journal of Primary Prevention, 22*(3), 263-298.

Hughes, T.L., Haas, A.P., & Avery, L. (1997). Lesbians and mental health: Preliminary results from the Chicago Women's Health Survey. *Journal of Gay and Lesbian Medical Association, 1,* 133-144.

Hughes, T.L., Haas, A.P., Razzano, L., Cassidy, R., & Matthews, A.K. (2000). Comparing lesbians' and heterosexual women's mental health: Findings from a multi-site study. *Journal of Gay and Lesbian Social Services, 11*(1), 57-76.

Hughes, T.L., Matthews, A.K., Razzano, L., & Aranda, F. (2003). Psychological distress in African American lesbians and heterosexual women. *Journal of Lesbian Studies, 7*(1), 51-68.

Hughes, T.L., & Wilsnack, S.C. (1994). Research on lesbians and alcohol: Gaps and implications. *Alcohol, Health, & Research World, 18,* 202-205.

Hughes, T.L., & Wilsnack, S.C. (1997). Use of alcohol among lesbians: Research and clinical implications. *American Journal of Orthopsychiatry, 66,* 20-36.

Hughes, T.L., Wilsnack, S.C., & Johnson, T. (2005). Investigating lesbians' mental health and alcohol use: What is an appropriate comparison group? In A. Omoto & H. Kurtzman (Eds.), *Sexual orientation and mental health: Examining Identity and Development in Lesbian, Gay, and Bisexual People.* Washington, DC: APA Books.

Institute of Medicine. (1999). *Lesbian health: Current assessment and directions for the future,* A.L. Solarz (Ed.). Washington, DC: National Academy Press.

Island, D., & Letellier, P. (1991). *Men who beat the men who love them.* Binghamton, NY: The Haworth Press.

Jordan, K.M., & Deluty, R.H. (1998). Coming out for lesbian women: Its relation to anxiety, positive affectivity, self-esteem, and social support. *Journal of Homosexuality, 35*(2), 41-63.

Jorm, A.F., Korten, A.E., Rodgers, B., Jacomb, P.A., & Christensen, H. (2002). Sexual orientation and mental health: Results from a community survey of young and middle aged adults. *British Journal of Psychiatry, 180,* 423-427.

Kellock, D.J., & O'Mahony, C.P. (1996). Sexually acquired metronidazole-resistant trichomoniasis in a lesbian couple. *Genitourinary Medicine, 72,* 60-61.

Koh, A.S. (2000). Use of preventive health behaviors by lesbian, bisexual, and heterosexual women: Questionnaire survey. *Western Journal of Medicine, 172,* 379-384.

Kurdek, L.A., & Schmitt, J.P. (1986). Relationship quality of partners in heterosexual married, heterosexual cohabiting, and gay and lesbian relationships. *Journal of Personality and Social Psychology, 51,* 711-720.

Kwakwa, H.A., & Ghobrial, M.W. (2003). Female-to-female transmission of human immunodeficiency virus. *Clinical Infectious Diseases, 36,* e40-41.

Lee, C.D., Blair, S.N., & Jackson, A.S. (1999). Cardiorespiratory fitness, body composition, and all-cause and cardiovascular disease mortality in men. *American Journal of Clinical Nutrition, 69,* 373-380.

Lemp, G.F., Jones, M., Kellogg, T.A., Nieri, G.N., Anderson, L., Withum, D., & Katz, M. (1995). HIV seroprevalence and risk behaviors among lesbians and bisexual women in San Francisco and Berkeley, California. *American Journal of Public Health, 85*(11), 1549-1552.

Leonard, K.E., & Mudar, P.J. (2000). Alcohol use in the year before marriage: Alcohol expectancies and peer drinking as proximal influences on husband and wife alcohol involvement. *Alcoholism: Clinical and Experimental Research, 24*(11), 1666-1679.

Leventhal, B., & Lundy, S.E. (Eds.). (1999). *Same-sex domestic violence: Strategies for change.* Thousand Oaks, CA: Sage Publications.

Lobel, K. (Ed.). (1986). *Naming the violence: Speaking out about lesbian battering.* Seattle, WA: Seal Press.

Manolio, T.A., Pearson, T.A., & Wenger, N.K. (1992). Cholesterol and heart disease in older persons and women: Review of an NHLBI workshop. *Annals of Epidemiology, 2,* 161-176.

Manson, J.E., & Spelsbert, A. (1996). Risk modification in the diabetic patient. In J.E. Manson, P.M. Ridker, J.M. Gaziano, & C.H. Hennekens (Eds.), *Prevention of myocardial infarction* (pp. 241-243). New York: Oxford University Press.

Manson, J.E., Stampfer, M.J., & Colditz, G.A. (1990). A prospective study of obesity and risk of coronary heart disease in women. *New England Journal of Medicine, 322,* 882-889.

Marrazzo, J.M., Koutsky, L.A., Eschenbach, D.A., Agnew, K., Stine, K., & Hillier, S. (2002). Characterization of vaginal flora and bacterial vaginosis in women who have sex with women. *Journal of Infectious Diseases, 185,* 1307-1313.

Marrazzo, J.M., Koutsky, L.A., & Handsfield, H.H. (2001). Characteristics of female sexually transmitted disease clinic clients who report same-sex behaviour. *International Journal of STD & AIDS, 12*(1), 41-46.

Marrazzo, J.M., Koutsky, L.A., Kiviat, N.B., Kuypers, J.M., & Stine, K. (2001). Papanicolaou test screening and prevalence of genital human papillomavirus among women who have sex with women. *American Journal of Public Health, 91*(6), 947-952.

Marrazzo, J.M., Koutsky, L.A., Stine, K.L., Kuypers, J.M., Grubert, T.A., Galloway, D.A., Kiviat, N.B., & Handsfield, H.H. (1998). Genital human papillomavirus infection in women who have sex with women. *The Journal of Infectious Diseases, 178*(6), 1604-1609.

Marrazzo, J.M., Stine, K., & Koutsky, L.A. (2000). Genital human papillomavirus infection in women who have sex with women: A review. *American Journal of Obstetrics and Gynecology, 183,* 770-774.

Marrazzo, J.M., Stine, K., & Wald, A. (2003). Prevalence and risk factors for infection with herpes simplex virus type-1 and type-2 among lesbians. *Sexually Transmitted Diseases, 30*(12), 890-895.

Matthews, A.K., Brandenburgh, D.L., Johnson, T., & Hughes, T.L. (2004). Correlates of underutilization of gynecological cancer screening among lesbian and heterosexual women. *Preventive Medicine, 38,* 105-113.

McGinnis, J.M., & Foege, W.H. (1993). Actual causes of death in the United States. *Journal of the American Medical Association, 270,* 2207-2212.

McKirnan, D.J., & Peterson, P.L. (1989). Alcohol and drug use among homosexual men and women: Epidemiology and population characteristics. *Addictive Behaviors, 14,* 545-553.

McLaughlin, E.M., & Rozee, P.D. (2001). Knowledge about heterosexual versus lesbian battering among lesbians. *Women & Therapy, 23*(3), 39-58.

Meyer, I.H. (2003). Prejudice, social stress, and mental health in lesbian, gay, and bisexual populations: Conceptual issues and research evidence. *Psychological Bulletin, 129*(5), 674-697.

Moran, N. (1996). Lesbian health care needs. *Canadian Family Physician, 42,* 879-884.

Morgan, K.S. (1992). Caucasian lesbians' use of psychotherapy: A matter of attitude. *Psychology of Women Quarterly, 16,* 127-130.

National Coalition Against Domestic Violence. (2002). From our lives, for our lives: Culturally appropriate responses to relationship violence in lesbian, bisexual, and transgender women of color communities. Workshop packet handed out at the National Coalition Against Domestic Violence Conference, San Francisco, California.

National Coalition of Anti-Violence Programs. (1998). *Annual report on lesbian, gay, bisexual, transgendered domestic violence.* Washington, DC: Author.

Niolan, R. (2000). Domestic violence in gay and lesbian couples. Retrieved December 10, 2003, from http://www.psychpage.com/learning/library/gay/gayvio.html.

Ocamb, K. (2000). The crisis of same-sex domestic violence. *Lesbian News, 25*(6), 45.

O'Hanlan, K.A., & Crum, C.P. (1996). Human papillomavirus-associated cervical intraepithelial neoplasia following exclusive lesbian sex. *Obstetrics and Gynecology, 88,* 702-703.

O'Hanlan, K.A., Dibble, S.L., Hafan, H.J., & Davids, R. (2004). Advocacy for women's health should include lesbian health. *Journal of Women's Health, 13,* 227-234.

Owens, J.F., Matthews, K.A., Wing, R.R., & Kuller, L.H. (1990). Physical activity and cardiovascular risk: A cross-sectional study of middle-aged premenopausal women. *Preventive Medicine, 1,* 147-157.

Paffenbarger, R.S., Jr., & Lee, I.-M. (1996). Exercise and fitness. In J.E. Manson, P.M. Ridker, J.M. Gaziano, & C.H. Hennekens (Eds.), *Prevention of myocardial infarction* (pp. 172-202). New York: Oxford University Press.

Patterson, C.J., & Friel, L.V. (1998). Sexual orientation and fertility. In G.R. Bentley & C.G.N. Mascie-Taylor (Eds.), *Infertility in the modern world: Present and future prospects* (pp. 238-260). Cambridge, U.K.: Cambridge University Press.

Patton, C.L., Millard, P.S., & Kessenich, C.R. (1998). Screening calcaneal ultrasound and risk factors for osteoporosis among lesbians and heterosexual women. *Journal of Women's Health, 7,* 909-915.

Peplau, L.A., Cochran, S.D., & Mays, V. (1997). A national survey of the intimate relationships of African American lesbians and gay men. In B. Greene (Ed.), *Ethnic and cultural diversity among lesbians and gay men* (pp. 11-38). Thousand Oaks, CA: Sage.

Poorman, P.B., & Seelau, S.M. (2001). Lesbians who abuse their partners: Using the FIRO-B to assess interpersonal characteristics. *Women & Therapy, 23*(3), 87-105.

Prentice, D.A., & Carranza, E. (2002). What women and men should be, shouldn't be, are allowed to be, and don't have to be: The contents of prescriptive gender stereotypes. *Psychology of Women Quarterly, 26,* 269-281.

Rankow, E.J., & Tessaro, R.N. (1998). Cervical cancer risk and papanicolaou screening in sample of lesbian and bisexual women. *Journal of Family Practice, 47,* 139-143.

Renzetti, C. (1988). Violence in lesbian relationships: A preliminary analysis of causal factors. *Journal of Interpersonal Violence, 3*(4), 381-399.

Rich, J.D., Buck, A., Tuomala, R.E., & Kazanjian, P.H. (1993). Transmission of human immunodeficiency virus infection presumed to have occurred via female homosexual contact. *Clinical Infectious Diseases, 17,* 1003-1005.

Ristock, J.L. (2001). Decentering heterosexuality: Responses of feminist counselors to abuse in lesbian relationships. *Women & Therapy, 23*(3), 59-72.

Roberts, S.A., Dibble, S.L., & Scanlon, C. (1998). Differences for risk factors for breast cancer: Lesbians and heterosexual women. *Journal of the Gay and Lesbian Medical Association, 2,* 93-101.

Ryan, H., Wortley, P.M., Easton, A., Pederson, L., & Greenwood, G. (2001). Smoking among lesbians, gays, and bisexuals: A review of the literature. *American Journal of Preventive Medicine, 21,* 142-149.

Saltzberg, S., Stroh, J.A., & Frishman, W.H. (1988). Isolated systolic hypertension in the elderly: Pathophysiology and treatment. *The Medical Clinics of North America, 72,* 523-547.

Saulnier, C.F. (2002). Deciding who to see: Lesbians discuss their preferences in health and mental health care providers. *Social Work, 47*(4), 355-367.

Scheer, S., Peterson, I., Page-Shafer, K., Delgado, V., Gleghorn, A., Ruiz, J., Molitor, F., McFarland, W., & Klausner, J. (2002). The Young Women's Survey Team. Sexual and drug use behavior among women who have sex with both women and men: Results of a population-based survey. *American Journal of Public Health, 92*(7), 1110-1112.

Schneider, M.S. (1986). The relationships of cohabiting lesbian and heterosexual couples: A comparison. *Psychology of Women Quarterly, 10,* 234-239.

Sempos, C.T., Cleeman, J.I., & Carroll, M.D. (1993). Prevalence of high blood cholesterol among U.S. adults: An update based on guidelines from the Second Report of the National Cholesterol Education Program Adult Treatment Panel. *Journal of the American Medical Association, 269,* 3009-3014.

Shotsky, W.J. (1996). Women who have sex with other women: HIV seroprevalence in New York State counseling and testing programs. *Women & Health, 24*(2), 1-15.

Siever, M.D. (1994). Sexual orientation and gender as factors in socioculturally acquired vulnerability to body dissatisfaction and eating disorders. *Journal of Consulting and Clinical Psychology, 62*(2), 252-260.

Skinner, C.J., Stokes, J., Kirlew, Y., Kavanagh, J., & Forster, G.E. (1996). A case-controlled study of the sexual health needs of lesbians. *Genitourinary Medicine, 72*(4), 277-280.

Sorensen, L., & Roberts, S.J. (1997). Lesbian uses of and satisfaction with mental health services: Results from the Boston Lesbian Health Project. *Journal of Homosexuality, 33*(1), 35-49.

Stuehling, J.E. (2001). Crime victims compensation for battered women: Advocating for economic justice. Pennsylvania Coalition Against Domestic Violence. Pennsylvania Commission on Crime and Delinquency (PCCD), Bureau of Victims' Services.

Tigert, L.M. (2001). The power of shame: Lesbian battering as a manifestation of homophobia. *Women & Therapy, 23*(3), 73-85.

Valanis, B.G., Bowen, D.J., Bassford, T., Whitlock, E., Charney, P., & Carter, R.A. (2000). Sexual orientation and health: Comparisons in the Women's Health Initiative sample. *Archives of Family Medicine, 9*(9), 843-853.

Walker, L.E. (2000). *Battered women syndrome.* New York: Springer.

Wei, M., Kampert, J.B., & Barlow, C.E. (1999). Relationship between low cardiorespiratory fitness and mortality in normal-weight, overweight, and obese men. *Journal of the American Medical Association, 282,* 1547-1553.

Weinberg, T.S. (1994). *Gay men, drinking, and alcoholism.* Carbondale: Southern Illinois University Press.

Whelton, P.K., He, J., & Appel, L.F. (1996). Treatment and prevention in hypertension. In J.E. Manson, P.M. Ridker, J.M. Gaziano, & C.H. Hennekens (Eds.), *Pre-*

vention of myocardial infarction (pp. 154-171). New York: Oxford University Press.

Willett, W.C., Green, A., & Stampfer, M.J. (1987). Relative and absolute excess risks of coronary heart disease among women who smoke cigarettes. *New England Journal of Medicine, 317,* 1303-1309.

Wilsnack, S.C. (1995). Alcohol use and alcohol problems in women. In A.L. Stanton & S.J. Gallant (Eds.), *The psychology of women's health: Progress and challenges in research and application* (pp. 457-498). Washington, DC: American Psychological Association.

Wing, R.R., Kuller, L.H., & Bunker, C.H. (1989). Obesity, obesity-related behaviors and coronary heart disease risk factors in black and white premenopausal women. *International Journal of Obesity, 13,* 511-519.

Younglove, J.A., Kerr, M.G., & Vitello, C.J. (2002). Law enforcement officers' perceptions of same sex domestic violence. *Jounal of Interpersonal Violence, 17*(7), 760-772.

Zak, A., & McDonald, C. (1997). Satisfaction and trust in intimate relationships: Do lesbians and heterosexual women differ? *Psychological Reports, 80*(3), 904-906.

Chapter 6

Public Health and Gay and Bisexual Men: A Primer for Practitioners, Clinicians, and Researchers

Scott D. Rhodes
Leland J. Yee

INTRODUCTION

The diversity among gay and bisexual men mirrors the expansive diversity of society as a whole. Gay and bisexual men vary in their race, ethnicity, culture, educational and income levels, and physical ability, and come from every religious, political, and family background. Each gay and bisexual man is an individual with specific characteristics and health needs that, similar to members of any community or population, should not be assumed based on generalizations or stereotypes. Whether exploring needs through basic behavioral and epidemiologic research or planning, offering, providing, or evaluating one-on-one counseling or support services, referrals, clinical services, or group- or community-level interventions designed to affect health-related outcomes or behavior, one must move beyond one's own assumptions about gay or bisexual men. One must develop a comprehensive understanding of the individual existing within a variety of influencing contexts. These contexts include a variety of family systems, spatial neighborhoods, and social networks; institutions (schools, workplaces, and religious organizations); racial and ethnic communities; and other influencing contexts from the larger society. These contexts have unique norms and cultures and impose expectations that create and interact with the gay or bisexual man's sense of self and identity. These influencing contexts vary in the messages that are overtly and covertly relayed about being a gay or bisexual man. These messages are internalized and affect each individual differently.

Because of this diversity, describing best practices is complex, and generalizations may offer a false sense of understanding and unwarranted confidence among practitioners, clinicians, and researchers who seek quick answers. The important lesson is that all gay and bisexual men are not the same. They do not fit preconceived notions of what being a gay or bisexual man entails. Similarly, approaches that are effective in one situation may not prove successful in another.

Although much public health dialogue currently is occurring regarding the immense and growing health disparities that exist by race and ethnicity, less discussion has been focused on the health disparities that exist by sexual orientation. Of course, a discussion on the disproportionate HIV infection rates by race and ethnicity inherently includes sexual orientation; however, what about differential rates in certain types of cancer among gay and bisexual men? Although public health recognizes and finally is exploring the role of racism as a determinant of health in order to reduce and ultimately eliminate health disparities based on race and ethnicity, research about homophobia as a determinant of health is much less common. Such omission in the current public health dialogue should not be taken as license to ignore the role of homophobia in affecting the health of gay and bisexual men, but rather a call for recognition and action by those who plan programs and provide services (e.g., practitioners and clinicians) as well as those who explore health needs and outcomes (e.g., researchers).

This chapter briefly examines gay and bisexual men as a group; summarizes some of the major public health issues affecting gay and bisexual men, as evidenced in empirical research; highlights an example of an effective intervention strategy designed to address their health needs; and provides key approaches and consideration for practitioners, clinicians, and researchers to use as tools. A single chapter cannot provide sufficient guidance for improving public health services to gay and bisexual men. Therefore, we assert that a thorough understanding and appreciation of specific concerns, challenges, and strengths of the individual or specific community are necessary in order to achieve desired outcomes effectively, efficiently, and as respectfully as possible. The approaches and considerations outlined at the conclusion of this chapter are fundamental to working to reduce health disparities and improve the health of gay and bisexual men. These approaches are transferable and not necessarily exclusive to meeting the health needs of gay and bisexual men.

WHO ARE GAY AND BISEXUAL MEN?

Calculating an exact number of gay and bisexual men in a community, state, region, or country is challenging for two main reasons. First, defining what constitutes gay and bisexual is problematic. Profound differences can exist among (1) how individuals define and describe themselves, (2) how they feel, and (3) their behaviors. Furthermore, how men define and describe themselves, how they feel, and their behaviors may change during their life course. Some men will report being gay or bisexual, while others may not. Some men may be attracted to other men but not engage in same-sex sexual behavior. Still other men may engage in same-sex sexual behavior but not identify themselves or describe themselves as gay or bisexual. Currently, the trend is to label men who do not self-identify as gay or bisexual but engage in same-sex behavior as "men who have sex with men" (MSM). For the purposes of sexual risk and sexual-risk reduction, the use of the term MSM is an attempt to move beyond labels and identity toward a focus on behavior. For the purposes of human immunodeficiency virus (HIV) infection and acquired immune deficiency syndrome (AIDS) prevention and surveillance, focusing on sexual behavior has been viewed as a method to avoid the debates regarding identity and stigma. The focus becomes not who an individual is or how he identifies himself, but rather the sexual behavior that may put him at risk for HIV or other sexually transmitted diseases (STDs).

Second, because of the fear of social reprisal resulting from disclosing a gay or bisexual orientation or desire, men who may be gay or bisexual are likely to underreport their same-sex orientation or same-sex behavior. Thus, the number of men who identify as gay or bisexual is difficult to estimate. However, researchers have attempted to estimate the number of men who identify as gay and bisexual and who engage in same-sex sexual behavior.

In the 1940s, Alfred Kinsey and his colleagues found that among men 37 percent reported some homosexual contact, 13 percent reported more homosexual than heterosexual contact, and 4 percent reported exclusively homosexual contact (Kinsey, Pomeroy, & Martin, 1948). Although his research has been criticized, Kinsey's work in sexuality remains a rare and relatively authoritative study of sexual behavior in the United States. Subsequent national and international studies have found rates of same-sex sexual behavior among men ranging from 2.7 percent to 9.8 percent (ACSF Investigators, 1992; Johnson, Wadsworth, Wellings, Bradshaw, & Field, 1992; Laumann, Gagnon, Michael, & Michaels, 1994; Melbye & Biggar, 1992; Michaels, 1996).

THE HEALTH OF GAY AND BISEXUAL MEN

Limited data on this population makes the study of the health of gay and bisexual men difficult. Only recently have some population-based studies attempted to incorporate measures (both direct or, more often, proxy measures) of sexual orientation among study participants (Cochran & Mays, 2000; Gilman et al., 2001). Without data on sexual orientation, assessing the health needs of gay and bisexual men is problematic. However, it is clear that gay and bisexual men are disproportionately affected by some infectious diseases, such as HIV and types of viral hepatitis, and by some noncommunicable diseases, such as lung cancer from increased rates of smoking and AIDS-related malignancies. The list of diseases provided in this chapter is not meant to be exhaustive, but it provides a brief introduction to a few of the major health issues facing gay and bisexual men.

INFECTIOUS DISEASES AMONG GAY AND BISEXUAL MEN

A number of communicable diseases are of paramount importance within the gay and bisexual male communities. These communicable diseases include HIV, hepatitis, and STDs.

Human Immunodeficiency Virus (HIV)

Although a number of infectious diseases are especially serious for gay and bisexual men by virtue of their prevalence and incidence, HIV infection is arguably the most critical. Spread effectively by sex or parenteral (blood to blood) means, HIV destroys the immune systems of infected individuals over time. With impaired immune responses, infected individuals may die of an opportunistic infection or malignancy, such as toxoplasmic encephalitis, *Pneumocystis* pneumonia, extrapulmonary *Cryptococcosis, Mycobacterium avium intracellulare* (MAI), or *Mycobacterium avium* complex (MAC), and candidiasis of the esophagus, trachea, bronchi, or lungs. The clinical management of HIV infection has greatly improved over the past few years through the use of highly active antiretroviral therapy (HAART) to slow the progression of HIV and the introduction of other prophylactic therapies to prevent or control opportunistic infections. Although neither a vaccine against HIV nor a cure for AIDS exists, the lives of persons living with HIV/AIDS (PLWH/A) have been greatly extended through the development of medical regimens to reduce viral replication and slow disease progression.

HIV continues to disproportionately affect gay men, with an estimated 365,000 to 535,000 currently infected with HIV in the United States (Blair, Fleming, & Karon, 2002; Catania et al., 2001; Wolitski, Valdiserri, Denning,

& Levine, 2001). A 1997 study of urban MSM* suggested HIV prevalence of 17 percent overall, with the prevalence ranging from 29 percent among African-American MSM to 40 percent among MSM who used injected drugs (Catania et al., 2001). Although there has been a decline in the prevalence and incidence of HIV infection among gay men in the United States during the past ten to fifteen years, data suggest that gay men still account for a significant proportion of all new infections (Karon, Fleming, Steketee, & DeCock, 2001). Moreover, recent reports suggest that the rates of new infections among gay men, after this period of decline, may be on the rise (Centers for Disease Control and Prevention, 2001; Kellogg, McFarland, & Katz, 1999). Black and Latino subgroups of the gay community have been particularly affected by the HIV epidemic (Centers for Disease Control and Prevention, 2001; Malebranche, 2003), with these two groups comprising 53 percent of all gay men diagnosed with AIDS in 1999 (Wolitski et al., 2001). HIV is prominent in the gay community not just among young men, but across many age groups. In a recent probability survey of 2,881 MSM over the age of fifty from several urban centers in the United States (New York, Los Angeles, Chicago, and San Francisco), the prevalence of HIV was 19 percent for men in their fifties and 3 percent for men in their sixties (Dolcini, Catania, Stall, & Pollack, 2003). In order to effectively meet the prevention, care, service, and treatment needs of the MSM community, efforts must take these epidemiologic factors into account.

Viral Hepatitis

The term "hepatitis" simply means inflammation of the liver. A number of factors may cause this condition. In addition to the ingestion of drugs toxic to the liver, some noncommunicable types of hepatitis occur, such as autoimmune diseases in which the liver is the primary organ affected. Communicable viruses that primarily affect the liver also may cause hepatitis. Among the viral hepatitidies, hepatitis A virus (HAV) and hepatitis B virus (HBV) are important with respect to the health of gay and bisexual men. As defined by the Centers for Disease Control and Prevention (CDC), MSM are considered to be at increased risk for HAV and HBV (Centers for Disease Control and Prevention, 2002), and outbreaks of both HAV and HBV have been reported among MSM (Bell et al., 2001; Diamond et al., 2003; Henning, Bell, Braun, & Barker, 1995; Kahn, 2002).

---

*Given the differences in interpreting the terms "gay," "bisexual," and "MSM," we have chosen to maintain the integrity of the original research by using the reported terminology throughout this chapter.

Hepatitis A is spread through fecal-oral contact (Chin, 2000). Sexual transmission may occur via direct anal-oral contact (rimming) or by contact with fingers, sex toys, or condoms that have been in or near the anus of an infected sex partner. Although infection with HAV does not become chronic (persistent) and rarely results in death, infection with HAV may result in symptoms that may be debilitating, including jaundice, nausea, vomiting, fatigue, weakness, and fever (Zachoval & Deinhardt, 1998). The morbidity associated with infection exerts a significant human as well as financial toll, including medical expenditures and productivity lost as a result of the infected individual's inability to work. On average, adults with hepatitis A lose twenty-seven days of work, and between 11 and 22 percent of persons with hepatitis A are hospitalized. Average medical costs associated with hepatitis A infection range from $1,817 to $2,459 per case for adults (Centers for Disease Control and Prevention, 1999b). In one common-source outbreak in the United States among forty-three persons, the estimated cost was approximately $800,000 (Dalton, Haddix, Hoffman, & Mast, 1996). The estimated annual direct and indirect costs of HAV infection in the United States in 1989 was more than $200 million (Hadler, 1991).

In developed countries such as the United States, HBV is mainly spread via sexual contact. Unlike hepatitis A, infection with hepatitis B becomes chronic in a portion of individuals and may lead to liver cancer. An estimated 1.25 million persons in the United States are chronically infected with HBV, and 128,000 to 300,000 new infections occur annually (Lee, 1997). HBV is transmitted by body fluids such as blood, semen, saliva, and vaginal secretions, or parenterally through exposure to contaminated needles, body-piercing equipment, or medical equipment. Although HBV infection in the general population is quite low, HBV is quite prevalent in the MSM community. Estimates of the prevalence of previous HBV infection in this population range from 5 to 81 percent, with the prevalence of hepatitis B surface antigen (HBsAg), which is indicative of persistent hepatitis B infection, ranging from 1 to 11 percent (Brook, 2002; Seage et al., 1997).

In 1982, the FDA licensed a three-dose vaccine against HBV, and a two-dose vaccine against HAV was licensed in 1996. More recently, a combined HBV and HAV vaccine has become available. The CDC recommends vaccination against both HAV and HBV for all gay and bisexual men (Centers for Disease Control and Prevention, 1991). However, many gay and bisexual men remain unvaccinated, and health care providers do not adequately assess risk and suggest vaccination for those at high risk (Institute of Medicine & Committee on Prevention and Control of Sexually Transmitted Diseases, 1997; Kahn, 2002). Just why some individuals obtain the HBV vaccine and others do not, and why some individuals complete the vaccine series and others do not is not fully understood, although this is currently a topic of research (Rhodes & Hergenrather, 2003; Yee & Rhodes, 2002). An understanding of these behavioral factors will allow for more efficient and effective targeted interventions to increase vaccination initiation and completion among gay and bisexual men.

Viral hepatitis is an important public health issue for gay and bisexual men both because of the morbidity and mortality it inflicts and because HAV and HBV vaccination forms the most analogous paradigm for the effective delivery of vaccines to this population. Should a future vaccine for other diseases that affect gay and bisexual men, such as HIV, become available, understanding hepatitis vaccination behavior will provide insight into the effective delivery of vaccine to this population (Rhodes, Yee, & Hergenrather, 2003; Yee & Rhodes, 2002).

Other Sexually Transmitted Diseases Among Gay and Bisexual Men

Beyond HIV and hepatitis, other sexually transmitted diseases (STDs) such as syphilis, gonorrhea, herpes, and chlamydia also are major public health concerns affecting gay and bisexual men because of their immediate medical impact and the fact that STDs serve as a surrogate marker of high-risk sexual activity. Recent studies have observed an increasing incidence of STDs among MSM in the United States (Centers for Disease Control and Prevention, 1999a, 2001; Fox et al., 2001; Williams et al., 1999). These reports parallel reported increases in risky sexual behaviors among MSM (Centers for Disease Control and Prevention, 1999a; Chen et al., 2002). These observations have important public health ramifications, as they highlight the need for more effective prevention strategies. Another important factor is that ulcerative STDs, such as genital herpes, may facilitate the spread of HIV infection (Renzi et al., 2003).

NONCOMMUNICABLE DISEASES AMONG GAY AND BISEXUAL MEN

Several noninfectious diseases are particularly salient to gay and bisexual men as a result of their being affected disproportionately. These include some types of cancer as well as psychosocial issues.

Cancer

Lung Cancer and Smoking

The association of tobacco use with a number of health issues, including cardiovascular disease and cancer, is well documented (Doll & Hill, 1952; Shaper, Wannamethee, & Walker, 2003). Concern has been expressed that tobacco companies have turned to target-marketing tobacco to gay and bisexual consumers (Offen, Smith, & Malone, 2003; Smith & Malone, 2003; Yamey, 2003). Although information on the smoking trends of gay and bisexual men is extremely limited, a higher prevalence of smoking among gay men compared to the population as a whole has been found (Ryan, Wortley, Easton, Pederson, & Greenwood, 2001; Skinner, 1994; Stall, Greenwood, Acree, Paul, & Coates, 1999; Valanis et al., 2000). In 1992, a study that used household and bar-based sampling found 48 percent of MSM surveyed reported smoking, compared to only 27 percent of U.S. men who reported smoking (Stall et al., 1999). Such increased rates of smoking result in increased morbidity and mortality among gay and bisexual men.

Human Papillomavirus Infection and Cancer

Human papillomavirus (HPV) is a virus associated with genital warts. Over 100 types of HPV exist; approximately forty are spread sexually and several strains are considered to generate a high risk for the development of cancer. HPV is considered to be one of the most common STDs. Although most individuals do not develop symptoms, some studies estimate that the majority of the sexually active U.S. population is exposed to at least one or more types of HPV over their lifetimes. Because HPV is highly prevalent, an individual does not need have to have many sexual partners to be exposed to this virus (Gottlieb, 2002).

A strong association has been observed between infection with HPV and cervical cancer among women. In particular, infection with two strains of HPV, HPV-16 and HPV-18, are strongly associated with cervical cancer (Palefsky, Holly, Ralston, & Jay, 1998). Although anal cancer is rare in the general population, studies have suggested that the risk of anal cancers among men with a history of anal intercourse could be as much as thirty times higher (Frisch, Smith, Grulich, & Johansen, 2003; Palefsky et al., 1998). More research is needed to confirm these observations.

An important corollary of this issue is the possible use of an anal pap test (pap smear) as a cancer-screening tool. The pap test has been successfully used as a tool among women. The potential use of this test as a screening tool for anal cancer is now being explored. However, the use of the anal pap test is not a widely accepted standard medical procedure, and most clinicians are neither familiar with nor trained in anal pap test administration and interpretation.

AIDS-Related Malignancies

The immunosuppression that results from HIV infection facilitates the development of a number of AIDS-related malignancies. Given the disproportionate occurrence of HIV among gay and bisexual men, AIDS-related malignancies form a central public health concern for gay and bisexual men.

Kaposi's Sarcoma

Kaposi's sarcoma (KS) is a rare neoplasm that was first described by Mortiz Kaposi in the 1870s as affecting elderly Mediterranean and Jewish men. This vascular neoplasm that affects spindle cells manifests as reddish-purple skin lesions on the skin or mucosal surfaces, but may also occur in the internal organs. There are four main forms of KS. The "classic form" was described by Moritz Kaposi and is primarily found in older men of Mediterranean descent. A second "endemic form" is found in parts of Africa in varied age groups. The third form involves individuals who have received organ transplants and are undergoing immunosuppressive therapy. Finally, the fourth form, also called the "epidemic form," affects individuals with HIV infection (Cannon, Laney, & Pellett, 2003; Chin, 2000).

KS is now believed to be caused by infection with the newly identified human herpes virus-8 (HHV-8) (Antman & Chang, 2000; Chang et al., 1994; Martin et al., 1998; O'Brien et al., 1999). Immunosuppression is likely an important factor in the pathogenesis of epidemic KS. In healthy individuals infected with HHV-8, the immune response is able to control it. The impaired immune systems of individuals with advanced HIV potentially hinders the ability for an effective immune response to control HHV-8 pathogenesis (Wang et al., 2001). KS is likely spread easily via sexual means, and this route of transmission may explain the higher incidence among individuals who acquired their HIV sexually than among those with exposure to blood products (Chin, 2000).

Lymphomas

Lymphoma is a type of cancer that can occur when an error occurs in the way a lymphocyte is produced, resulting in an abnormal cell. These abnormal cells can accumulate by two mechanisms: (1) they can duplicate faster than normal cells or (2) they can live longer than normal lymphocytes. A lymphoma is a cancer of the lymphoid tissue and is generally divided into two types. Hodgkin's disease tumors contain giant cells of unknown origin, although B lymphocytes (often called B-cells) are believed to play a role. Non-Hodgkin's lymphoma tumors lack giant cells and may arise from T lymphocytes (often called T-cells), B-cells, or monocytes and are more common than Hodgkin's tumors in HIV disease. Lymphomas are approximately 50 to 100 times more common among individuals with HIV infection than in the general population (Chin, 2000), and lymphomas rank as one of the most common cancers associated with HIV infection (Stine, 2003).

HOMOPHOBIA AND HEALTH

Just as racism has been identified as a cause for decreased health status among racial and ethnic minorities (Institute of Medicine, 2003), homophobia also exists within a broad historical and contemporary context and has far-reaching ramifications, including how programs are designed and delivered and how research is prioritized and funded. Thus, opportunities to explore, understand, and improve the health of gay and bisexual men are missed. Although the effects of homophobia are not sufficiently explored, at least two main outcomes of homophobia are distinguishable. These outcomes pertain to reduced access to and quality of services, care, and programs and reduced physical health resulting from the mind-body interaction.

First, because of the influences of homophobia, gay and bisexual men may have reduced access to health services, care, and programs and thus receive inadequate prevention education, prevention intervention, health screenings, and diagnosis and treatment. Gay and bisexual men may not relay accurate information to practitioners, clinicians, and researchers who are exploring needs through basic behavioral and epidemiologic research, or those who are planning, offering, providing, or evaluating one-on-one counseling or support services, referrals, clinical services, or group- or community-level interventions. For example, within a public health clinic, available care may not be conducive to disclosure of a gay or bisexual orientation, and thus the gay or bisexual man may not receive the full benefit of HAV and HBV vaccination services. Thus, a potential opportunity to prevent disease has been missed.

Second, current research is exploring mind-body connections. The role of homophobia in the health of gay and bisexual men goes beyond predicting access to and the quality of health care received and the lower priority given to gay and bisexual men's health. Homophobia also may increase rates of stress, depression, and anxiety; attempted suicide; substance use; and health-compromising behaviors (Catania et al., 2001; Cochran & Mays, 2000; Garofalo, Wolf, Wissow, Woods, & Goodman, 1999; Gilman et al., 2001; Stall & Wiley, 1988). Innovative research in psychoneuroimmunology has found associations between psychological phenomena and decreased health status. For example, studies among gay and bisexual HIV-positive men suggest that stressful life events, dysphoria, and limited social support are associated with more rapid clinical HIV progression (Leserman et al., 1999, 2002). Furthermore, research is beginning to examine the associations between low self-esteem and psychological distress resulting from homophobia with behavioral risk (Herek, 1994; Malebranche, 2003; Stokes & Peterson, 1998).

Another important consideration is the role of homophobia in risk behavior associated with non-gay-identified men. The term "down low" has increased in use, especially in the media, to describe men who may not self-identify as gay and in fact who may have girlfriends or female spouses but have sexual intercourse with other men. Men "on" the down low, or on the "DL" as is heard, live a complex existence, juggling sexual identity, desire, and behavior within influencing homophobic contexts that dictate adherence to traditional hegemonic masculinity that is characterized by the avoidance of feminine behaviors, the display of dominance and power, the portrayal of independence and stoicism, and the embrace of risk behaviors. Use of the term DL may not be universally accepted; in fact, men who do not want to be labeled as gay may be just as wary of being labeled DL. The term is included here because of the attention that this concept is being given currently. Caution should be used in labeling people.

Although the complete etiology of homophobia's effect on the health of gay and bisexual men remains imprecise to date, homophobia clearly affects the health of gay and bisexual men (Gilman et al., 2001; Savin-Williams, 1994). Although much more research is needed to understand the health outcomes of gay and bisexual men, slow but important strides have been made to improve their health behaviors. The following section moves from the current health status and potential causes of compromised health among gay and bisexual men to explore the theoretic basis of a widely disseminated and successfully evaluated intervention approach for self-identified gay and bisexual men. A number of efficacious interventions have been developed to change sexual risk behavior among gay and bisexual men; however, there is a dearth of interventions targeting other health issues that are of particular importance for gay and bisexual men. In fact, little research literature exists that tests, much less suggests, scientifically sound interventions to positively affect the health of gay and bisexual men. What does exist has, in many cases, not been evaluated and/or shown to be scientifically sound. Thus, we now turn to an intervention that has proven to be effective in reducing sexual risk behaviors among gay and bisexual men.

AN EFFECTIVE HIV-PREVENTION STRATEGY

A Natural-Helper Model for HIV Prevention

In recent years, public health professionals have introduced a number of approaches based on natural helpers, or indigenous leaders, to address a variety of health issues, often in traditionally underserved or more vulnerable communities (U.S. Department of Health and Human Services, 1994a,b). Natural helpers, also commonly known as community health advocates, lay health advisors or educators, community-health representatives, community health outreach workers, *promotores de salud,* peer educators, peer leaders, indigenous leaders, and opinion leaders, among other titles, are "individuals to whom others naturally turn to for advice, emotional support, and tangible aid" (Eng & Parker, 2002, p. 126). Respected, trusted, and responsive to the needs of others, natural helpers are identified, recruited, and trained within a narrowly defined health focus. They are "community members who work almost exclusively in community settings" (Witmer, Seifer, Finocchio, Leslie, & O'Neil, 1995, p. 1055). They relay health information and connect friends, family members, and acquaintances to resources to promote health while strengthening preexisting community networks and ties (Eng, Parker, & Harlam, 1997; Eng & Parker, 2002; Institute of Medicine, 2003; Israel, 1985). Natural helpers are uniquely qualified to reach the members of their social networks because they are members of the communities in which they interact; are among the first resources used when members of their social networks need advice, support, or assistance; possess an intimate understanding of the community's networks as well as the community's strengths and health needs; understand what is meaningful to those communities; communicate in the language of community members; and recognize and incorporate cultural buffers (e.g., identity, coping, health practices) to promote positive health outcomes (Altpeter, Earp, Bishop, & Eng, 1999; Bishop, Earp, Eng, & Lynch, 2002; Giblin, 1989; Jackson & Parks, 1997; Love, Gardner, & Legion, 1997; Thomas, Eng,

Clark, Robinson, & Blumenthal, 1998). Natural helpers serve to build partnerships with formal health care delivery systems to connect people with the services they need and to stimulate social action that promotes community participation in the health system and political dynamics to affect health status (Eng et al., 1997; Eng & Parker, 2002). Natural helpers also may coordinate with service providers to understand and address the community's health needs and increase the cultural relevancy of interventions by helping providers and health care systems build their cultural competence and develop programs that are asset oriented (Altpeter et al., 1999; Earp & Flax, 1999; Eng & Parker, 2002; Institute of Medicine, 2003; Wilkenson, 1992; Witmer et al., 1995). Rather than using a deficits approach to health, using a natural-helper approach builds on the strengths of the community. Using their position, expanded knowledge base, and skills, natural helpers reduce morbidity and mortality while improving health outcomes in their communities (Eng & Parker, 2002).

The Popular-Opinion-Leader Intervention

A bar-based HIV-prevention intervention using natural helpers, the popular-opinion-leader (POL) intervention developed at the Center for AIDS Intervention Research (CAIR) has been found to be effective in HIV-risk-behavior reduction, including decreasing unprotected anal intercourse among gay bar patrons (Kelly et al., 1992). This community-level intervention is based on theories of peer influence (Hallinan, 1982), social support (House, 1981), and diffusion of innovations (Rogers, 1983). As it was originally tested, using the naturally occurring social network of the bar, natural helpers known as POLs were selected based on their popularity. They attended four weekly ninety-minute sessions that led them through a colearning process of exploring and thoroughly understanding HIV prevention (both facts and skills) and practicing effective communication and leadership strategies. The training of these POLs covered basic epidemiology and transmission of HIV/AIDS, behavioral strategies for risk reduction, misconceptions about HIV/AIDS, characteristics of effective health-promotion messages, and role-plays of conversations endorsing safer sex. Community-level triggers in the form of posters within the bar and buttons worn by POLs promoted the intervention and encouraged dialogue between bar patrons and opinion leaders; many times these POLs were bartenders. Bartenders have more- and less-busy moments, are often casual yet well-trusted confidantes, and are "on-site" regularly.

The use of a natural-helper approach is especially appropriate for HIV prevention because opinion leaders can reach populations not easily accessed by traditional health professionals. For example, this approach may reach individuals with asymptomatic infections and people who encounter barriers to HIV/AIDS care. Popular opinion leaders provide information and teach skills regarding safer sex and risk reduction and can participate in the development and distribution of culturally relevant educational materials that use culturally relevant channels, affecting the norms regarding sexual risk within their own social networks. Implicit in this approach is the exchange of social support (Eng & Parker, 2002). Although social support has been widely defined, some of the most persistent and empirically observed subconstructs include four broad types of supporting behaviors or acts:

1. emotional support, which involves the provision of trust, caring, empathy, and love;
2. instrumental support, which involves the provision of tangible aid and services that directly assist an individual;
3. informational support, which involves the provision of advice, suggestions, and information that an individual can use; and
4. appraisal support, which involves the provision of information that is useful for self-evaluation purposes (constructive feedback, affirmation, and social comparison and influence) (Heaney & Israel, 2002).

From a public health perspective, the empirical associations found between social support and health (Berkman, Glass, Brissette, & Seeman, 2000; Broadhead et al., 1983; Cassel, 1976; Kaplan, Cassel, & Gore, 1977) hold substantial potential for translating the health-enhancing effects of social support into interventions (Heaney & Israel, 2002). Although the POL intervention has been empirically tested as an approach to reduce HIV infection exposure and transmission, its potential use in other health issues has yet to be sufficiently explored.

SUGGESTED APPROACHES AND CONSIDERATIONS FOR PRACTITIONERS, CLINICIANS, AND RESEARCHERS

The Importance of Partnering with Community Members

Many of the complex health problems that persist into the twenty-first century have proven to be ill-suited for traditional "outside expert" approaches to intervention development and implementation, as evidenced by the often disappointing outcomes they have yielded (Centers for Disease Control and Prevention & Agency for Toxic Substances and Disease Registry Committee on Community Engagement, 1997; Green, 2001; Israel, Schulz, Parker, & Becker, 1998; Minkler & Wallerstein, 2003; O'Toole, Aaron, Chin, Horowitz, & Tyson, 2003). Instead, promoting a community's health through community partnership is viewed as a more viable mechanism for health promotion and disease prevention (Institute of Medicine, 2003; Israel et al., 1998; Minkler & Wallerstein, 2003; O'Toole et al., 2003; Wallerstein & Duran, 2003; Wandersman, 2003). Practitioners, clinicians, and researchers are currently exploring how to best partner with community representatives and lay community members in order to increase the quality and validity of efforts through the incorporation of local knowledge and local theory based on the lived experience of communities involved. Emerging evidence within other populations suggests that through this process of partnership with the community representatives and lay community members, advances in health can occur as health promotion and disease prevention approaches, strategies, and efforts increase in authenticity (Viswanathan et al., 2003). This point is especially important, as interventions are disseminated with the expectation that what worked with gay or bisexual men in one geographic location will work in another location. The movement toward strict intervention fidelity may in fact jeopardize effectiveness because of the lack of appropriateness and suitability for local context. Practitioners, clinicians, and researchers must establish authentic co-learning partnerships with gay and bisexual men if improvements in health are to occur within these communities.

The Importance of Community

Partnering with community members leads to two questions: (1) Who comprises a community? and (2) Does the current focus on MSM promote or hinder community approaches to the planning, provision, and evaluation of one-on-one counseling or support services, referrals, clinical services, or group- or community-level interventions? Community is a unit of identity, and for many gay and bisexual men that identity is as a gay or bisexual man. A sense of community contributes to the success of the POL intervention, for example. In most public health practice and research, the language used is related to sexual risk. As mentioned, by using the term "men who have sex with men" or "MSM," practitioners, clinicians, and researchers have tried to focus on the behaviors associated with sexual risk. Unfortunately, this approach may limit health-promotion and disease-prevention efforts. The focus is placed on the individual, an MSM, rather than on community; self-identified gay and bisexual men are taken out of their contexts, and intervention strategies are founded on individual behavior change. Rather than understanding a community of gay and bisexual men and building on social networks, the MSM approach leads to interventions that are deficit oriented. For many gay and bisexual men, public health approaches may be more successful if they build community. Thus, an all-or-nothing approach must be revised to consider gay and bisexual men and MSM within community contexts. This community approach differs from a social control model in which practitioners, clinicians, and researchers ask, "How can we motivate people to change?" Yet, we cannot "give" individuals motivation. Rather, the flip side may be more effective. From a social-change model, the question is reworked and becomes, "What are people's motives for changing or not changing?" Thus, effective interventions build on what is important to individuals, and in many cases what is important to individuals is a connection to social networks and communities (Eng, Salmon, & Mullan, 1992).

Individuals and Communities Are Complex

It has been rhetorically asked, "Where did the field get the idea that evidence of an intervention's efficacy from carefully controlled trials could be generalized as the 'best practice' for widely varied populations and situations?" (Green, 2001, p. 167). Human behavior is most often approached from a positivist or postpositivist assumption; we assume that experimental interventions shown to work in one setting can be repeated in another. A medical intervention can be counted on to have a similar efficacy on a variety of individuals, with minor adjustments of dosage by age and sex. However, human behavior is more unpredictable. Behavior change occurs within a rich fabric of culture, socioeconomic condition, social customs, laws, and policies. Thus, as was asserted in the chapter introduction, to work with gay and bisexual men, to work with any group of individuals or members from any self-identified community, one must move beyond one's own assumptions to develop a comprehensive understanding of the individual within a variety of influencing structures. Public health practitioners, clinicians, and researchers must not assume that the gay or bisexual male community is monolithic; communities vary and individuals within communities vary. The *generalizability* of knowledge about one community to the next may be limited; however, the *transferability* of processes to develop knowledge and understanding may be a more reasonable expectation. Furthermore, the emphasis on fidelity to the implementation of efficacious interventions also may be misplaced; each community is unique, and the appropriateness of intervention approaches may require variations by geographic location, individual and community experience, and community context and subcontext, among other variables.

CONCLUSION

Many of the important public health concerns facing our country affect gay and bisexual men disproportionately, including infectious diseases such as HIV, HAV, HBV, and other STDs, and noncommunicable diseases such as types of cancers and AIDS-related malignancies. Although in this chapter we delineated these health conditions and provided data to document the public health impact, overall limited research exists to identify, explore, and intervene in the health status of gay and bisexual men. Disproportionate rates of disease burden carried by gay and bisexual men are not well documented, understood, or characterized, and factors that contribute to these rates are not well defined. Although it has been hypothesized that violence (Harper & Schneider, 2003; Willis, 2004), unhealthy body images (Boroughs & Thompson, 2002), and substance use (Lee, Galanter, Dermatis, & McDowell, 2003) potentially affect gay and bisexual men disproportionately, the public health impact of this requires further empirical clarification and evaluation.

Furthermore, few interventions for identifiable health disparities (e.g., HIV) have been developed and found effective in improving the health of gay and bisexual men. Current HIV-prevention efforts among gay and bisexual men are insufficient, and creative strategies are desperately needed. In part, the current lack of understanding of gay and bisexual men's health may be a symptom of overt and covert homophobia at multiple levels that limits behavioral, epidemiologic, and intervention research.

Although the marketing of tobacco products to the gay community is well documented and ongoing, the prevention and treatment interventions for gay and bisexual men are virtually nonexistent (Ryan et al., 2001). Even among existing interventions to affect health behavior, few have been rigorously evaluated. For example, while hepatitis A and hepatitis B are diseases recognized as disproportionately affecting gay and bisexual men, and gay and bisexual men constitute a prioritized group for targeted vaccination (Centers for Disease Control and Prevention, 2002; Gay and Lesbian Medical Association, 2001), only one U.S.-based intervention (Sansom, Rudy, Strine, & Douglas, 2003) can be found in the published peer-reviewed literature.

Research priorities include

1. further research to understand sexual orientation in terms of identity, desire, and behavior throughout the life course;

2. more comprehensive surveillance and data collection to identify and understand disproportionate rates of disease burden borne by gay and bisexual men;
3. exploration of such ecologic risk factors as homophobia on health behavior and health outcomes; and
4. the development, implementation, and evaluation of creative yet scientifically sound interventions to reach a variety of gay and bisexual men for a variety of health issues.

QUESTIONS TO CONSIDER

1. Many concerns about privacy issues have been expressed concerning research studies. Would it be useful to systematically collect sexual orientation data in future research studies? Why would these data be useful? How can these data be properly collected and stored to ensure the protection of the privacy of study participants?
2. Some people argue that the health and well-being of individuals are in the individual's control. How would homophobia affect one's health and well-being? What are some of the ways that the larger community and society as a whole influence the health, access to health care, and health-seeking behaviors of individuals?
3. What steps can you take to make your own work more directly applicable and accessible for gay and bisexual men?
4. Of which community or communities do you consider yourself a member? What do you gain from community membership and affiliation? Why would a sense of community be important for gay and bisexual men? How can the communities be better utilized for improving the effectiveness of public health interventions?
5. Can strengthening the gay and bisexual community and fostering positive identification within this community improve health? How can interventions better utilize community identification to improve effectiveness?

REFERENCES

ACSF Investigators. (1992). AIDS and sexual behaviour in France. *Nature, 360* (6403), 407-409.
Altpeter, M., Earp, J. A., Bishop, C., & Eng, E. (1999). Lay health advisor activity levels: Definitions from the field. *Health Education & Behavior, 26*(4), 495-512.
Antman, K., & Chang, Y. (2000). Kaposi's sarcoma. *New England Journal of Medicine, 342*(14), 1027-1038.

Bell, A., Ncube, F., Hansell, A., Davison, K. L., Young, Y., Gilson, R., Macdonald, N., Heathcock, R., Warburton, F., & Maguire, H. (2001). An outbreak of hepatitis A among young men associated with having sex in public venues. *Communicable Disease and Public Health, 4*(3), 163-170.

Berkman, L. F., Glass, T., Brissette, I., & Seeman, T. E. (2000). From social integration to health: Durkheim in the new millennium. *Social Science Medicine, 51*(6), 843-857.

Bishop, C., Earp, J. A., Eng, E., & Lynch, K. S. (2002). Implementing a natural helper lay health advisor program: Lessons learned from unplanned events. *Health Promotion Practice, 3*(2), 233-244.

Blair, J. M., Fleming, P. L., & Karon, J. M. (2002). Trends in AIDS incidence and survival among racial/ethnic minority men who have sex with men, United States, 1990-1999. *Journal of Acquired Immune Deficiency Syndromes, 31*(3), 339-347.

Boroughs, M., & Thompson, J. K. (2002). Exercise status and sexual orientation as moderators of body image disturbance and eating disorders in males. *The International Journal of Eating Disorders, 31*(3), 307-311.

Broadhead, W. E., Kaplan, B. H., James, S. A., Wagner, E. H., Schoenbach, V. J., Grimson, R., Heyden, S., Tibblin, G., & Gehlbach, S. H. (1983). The epidemiologic evidence for a relationship between social support and health. *American Journal of Epidemiology, 117*(5), 521-537.

Brook, M. G. (2002). Sexually acquired hepatitis. *Sexually Transmitted Infections, 78*(4), 235-240.

Cannon, M. J., Laney, A. S., & Pellett, P. E. (2003). Human herpesvirus 8: Current issues. *Clinical Infectious Diseases, 37*(1), 82-87.

Cassel, J. C. (1976). The contribution of the social environment to host resistance: The Fourst Wade Hampton Frost Lecture. *American Journal of Epidemiology, 104,* 107-123.

Catania, J. A., Osmond, D., Stall, R. D., Pollack, L., Paul, J. P., Blower, S., Binson, D., Canchola, J. A., Mills, T. C., Fisher, L., Choi, K. H., Porco, T., Turner, C., Blair, J., Henne, J., Bye, L. L., & Coates, T. J. (2001). The continuing HIV epidemic among men who have sex with men. *American Journal of Public Health, 91*(6), 907-914.

Centers for Disease Control and Prevention. (1991). Update on adult immunization recommendations of the Immunization Practices Advisory Committee (ACIP). *Morbidity and Mortality Weekly Report, 40*(RR-12), 1-52.

Centers for Disease Control and Prevention. (1999a). Increases in unsafe sex and rectal gonorrhea among men who have sex with men—San Francisco, California: 1994-1997. *Morbidity and Mortality Weekly Report, 48,* 45-48.

Centers for Disease Control and Prevention. (1999b). Prevention of hepatitis A through active or passive immunization: Recommendations of the Advisory Committee on Immunization Practices (ACIP). *Morbidity and Mortality Weekly Report, 48*(RR-12), 1-37.

Centers for Disease Control and Prevention. (2001). HIV incidence among young men who have sex with men—Seven U.S. cities, 1994-2000. *Morbidity and Mortality Weekly Report, 50*(21), 440-444.

Centers for Disease Control and Prevention. (2002). Sexually transmitted diseases treatment guidelines. *Morbidity and Mortality Weekly Report, 51*(RR-6), 59-63.

Centers for Disease Control and Prevention, & Agency for Toxic Substances and Disease Registry Committee on Community Engagement. (1997). *Principles of community engagement.* Atlanta, GA: U.S. Department of Health and Human Services.

Chang, Y., Cesarman, E., Pessin, M. S., Lee, F., Culpepper, J., Knowles, D. M., & Moore, P. S. (1994). Identification of herpesvirus-like DNA sequences in AIDS-associated Kaposi's sarcoma. *Science, 266*(5192), 1865-1869.

Chen, S. Y., Gibson, S., Katz, M. H., Klausner, J. D., Dilley, J. W., Schwarcz, S. K., Kellogg, T. A., & McFarland, W. (2002). Continuing increases in sexual risk behavior and sexually transmitted diseases among men who have sex with men: San Francisco, California, 1999-2001, USA. *American Journal of Public Health, 92*(9), 1387-1388.

Chin, J. (2000). *Control of communicable diseases manual.* Washington, DC: American Public Health Association.

Cochran, S. D., & Mays, V. M. (2000). Lifetime prevalence of suicide symptoms and affective disorders among men reporting same-sex sexual partners: Results from NHANES III. *American Journal of Public Health, 90*(4), 573-578.

Dalton, C. B., Haddix, A., Hoffman, R. E., & Mast, E. E. (1996). The cost of a foodborne outbreak of hepatitis A in Denver, Colorado. *Archives of Internal Medicine, 156*(9), 1013-1016.

Diamond, C., Thiede, H., Perdue, T., Secura, G. M., Valleroy, L., Mackellar, D., & Corey, L. (2003). Viral hepatitis among young men who have sex with men: Prevalence of infection, risk behaviors, and vaccination. *Sexually Transmitted Disease, 30*(5), 425-432.

Dolcini, M. M., Catania, J. A., Stall, R. D., & Pollack, L. (2003). The HIV epidemic among older men who have sex with men. *Journal of Acquired Immune Deficiency Syndromes, 33*(2 Suppl), S115-S121.

Doll, R., & Hill, A. B. (1952). A study of the aetiology of carcinoma of the lung. *British Medical Journal, 2*(4797), 1271-1286.

Earp, J. A., & Flax, V. L. (1999). What lay health advisors do: An evaluation of advisors' activities. *Cancer Practice, 7*(1), 16-21.

Eng, E., & Parker, E. A. (2002). Natural helper models to enhance a community's health and competence. In R. J. DiClemente, R. A. Crosby, & M. C. Kegler (Eds.), *Emerging theories in health promotion practice and research: Strategies for improving public health* (pp. 126-156). San Francisco, CA: Jossey-Bass.

Eng, E., Parker, E., & Harlan, C. (1997). Lay health advisor intervention strategies: A continuum from natural helping to paraprofessional helping. *Health Education & Behavior, 24*(4), 413-417.

Eng, E., Salmon, M., & Mullan, F. (1992). Community empowerment: The critical base for primary care. *Journal of Family and Community Health, 15*(1), 1-12.

Fox, K. K., del Rio, C., Holmes, K. K., Hook, E. W., III, Judson, F. N., Knapp, J. S., Procop, G. W., Wang, S. A., Whittington, W. L., & Levine, W. C. (2001). Gonorrhea in the HIV era: A reversal in trends among men who have sex with men. *American Journal of Public Health, 91*(6), 959-964.

Frisch, M., Smith, E., Grulich, A., & Johansen, C. (2003). Cancer in a population-based cohort of men and women in registered homosexual partnerships. *American Journal of Epidemiology, 157*(11), 966-972.

Garofalo, R., Wolf, R. C., Wissow, L. S., Woods, E. R., & Goodman, E. (1999). Sexual orientation and risk of suicide attempts among a representative sample of youth. *Archives of Pediatric & Adolescent Medicine, 153*(5), 487-493.

Gay and Lesbian Medical Association. (2001). *Healthy people 2010: Companion document for lesbian, gay, bisexual, and transgender (LGBT) health.* San Francisco, CA: Gay and Lesbian Medical Association.

Giblin, P. T. (1989). Effective utilization and evaluation of indigenous health care workers. *Public Health Reports, 104*(4), 361-368.

Gilman, S. E., Cochran, S. D., Mays, V. M., Hughes, M., Ostrow, D., & Kessler, R. C. (2001). Risk of psychiatric disorders among individuals reporting same-sex sexual partners in the National Comorbidity Survey. *American Journal of Public Health, 91*(6), 933-939.

Gottlieb, N. (2002). *A primer on HPV.* National Cancer Institute. Retrieved December 1, 2003, from http://newscenter.cancer.gov/newscenter/benchmarks-vol2-issue4/page2.

Green, L. W. (2001). From research to "best practices" in other settings and populations. *American Journal of Health Behavior, 25*(3), 165-178.

Hadler, S. (1991). Global impact of hepatitis A virus infection: Changing patterns. In F. Hollinger, S. Lemon, & H. Margolis (Eds.), *Viral hepatitis and liver diseases* (pp. 14-20). Baltimore, MD: Williams and Wilkins.

Hallinan, M. T. (1982). The peer influence process. *Studies in educational evaluation, 7*(3), 285-306.

Harper, G. W., & Schneider, M. (2003). Oppression and discrimination among lesbian, gay, bisexual, and transgendered people and communities: A challenge for community psychology. *American Journal of Community Psychology, 31*(3-4), 243-252.

Heaney, C. A., & Israel, B. A. (2002). Social networks and social support. In K. Glanz, F. M. Lewis, & B. K. Rimer (Eds.), *Health behavior and health education: Theory, research and practice* (pp. 185-209). San Francisco, CA: Jossey-Bass.

Henning, K. J., Bell, E., Braun, J., & Barker, N. D. (1995). A community-wide outbreak of hepatitis A: Risk factors for infection among homosexual and bisexual men. *American Journal of Medicine, 99*(2), 132-136.

Herek, G. M. (1994). Assessing heterosexuals' attitudes toward lesbian and gay men. In B. Greene & G. M. Herek (Eds.), *Psychological perspectives on lesbian and gay issues* (pp. 206-228). Thousand Oaks, CA: Sage Publication.

House, J. S. (1981). *Work stress and social support.* Reading, MA: Addison-Wesley.

Institute of Medicine. (2003). *Unequal treatment: Confronting racial and ethnic disparities in health care.* Washington, DC: National Academy Press.

Institute of Medicine, & Committee on Prevention and Control of Sexually Transmitted Diseases. (1997). *The hidden epidemic: Confronting sexually transmitted diseases.* Washington, DC: National Academy Press.

Israel, B. A. (1985). Social networks and social support: Implications for natural helper and community level interventions. *Health Education Quarterly, 12*(1), 65-80.

Israel, B. A., Schulz, A. J., Parker, E. A., & Becker, A. B. (1998). Review of community-based research: Assessing partnership approaches to improve public health. *Annual Review of Public Health, 19,* 173-202.

Jackson, E. J., & Parks, C. P. (1997). Recruitment and training issues from selected lay health advisor programs among African Americans: A 20-year perspective. *Health Education & Behavior, 24*(4), 418-431.

Johnson, A. M., Wadsworth, J., Wellings, K., Bradshaw, S., & Field, J. (1992). Sexual lifestyles and HIV risk. *Nature, 360*(6403), 410-412.

Kahn, J. (2002). Preventing hepatitis A and hepatitis B virus infections among men who have sex with men. *Clinical Infectious Diseases, 35*(11), 1382-1387.

Kaplan, B. H., Cassel, J. C., & Gore, S. (1977). Social support and health. *Medical Care, 15*(5 Suppl), 47-58.

Karon, J. M., Fleming, P. L., Steketee, R. W., & De Cock, K. M. (2001). HIV in the United States at the turn of the century: An epidemic in transition. *American Journal of Public Health, 91*(7), 1060-1068.

Kellogg, T., McFarland, W., & Katz, M. (1999). Recent increases in HIV seroconversion among repeat anonymous testers in San Francisco. *AIDS, 13*(16), 2303-2304.

Kelly, J. A., St. Lawrence, J. S., Stevenson, L. Y., Hauth, A. C., Kalichman, S. C., Diaz, Y. E., Brasfield, T. L., Koob, J. J., & Morgan, M. G. (1992). Community AIDS/HIV risk reduction: The effects of endorsements by popular people in three cities. *American Journal of Public Health, 82*(11), 1483-1489.

Kinsey, A. C., Pomeroy, W. B., & Martin, C. E. (1948). *Sexual behavior in the human male.* Philadelphia, PA: W. B. Saunders.

Laumann, E. G., Gagnon, J. H., Michael, R. T., & Michaels, S. (1994). *The social organization of sexuality: Sexual practices in the United States.* Chicago, IL: University of Chicago Press.

Lee, S. J., Galanter, M., Dermatis, H., & McDowell, D. (2003). Circuit parties and patterns of drug use in a subset of gay men. *Journal of Addictive Diseases, 22*(4), 47-60.

Lee, W. M. (1997). Hepatitis B virus infection. *New England Journal of Medicine, 337*(24), 1733-1745.

Leserman, J., Jackson, E. D., Petitto, J. M., Golden, R. N., Silva, S. G., Perkins, D. O., Cai, J., Folds, J. D., & Evans, D. L. (1999). Progression in AIDS: The effects of stress, depressive symptoms, and social support. *Psychosomatic Medicine, 61*(3), 397-406.

Leserman, J., Petitto, J. M., Gu, H., Gaynes, B. N., Barroso, J., Golden, R. N., Perkins, D. O., Folds, J. D., & Evans, D. L. (2002). Progression to AIDS, a clinical AIDS condition and mortality: Psychosocial and physiological predictors. *Psychological Medicine, 32*(6), 1059-1073.

Love, M. B., Gardner, K., & Legion, V. (1997). Community health workers: Who they are and what they do. *Health Education & Behavior, 24*(4), 510-522.

Malebranche, D. J. (2003). Black men who have sex with men and the HIV epidemic: Next steps for public health. *American Journal of Public Health, 93*(6), 862-865.

Martin, J. N., Ganem, D. E., Osmond, D. H., Page-Shafer, K. A., Macrae, D., & Kedes, D. H. (1998). Sexual transmission and the natural history of human herpesvirus 8 infection. *New England Jounal of Medicine, 338*(14), 948-954.

Melbye, M., & Biggar, R. J. (1992). Interactions between persons at risk for AIDS and the general population in Denmark. *American Journal of Epidemiology, 135*(6), 593-602.

Michaels, S. (1996). The prevalence of homosexuality in the United States. In R. P. Cabaj & T. S. Stein (Eds.), *Textbook of homosexuality and mental health* (pp. 43-63). Washington, DC: American Psychiatric Press.

Minkler, M., & Wallerstein, N. (2003). Introduction to community-based participatory research. In M. Minkler & N. Wallerstein (Eds.), *Community-based participatory research for health* (pp. 3-26). San Francisco, CA: Jossey-Bass.

O'Brien, T. R., Kedes, D., Ganem, D., Macrae, D. R., Rosenberg, P. S., Molden, J., & Goedert, J. J. (1999). Evidence for concurrent epidemics of human herpesvirus 8 and human immunodeficiency virus type 1 in U.S. homosexual men: Rates, risk factors, and relationship to Kaposi's sarcoma. *The Journal of Infectious Diseases, 180*(4), 1010-1017.

Offen, N., Smith, E. A., & Malone, R. E. (2003). From adversary to target market: The ACT UP boycott of Philip Morris. *Tobacco Control, 12*(2), 203-207.

O'Toole, T. P., Aaron, K. F., Chin, M. H., Horowitz, C., & Tyson, F. (2003). Community-based participatory research: Opportunities, challenges, and the need for a common language. *Journal of General Internal Medicine, 18,* 592-594.

Palefsky, J. M., Holly, E. A., Ralston, M. L., & Jay, N. (1998). Prevalence and risk factors for human papillomavirus infection of the anal canal in human immunodeficiency virus (HIV)-positive and HIV-negative homosexual men. *The Journal of Infectious Diseases, 177*(2), 361-367.

Renzi, C., Douglas, J. M., Jr., Foster, M., Critchlow, C. W., Ashley-Morrow, R., Buchbinder, S. P., Koblin, B. A., McKirnan, D. J., Mayer, K. H., & Celum, C. L. (2003). Herpes simplex virus type 2 infection as a risk factor for human immunodeficiency virus acquisition in men who have sex with men. *The Journal of Infectious Diseases, 187*(1), 19-25.

Rhodes, S. D., & Hergenrather, K. C. (2003). Using an integrated approach to understand vaccination behavior among young men who have sex with men: Stages of change, the health belief model, and self-efficacy. *Journal of Community Health, 28*(5), 347-362.

Rhodes, S. D., Yee, L. J., & Hergenrather, K. C. (2003). Hepatitis A vaccination among young African American men who have sex with men in the deep south: Psychosocial predictors. *Journal of the National Medical Association, 95*(4 Suppl), 31S-36S.

Rogers, E. M. (1983). Diffusion of innovations. New York: The Free Press.

Ryan, H., Wortley, P. M., Easton, A., Pederson, L., & Greenwood, G. (2001). Smoking among lesbians, gays, and bisexuals: A review of the literature. *American Journal of Preventive Medicine, 21*(2), 142-149.

Sansom, S., Rudy, E., Strine, T., & Douglas, W. (2003). Hepatitis A and B vaccination in a sexually transmitted disease clinic for men who have sex with men. *Sexually Transmitted Diseases, 30*(9), 685-688.

Savin-Williams, R. C. (1994). Verbal and physical abuse as stressors in the lives of lesbian, gay male, and bisexual youths: Associations with school problems, running away, substance abuse, prostitution, and suicide. *Journal of Consulting and Clinical Psychology, 62*(2), 261-269.

Seage, G. R., III, Mayer, K. H., Lenderking, W. R., Wold, C., Gross, M., Goldstein, R., Cai, B., Heeren, T., Hingson, R., & Holmberg, S. (1997). HIV and hepatitis B infection and risk behavior in young gay and bisexual men. *Public Health Reports, 112*(2), 158-167.

Shaper, A. G., Wannamethee, S. G., & Walker, M. (2003). Pipe and cigar smoking and major cardiovascular events, cancer incidence and all-cause mortality in middle-aged British men. *International Journal of Epidemiology, 32*(5), 802-808.

Skinner, W. F. (1994). The prevalence and demographic predictors of illicit and licit drug use among lesbians and gay men. *American Journal of Public Health, 84*(8), 1307-1310.

Smith, E. A., & Malone, R. E. (2003). The outing of Philip Morris: Advertising tobacco to gay men. *American Journal of Public Health, 93*(6), 988-993.

Stall, R. D., Greenwood, G. L., Acree, M., Paul, J., & Coates, T. J. (1999). Cigarette smoking among gay and bisexual men. *American Journal of Public Health, 89*(12), 1875-1878.

Stall, R., & Wiley, J. (1988). A comparison of alcohol and drug use patterns of homosexual and heterosexual men: The San Francisco Men's Health Study. *Drug and Alcohol Dependence, 22*(1-2), 63-73.

Stine, G. (2003). *AIDS update 2003.* Upper Saddle River, NJ: Prentice Hall.

Stokes, J. P., & Peterson, J. L. (1998). Homophobia, self-esteem, and risk for HIV among African American men who have sex with men. *AIDS Education and Prevention, 10*(3), 278-292.

Thomas, J. C., Eng, E., Clark, M., Robinson, J., & Blumenthal, C. (1998). Lay health advisors: Sexually transmitted disease prevention through community involvement. *American Journal of Public Health, 88*(8), 1252-1253.

U.S. Department of Health and Human Services. (1994a). *Community health advisors: Models, research and practice, selected annotations—United States* (Vol. 1). Atlanta, GA: Division of Chronic Disease Control and Community Intervention, National Center for Chronic Disease Prevention and Health Promotion, Centers for Disease Control and Prevention, Public Health Service, U.S. Department of Health and Human Services.

U.S. Department of Health and Human Services. (1994b). *Community Health Advisors: Models, research, and practice, selected annotations—United States* (Vol. 2). Atlanta, GA: Division of Chronic Disease Control and Community Intervention, National Center for Chronic Disease Prevention and Health Promotion, Centers for Disease Control and Prevention, Public Health Service, U.S. Department of Health and Human Services.

Valanis, B. G., Bowen, D. J., Bassford, T., Whitlock, E., Charney, P., & Carter, R. A. (2000). Sexual orientation and health: Comparisons in the women's health initiative sample. *Archives of Family Medicine, 9*(9), 843-853.

Viswanathan, M., Eng, E., Ammerman, A., Gartlehner, G., Lohr, K. N., Griffith, D., Rhodes, S. D., Webb, L., Sutton, S. F., Swinson, T., Jackman, A., & Whitener, L. (2003). *Community-based participatory research: Evidence report.* Research Triangle Park, NC: RTI International–University of North Carolina Evidence-Based Practice Center.

Wallerstein, N., & Duran, B. (2003). The conceptual, historical, and practice roots of community-based participatory research and related participatory traditions. In M. Minkler & N. Wallerstein (Eds.), *Community-based participatory research for health* (pp. 27-52). San Francisco, CA: Jossey-Bass.

Wandersman, A. (2003). Community science: Bridging the gap between science and practice with community-centered models. *American Journal of Community Psychology, 31*(3-4), 227-242.

Wang, Q. J., Jenkins, F. J., Jacobson, L. P., Kingsley, L. A., Day, R. D., Zhang, Z. W., Meng, Y. X., Pellett, P. E., Kousoulas, K. G., Baghian, A., Rinaldo, C. R., Jr., & Pellet, P. E. (2001). Primary human herpesvirus 8 infection generates a broadly specific CD8(+) T-cell response to viral lytic cycle proteins. *Blood, 97*(8), 2366-2373.

Wilkenson, D. Y. (1992). Indigenous community health workers in the 1960's and beyond. In R. L. Braithwaite & S. E. Taylor (Eds.), *Health issues in the black community* (pp. 255-266). San Francisco, CA: Jossey-Bass.

Williams, L. A., Klausner, J. D., Whittington, W. L., Handsfield, H. H., Celum, C., & Holmes, K. K. (1999). Elimination and reintroduction of primary and secondary syphilis. *American Journal of Public Health, 89*(7), 1093-1097.

Willis, D. G. (2004). Hate crimes against gay males: An overview. *Issues in Mental Health Nursing, 25*(2), 115-132.

Witmer, A., Seifer, S. D., Finocchio, L., Leslie, J., & O'Neil, E. H. (1995). Community health workers: Integral members of the health care work force. *American Journal of Public Health, 85*(8 Pt 1), 1055-1058.

Wolitski, R. J., Valdiserri, R. O., Denning, P. H., & Levine, W. C. (2001). Are we headed for a resurgence of the HIV epidemic among men who have sex with men? *American Journal of Public Health, 91*(6), 883-888.

Yamey, G. (2003). Gay tobacco ads come out of the closet. *British Medical Journal, 327,* 296.

Yee, L. J., & Rhodes, S. D. (2002). Understanding correlates of hepatitis B virus vaccination in men who have sex with men: What have we learned? *Sexually Transmitted Infections, 78*(5), 374-377.

Zachoval, R., & Deinhardt, F. (1998). Natural history and experimental models. In A. Zuckerman & H. C. Thomas (Eds.), *Viral hepatitis* (2nd ed.) (pp. 43-57). London: Churchill Livingstone.

Chapter 7

The Whole Person:
A Paradigm for Integrating the Mental
and Physical Health of Trans Clients

Sheila C. Kirk
Claudette Kulkarni

Few topics arouse such controversy as transsexualism: men who want
to be women, and women who want to be men. . . . Despite a deluge of
media coverage, *this remains the most misunderstood area of human
behavior.* (Ettner, 1999; emphasis ours)

INTRODUCTION

One of the reasons why transpeople are so misunderstood is because we,
their providers, sometimes forget the obvious: in most ways, transpeople
are really just like everybody else. They come to us because they need help
with something. They might be in pain, or they might simply need support
in transitioning to a point on the gender continuum where they can live
happy and meaningful lives. They might engage with us in an open and self-
reflective way, or they might believe that we are the "gatekeepers" for what
they want and so tell us what they think we want to hear rather than what we
need to know to help them. They might be focused on their "gender issues,"
or they might bring with them a number of problems unrelated to their
transness.

Sometimes we do have some of what they need: we can tell them how
and where to get hormones, explain what to expect from employers, explore
ways of coming out to family, give them information about local resources,
guide them in locating a reputable physician or surgeon, clarify state laws
relative to getting a legal name change, and so on. If we do not already have
the answers to such logistical questions, we can get them. We can do some
research, talk to a more knowledgeable colleague, locate a specialist in the

area, and use our common sense and professional skills to help transpeople find their way in this very inhospitable world.

Usually, however, we do *not* have all the answers. Often this is because one group of problems that plagues transpeople is far beyond any simple solution: problems that result from the social prejudice, discrimination, moral condemnation, and abuse (societal, cultural, religious, street violence) that transpeople face every day living in a transphobic society.

Transphobia is the irrational and unfounded fear, hatred, or discriminatory treatment of transpeople (i.e., people who transgress the boundaries of the binary sex/gender model established by society). A society that is transphobic typically condones and often promotes a range of behaviors, from simple discrimination in housing and employment to cruel acts of intolerance and prejudice, from demeaning verbal harassment to vicious sexual and physical assults, from the withholding of life-saving emergency services to outright murder. In a transphobic society, transpeople often live in fear for their lives, especially those who do not "pass" well. Transphobic attitudes and actions underlie the high rates of social isolation, self-hatred, and high-risk behaviors found in the trans community. According to some sources, the rate of violence against transpeople is on the rise in the United States and around the world.

Sometimes, the roots of these problems stretch from childhood into adulthood (e.g., the transperson who knew as a child that it was not safe to express feelings about being "different" may now be struggling with behaviors and defenses not unlike the symptoms of post-traumatic stress disorder). Other times, the source of these problems is in the present, where transpeople face a variety of the stresses reserved for the oppressed—for example, the literal threat of being bashed or even killed by bigoted people, the haunting anguish of being ridiculed by kids in the neighborhood, the frustration of losing jobs, the lack of legal recourse against discrimination, the risk of being refused care in a medical emergency—all simply because one is perceived as "odd." These are political and social problems that require political and social responses. We can all get involved in such actions, but most of the time any resulting benefits will not occur in time to help the person sitting across from us right now. Sometimes, all we can do is facilitate our clients' coming to terms with the realities of a transphobic society. That may not be the best solution, but it may be the only one at that moment.

Because transpeople *are* like everybody else, they are likely to bring with them a range of personal problems and inner conflicts that may or may not be related to gender. They may come to us complaining of the very same difficulties that others bring to us: feelings of anxiety, depression, anger, alienation, suicidal thoughts, personality disorders, questions about their sexual orientation, histories of childhood abuse, patterns of troubled relationships, homelessness, substance abuse, financial problems, concerns about HIV/AIDS, and so on. Some of these problems will absolutely hinder the transperson from moving toward his or her goals; some will merely complicate or compromise the process of transitioning.

Regardless of the sources of such problems, doing the necessary inner work and healing will enhance the transperson's chances of thriving in her or his new life. Any of these problems can be solved—or at least addressed—when all members of the team (the trans individual, mental health provider, caseworkers, physicians, public health practitioner, etc.) work together with the sole intent of helping the transperson achieve her or his overall goal: living successfully in a new gender role. This kind of collaboration, or integrated model of providing care, requires mutual respect, communication, an openness to exchanging information, and an appreciation for one another's roles. The relationship between the client's mental health professional and his or her physician is particularly central to the client's success in transitioning to a new gender role.

Of course, helping someone does not mean simply submitting to the desperate demands of sometimes desperate people. Rather, it means helping transpeople be *successful in the long term*. It means accepting *their* sense of their gender identity and supporting *their* right to make their own decisions. It means facilitating and supporting the transperson through the very thorny process of transitioning. *However,* it also means recognizing our ethical responsibility to provide thoughtful and effective care. We do not need to know everything to do this (i.e., to be "gender specialists"), but we do need to be willing to learn, to read, to consult with more experienced colleagues, and to otherwise educate ourselves. The burden for this is ours, *not* our clients'. We will learn from them, but it is not their job to teach us. We must do our own homework on our own time. Hopefully, reading this chapter will be a beginning (or a refresher) of that learning (see also Exhibit 7.1).

Finally, let us take a quick look at two overvalued issues: prevalence and etiology. Many studies related to transness have been conducted over the past forty years or so (especially in European countries). Most of these studies have focused on determining the prevalence of transsexualism versus other categories of transness. The findings have been inconclusive at best. No one really knows how many transpeople there are in the world. In addition, the issue of prevalence, although interesting, is somewhat irrelevant. Whether there are millions of transpeople in the world or just the one sitting in front of you, all people deserve to be treated with respect and to be appreciated for who they are and what they need rather than for whether they represent a significant portion of our society. Similarly, the question of etiology is both irrelevant and problematic. To ask about the *causes* of transness

> **EXHIBIT 7.1. The Harry Benjamin International Gender Dysphoria Association**
>
> The Harry Benjamin International Gender Dysphoria Association (HBIGDA) is an international organization of psychiatric, psychological, and medical professionals working to help transpeople transition to their new gender. One of the ways HBIGDA has done this is through its Standards of Care for Gender Identity Disorders (Meyer et al., 2001). Now in its sixth version, the Standards of Care provide practitioners with very basic and "flexible directions for the treatment of persons with gender identity disorders" (p. 1). The Overarching Treatment Goal of these guidelines is to help transpeople achieve "lasting personal comfort with the gendered self in order to maximize overall psychological well-being and self-fulfillment" (p. 1). HBIGDA recognizes the problem of labeling people with a "disorder," but argues that there are reasons to do this: "The designation of gender identity disorders as mental disorders is not a license for stigmatization, or for the deprivation of gender patients' civil rights. The use of a formal diagnosis is often important in offering relief, providing health insurance coverage, and guiding research to provide more effective future treatments" (p. 6). Although some in the trans community are inclined to criticize HBIGDA as being too conservative or too pathologizing, this international organization has played an invaluable role in creating a world safer for transpeople. We strongly suggest that anyone working with transsexuals review and become familiar with these guidelines (www.hbigda.org).

is to imply that something has gone *wrong* in an individual's development—that she or he is not "normal." Unfortunately, this kind of thinking is far too common, not only in society at large but also in the LGB portion of the LGBT community. This must stop if those of us charged with the public's health are to create a truly hospitable atmosphere for a truly diverse human community.

RELEVANT TERMS

Although the terms used in the trans community are continually changing, every practitioner should be familiar with a few basic ones. Please note that many of these terms continue to be hotly debated in the trans community, in feminist and postmodern theory, and among service providers.

Sex

Sex refers to anatomy and biology. Most societies promote the theory that there are only two "opposite" sexes and give physicians the authority to interpret and assign sex at birth based, by and large, on external genitalia. In reality, however, sex is best understood along a complex continuum that involves five sets of biological factors: genetic material (chromosomes and genes), hormones (testosterone and estrogen), gonads (testes and ovaries), genitals (internal and external), and a variety of secondary sex characteristics (e.g., body hair, fat distribution, breasts, facial features, etc.). Although all of these factors are biological, none of them is entirely free of cultural assumptions and implications. Our ideas about sex (what it means, what is allowed to members of each sex, what is thought to be "natural" to each sex) are shaped by the norms of the society in which we live.

Intersex

Intersex refers to people born with genitals or sexual anatomy that are ambiguous or with genitals of both sexes. Intersex people were formerly (and are still sometimes) called hermaphrodites. While intersexuality could be interpreted as a challenge to the fundamental assumption that there are only two sexes, the medical community tends to label intersexual conditions (adrenal hyperplasia, Klinefelter's syndrome, Turner syndrome, etc.) as "disorders" and "deformities"—in other words, as failed attempts at becoming male or female and thus in need of being "fixed." Therefore, many intersexed babies are surgically altered at birth. These controversial procedures involve surgically removing a baby's penis when it has been determined to be "too small" for a boy or doing a "clitoral reduction" when the clitoris is determined to be "too big" for a girl. (Various hormonal and other treatments, including further surgeries, may be required to support these surgeries, sometimes extending over the individual's entire lifetime.) All of this is done in order to keep intersex individuals "within the bounds of a two-sex gender system" (Fausto-Sterling, 2000, p. 66) and with the belief that a child can be raised as either gender as long as the parents "believe in the sex assignment" that the physicians have decided upon (Fausto-Sterling, 2000, p. 46). In other words, it is done to make the baby conform to societal ideals and to make the parents feel comfortable. Some intersex people and their supporters have organized to stop the medical community from performing sex reassignment surgery at birth, arguing that such surgeries are nothing but "cultural imperatives . . . disguised as medical necessity" (Intersex Society of North America, 1998, p. 1).

The Intersex Society of North America (ISNA), an activist organization, argues in its mission statement that "intersexuality is primarily a problem of stigma and trauma, not gender" and, therefore, that "all children should be assigned as boy or girl, without early surgery" (http://www.isna.org).

Most activists maintain that an intersex individual should have the right to choose to have (or not to have) surgery once she or he is in a position to make her or his own informed decision.

Sexual Orientation

Sexual orientation involves one's feeling of sexual attraction (revealed through fantasies, erotic and romantic feelings, etc.) and is distinguishable from **sexual behavior,** which involves sexual acts. Transpeople may identify as heterosexual, homosexual, bisexual, or asexual. Transsexuals often describe their sexual orientation from the position of their preferred gender, for example, a male-to-female transsexual who is attracted to women might describe herself as lesbian.

Gender

Gender is a complex phenomenon that some believe to be independent of sex and some believe to be interchangeable with sex. Like sex, it is generally assigned at birth based on one's visible genitalia and in the context of cultural norms. Although Western cultures tend to limit gender to two categories (man and woman), some cultures allow for a wider range of possibilities. **Gender identity** refers to a person's *inner* experience of gender: what a person *feels* she or he is, regardless of the gender attribution of others. Because gender identity is shaped by many factors (psychological considerations, cultural and social norms and taboos, family expectations, environmental forces, and so on), it can change over time for the individual. **Gender role** involves our public behavior—the role we take on in the world with others—and so it most often reflects our culture's expectations of that gender. Gender, gender identity, and gender role all reflect and support society's normative gender rules.

Transgender

Transgender is an umbrella term that designates someone who does not fit neatly into the societally accepted boxes called "male/man" and "female/woman," and who intentionally rejects the gender assigned to her or him at birth. Thus, it incorporates all persons who consciously transgress or violate gender norms, whether they intend or attempt to "pass" or not. Another phrase used to describe a transgender person is **gender variant,** though some in the trans community take exception to this term, contending that it portrays transpeople as a deviation from a norm.

Transsexual

Transsexual refers to an individual whose internally felt gender identity does not match the biological body she or he was born with and/or the gender she or he was assigned at birth. A phrase previously, and sometimes still, used with reference to transsexualism is **gender dysphoria**. Transsexuals meet the *Diagnostic and Statistical Manual*'s criteria for the diagnosis of "gender identity disorder" (a term highly disputed since it labels transsexualism as a "disorder"). Transsexuals can be male-to-female (**MTFs**; also called **transwomen**) and female-to-male (**FTMs**; also called **transmen**). Transsexuals may be "preoperative" (popularly referred to as "pre-op"), postoperative ("post-op"), or may not want surgery at all ("non-op") because they experience no internal conflict between their preferred gender and their genitals and feel that they can live in their chosen gender regardless of their genitals (e.g., transgenderists and she/males). While some transpeople argue that a person is a "true" transsexual only if she or he desires surgery, others argue that sex reassignment surgery should be abandoned altogether because it does not challenge "the gender binary" (i.e., the societal rule that limits all of us to only two choices: male or female).

Cross-Dressing

Cross-dressing refers to the act of dressing in the clothing conventionally worn by the other gender and may be used with reference to both transsexuals and cross-dressers. However, the term **cross-dresser** (formerly **transvestite**) is reserved for individuals who like to cross-dress but who do *not* experience a dissonance between their biologic body and their gender identity and who do *not* wish to permanently change their sex or gender (though some do want to take hormones to enhance their cross-dressing experience). Most cross-dressers are heterosexual men who cross-dress for purposes of amusement, role-playing, stress relief, or sexual gratification. Usually, biologic women are not called cross-dressers when they wear men's clothes because our culture allows females a much greater range of dressing behaviors (e.g., a woman generally is free to wear pants, have short hair, dress in a tuxedo, and so on). Some transsexuals go through periods of time believing or wondering if they are "just" cross-dressers.

Passing

Passing is the term used to assert that a transperson is so successful at presenting himself or herself in public as the "other" gender that she or he is perceived by nontranspeople as that gender. Passing is thus a benchmark achievement for most transsexuals and for some cross-dressers. When others do *not* see a transperson as the "other" gender, it is said that she or he is being **read, clocked,** or **made.**

Transitioning

Transitioning refers to the process of moving from one sex/gender to the opposite one. The process of transitioning involves a series of steps, nearly all of which may be accomplished with or without (though this may not be the wisest course) the involvement of various professionals—doctors, therapists, caseworkers, lawyers, and so on. In some ways, transitioning is a kind of developmental process: transpeople often start out rather awkwardly (given their previous socialization into the gender assigned at birth) and may take some time before they mature into their new roles. The HBIGDA Standards of Care (Meyer et al., 2001) outline the following process for transitioning.

Assessment and Psychotherapy

The Standards of Care strongly recommend that every transperson undergo a thorough psychological assessment by a mental health professional. Psychotherapy is not required unless it is recommended by that mental health professional and then only "to help the person to live more comfortably within a gender identity and to deal effectively with non-gender issues" (p. 12). At various points along the way, the mental health professional is expected to assess both the client's eligibility to proceed (i.e., Has the client met the specified criteria?) and his or her "readiness" to proceed (i.e., Is the client fully prepared to deal with the demands, responsibilities, and consequences of transitioning?).

Hormonal Therapy (HT)

The Standards of Care strongly suggest that the transperson be referred for hormones only after the psychological assessment and that hormonal therapy be undergone only under the care of a qualified physician. The mental health professional performing the assessment documents the referral in a "letter" to the physician who will be administering the hormonal treatment. However, the reality of the situation today is that many transpeople, intent on taking control of their own transitioning process, are already on hormones by the time they come to the mental health provider. Sometimes this has been done responsibly with a well-informed physician. Sometimes, however, desperate individuals put themselves at risk by securing hormones from unqualified doctors or even from questionable sources on the Internet. Since the taking of hormones is not without serious medical risks, it is imperative that every transperson taking hormones be seen regularly by a competent physician.

The Real-Life Experience

This consists of a period of time, usually up to one year, during which transsexual individuals are expected to live, work, and dress in their new role on a full-time basis. The decision to transition is almost always hugely difficult and may be experienced either as a relief or as a terrifying challenge. Generally, people contemplating or proceeding with transitioning will experience a variety of emotional and social reactions—some of which they may have anticipated, many they may not have.

Sex Reassignment Surgery (SRS)

Sex reassignment surgery (sometimes called gender confirmation surgery) can refer to any of a series of surgeries intended to help transgender individuals attain their desired sex/gender, though the term is used usually to refer to genital reconstruction surgery. The referral for surgery is documented in two "letters" to the surgeon, one from the primary mental health professional and the other (a second opinion) from another knowledgeable mental health professional. Most reputable surgeons, in fact, require these letters of referral. Unfortunately, some transpeople, again desperate to take control of their transitioning process, put themselves at risk by securing the services of unqualified surgeons or, in the cases of a few transwomen, even attempting to remove their own testicles.

MENTAL AND EMOTIONAL HEALTH

As a group, transpeople are among the most courageous people you will ever meet. They must make a variety of difficult decisions on a daily basis just to live their lives in ways that feel true to them. They must do this in the face of overwhelming prejudice and stressors. Many seek help only reluctantly, especially if they have had previous negative experiences with other providers. They fear being misunderstood by us, ridiculed by the rest of our staff, glared at by others in the waiting room, or "outed" by someone who might see them. Many arrive at our doors in crisis or, at least, in distress. It is critical, therefore, that we thoroughly assess the transperson's psychosocial history and current situation, both to ascertain how best to help the person determine her or his own needs *and* to gauge the very real risk of suicide that shadows many transpeople.

As noted previously, the problems that transpeople bring to us often do not have much to do with their transness as such, but rather are the result of growing up and living in a transphobic society. In addition, of course, whatever problems they do bring will be complicated by whatever personal experiences they have had unrelated to being transgender. Therefore, one of the responsibilities of the mental health provider will be to try to tease these things apart. For example: Is an individual having problems at work *because* she or he is transgender or because she or he has developed some problematic defenses? Is an individual having interpersonal difficulties *because* of the prejudice against transpeople or because she or he has unrealistic expectations of others? Is an individual having financial problems *because* she or he is being discriminated against or because she or he has made some poor decisions? Is an individual making impulsive decisions *because* she or he is a transsexual person frustrated with all of the delays in transitioning or because she or he does not have the skills to think things through? Sorting out all of these items may not be easy, but it may be essential to helping the individual transition.

Because transpeople *are* like everybody else, working with them therapeutically does not require special interventions or a different theoretical orientation than the one you already have—though it might require a more open mind and some additional knowledge. We can work with transpeople in whatever way we usually do, using our own conceptual framework, employing our usual interventions, and working with the therapeutic relationship however we usually do.

The dividing lines that separate transgender, transsexual, cross-dressers, and intersexed people are often blurred, confused, or blended—though, typically, each group wants something very different from us. Some transpeople are not sure which category they fit into; some are not sure they want to fit into any of them. We can only touch briefly on the needs of each here.

MENTAL HEALTH NEEDS OF TRANSSEXUALS

Many options are open to people who identify as transsexual: some may want more than anything to pass, while some may not care about passing at all; some may want hormones but not surgery; some may want surgery but are not in a place financially or medically to pursue that route; and some will not stop until they have achieved their surgery.

Most transsexuals tend to present in one of several typical ways or may start in one place and later move into another. The following groupings are not intended to be all-inclusive, but rather are meant to give practitioners who are new to working with transpeople a way of beginning to conceptualize the experiences of transsexuals.

Possible Mind-Sets of Transsexuals

Those who are certain about what they want and are determined to get it.

Some come in with "blinders" on, intent on getting what they believe they both need and have a right to get. Often, they do not want to think through the consequences and complications of transitioning, perhaps afraid that they will lose their momentum. The role of the mental health professional in these cases is to help these individuals transition while at the same time helping them ask the important questions they may be avoiding.

Those who feel convinced that they are transsexual and want to transition, but choose to take their time.

These individuals tend to go at their own pace, follow the Standards of Care, do everything "right." These clients often have fairly realistic ideas about transitioning: what it will take and what they might lose as a result. The role of the mental health professional in these cases is to support the client's process, provide resources, and identify any problematic areas.

Those who feel conflicted.

Some may be convinced that they are transsexual but feel confused, hopeless, or even terrified about what this means. They may wish it would all go away. Often, they cannot tolerate thinking about how much they will lose if they transition or how much they will lose if they do not. The role of the mental health professional in these cases is to help the trans individual explore these inner conflicts and come to a decision about whether to transition at all and how to go about it.

Those who are unsure whether they are transsexual.

Some might feel totally perplexed; some might simply be questioning their feelings. Some may have identified and lived as gay for years. More often than not, something has brought things to a head: a crisis of some sort, a dramatic increase in their desire to cross-dress, or a relationship that has ended because of their cross-dressing. The role of the mental health professional in these cases is, first, to work with the individual to identify and resolve any internal conflicts and, then, to help them make the most appropriate decisions about where to go from there.

Some Differences Between Transmen/FTMs and Transwomen/MTFs

The following will be huge generalizations; please use them *very* carefully. Transmen and transwomen share some experiences in relation to transitioning, but some significant differences exist between them, most of which do not appear to be biologically based, but rather are likely to be the result of socialization and social expectations.

Transmen usually are not focused on passing—partly because, as explained previously, our culture is more accepting of cross-dressing behaviors for biologic women and partly because testosterone will have a dramatic impact on their appearance and presentation, helping them to pass rather well. By and large, transmen do not report an association between wearing male clothing and sexual arousal. Most often they identify as heterosexual (i.e., they are attracted to women)—though they often identified previously as lesbians. For all of these reasons, transmen seem to adjust easily to transitioning and tend to have stable lives and relationships.

Transwomen, on the other hand, tend to be very focused on passing and to have had some experiences of sexual arousal related to the use of female clothing. Many transwomen are or have been married to women. Their sexual orientation appears to be more flexible than for transmen: many who had previously identified as heterosexual will find themselves attracted to men, some will adopt a bisexual orientation, and some will continue to feel attracted to women and thus identify as lesbian. It is not uncommon for transwomen to report one or more of the following experiences: periods of hypermasculinity (e.g., service in the armed forces, high-risk physical activities), periods of "purging" (i.e., discarding all of their female clothing only to go out and buy more), and a history of prostitution (or even to be engaged in prostitution currently, usually as a means of getting money for surgery). Although transwomen seem to have great difficulty establishing stable lives and relationships, they are more likely than transmen to gather together informally in support groups to help one another with transitioning.

Mental Health Services for Transsexuals

Most transsexuals are in search of medical interventions (hormones and/or surgery). A group modality (i.e., working in groups with other transsexuals) seems to offer the most advantages for most transsexuals. A group can be a sanctuary or oasis in the midst of an oppressive society, a place where many can, for the first time in their lives, talk freely, realize that they are not alone, and learn about the process that is ahead of them. There are times, however, when individual work might be called for—perhaps because it is the client's preference, perhaps because the client needs to work out some personal problems first (e.g., to do some healing from childhood sexual abuse, an issue which may have become intertwined with gender issues), or perhaps because we need to understand the client more deeply in order to help him or her better. Also, it is often rather frightening for transsexual people (especially MTFs) to begin cross-dressing in public. One simple way of helping them feel confident enough to negotiate this hurdle is to encourage them to cross-dress in session. Another is to give them a "travel letter" (a letter from the mental health professional that explains that the carrier of the letter is in the process of transitioning and what that means). This letter may be shown to police or others in times of need.

One may be wondering at this point whether there are any contraindications to helping a transsexual client transition. In our experience, the answer is *generally* no. Even those who suffer with significant mental disabilities (e.g., mental retardation), mental illnesses (e.g., schizophrenia), or significant personality disorders (often as a result of having had to split off an important part of themselves to survive) usually can be helped to make informed decisions about their bodies and their future. Are there exceptions? Of course—and that is when we must bring our skills to the task of helping clients come to terms with what is possible for them.

Another complicating factor in working with transsexuals is that, in spite of our most sincere efforts, some transsexual clients will insist on seeing us as the "gatekeeper" between them and their dream: getting the "letters" referring them for hormones and for surgery. They might feel that our only interest is in making them jump through hoops. The resulting implications for clinical practice can be huge and complex, often casting the therapist and client into a series of unavoidable dual relationships: the therapist as therapist, educator, adversary, and advocate, thus putting additional stresses on the work to be done. In addition, many transpeople have already had some kind of bad experience with a professional in the field and will come in already defensive or telling us what they think we want to hear so they can get what they need. This is when we must use our finest skills to convey our actual goal: helping the client transition *successfully*.

Mental Health Needs of Cross-Dressers

Cross-dressers are less likely than transsexuals to be involved in the mental health system since cross-dressers do not experience a conflict between their male identity and their desire to live out their "female side." Most appear to come to terms with their urge to cross-dress by finding safe outlets for doing this—alone and in private, with others in local groups, or by attending one of the many annual conferences held regularly in various parts of the country. Occasionally, some will come in search of help with relationship and family problems (e.g., how to deal with a less than understanding wife; whether and how to explain the situation to their children); or to get hormones (to augment the pleasure of cross-dressing); or as a result of some type of clash with a public structure (e.g., being arrested by a less than sympathetic legal system).

Mental Health Needs of Intersex Individuals

As explained previously, we are including a wide range of intersex individuals as transpeople—though some/many of them may not identify as transgender at all. Some intersex people report feeling neither entirely male nor entirely female. Some may have had no idea that they are intersex until something happens (e.g., something that should happen at puberty does not, or vice versa, or they are diagnosed as infertile). Some may take on a gay or lesbian identity because they feel that it allows them more latitude for gender expression. Some may endure a lifetime of suffering as a result of being incorrectly assigned to a sex/gender at birth.

While there are numerous Web sites, books, and groups devoted to learning more about or advocating for intersex individuals, there has been virtually no research, nor even much discussion, about the mental health needs of adult intersex people. There is a profound need for such research, not because intersex people are inherently more likely than others to have mental health problems, but because, although we have anecdotal accounts of the suffering experienced by some intersex people, we really do not have a body of knowledge that might guide us in developing compassionate and effective responses to their long-term needs. In the meantime, it would seem fitting to work with them as with any other person: with openness and compassion.

A Few Words About Partners and Family Members

In all likelihood, you are reading this chapter because you are concerned about the well-being of current or future transgender clients. You might wonder how their struggles affect their significant others (partners and spouses, children, other family members, friends, co-workers, and employers), but your focus is on your primary client, the transperson. That is both understandable and appropriate. However, having said that, we also urge you not to ignore or overlook the needs of the significant others of trans-people. Whether the transperson identifies as a cross-dresser, intersex, or transsexual, the struggles they experience and the changes they undertake will affect their family members and put stress on all of their relationships. The results may be devastating all around. We recommend offering family services wherever possible: couples' counseling, support groups for partners, and so on.

PHYSICAL HEALTH

As already discussed, both biologic male and female transgendered individuals exist on a spectrum or continuum. Some notable differences exist between them regarding how they occupy a place or move from a place on that continuum. One difference is that the greatest numbers of biologic male transgender individuals are cross-dressers only. They are frequently closeted and have no desire to transition to a transsexual mode of living. The numbers who move to adopt a gender role change are notably smaller.

In contrast, biologic females who are transgender and only cross-dress do exist (Stoller, 1982), but apparently are in small numbers. A significant number who have gender conflicts do move across the spectrum to transition and live in a male role. What must be kept in mind is that the medical and surgical experience of the cross-dresser will be vastly different from that which the MTF and FTM transsexual will experience. Biologic males and females who are cross-dressers only and never plan to take hormones or be operated upon will have potential for the same physical health disorders that affect nontransgender males and females. They will have good health or develop illness according to their genetics, the environment they live in, and the lifestyle they assume, just as other males and females do.

When the transgendered person assumes the role of a transsexual, while still having a genetic predisposition to good or poor health, they will have additional potential for particular illnesses because of hormone use, surgical interventions, and the lifestyle and behaviors they will enter into in their opposite gender role. They may engage in some of those behaviors without adequate and important knowledge. Some individuals, even with good information and education, may choose behavior patterns that are a threat and a detriment to their health. In addition, many MTFs and FTMs are extremely reluctant to have indicated and routine medical evaluations. They fear being embarrassed and ridiculed because of anatomic inconsistencies and, in the case of many FTM individuals, they have a strong aversion and repugnance to routine genital examinations. Added to all of this are three other factors that also have huge impact on the quality of life and longevity of the transsexual person. These three factors are significant barriers to good, sound medical care for the transgender/transsexual population and must be reversed:

1. *Health Care Providers:* Some doctors, nurses, and their assistants have little or no empathy for the needs of the transgender community. In addition, when medical care providers do have a desire to help, frequently they are without knowledge and experience. This is as much a barrier as discrimination in many instances.
2. *Insurance Companies, Third-Party Payers, and Governmental Agencies:* Without doubt, a lack of information and interest by health care payers has led to restriction of benefits and refusal of any support in obtaining adequate medical and surgical care for the transgender/transsexual person.
3. *Lack of Research:* Without sound and creditable research and the funding to support that research, information to reverse health disparities cannot be gathered. Lack of information and education leads right back to the ignorance of patients and their health care providers.

The discussion to follow will give insight into the physical health concerns that MTF and FTM transsexuals may experience. It is a brief discussion giving only an overview of the problems that can be encountered. The following will be divided into sections related to MTF and FTM transsexuals and will cover the following topics: contragender hormone therapy, body and facial/skull surgery, sexually transmitted infections, substance use, tumor disease, cardiovascular disease, metabolic disorders, and street and domestic violence.

MALE-TO-FEMALE TRANSSEXUALS

Contragender Hormone Therapy

When the biologic male body is feminized, many physiologic systems are reversed—systems that were first stimulated and then maintained for quite a period of time by testosterone. Estrogen administration for the MTF transsexual is by mouth, by injection, or by the transdermal route and is accompanied sometimes by progesterone and very frequently by an antiandrogen, a testosterone-inhibiting medication. Although most can use the regimen quite smoothly, safety cannot always be assured. Younger individuals manage quite well with such a drastic hormone alteration, but older individuals may not. If certain cardiovascular changes are already in place or if liver damage has occurred because of alcohol use or infection, the feminizing regimen could accelerate those processes and illness will result. Liver disease and electrolyte imbalances are possible with antiandrogen therapy. Hypertension can begin or existing elevated blood pressure can worsen in some individuals when taking estrogen. Diabetes can become evident on estrogen therapy, or an already-diagnosed diabetic can experience aggravation of the disease (Feldman, personal communication, 2002). Heart disease with fatality and central nervous system disease (e.g., stroke) are both reported with estrogen use (van Kesteren, Asscheman, Megens, & Gooren, 1997). Phlebitis, particularly when involving the deep vein system in the legs and abdomen, is a real concern for those who develop hypercoagulability of the blood. A severe complication of this disorder, pulmonary embolism (blood clots to the lungs), is sometimes a fatal event and is present in a number of estrogen users (Asscheman, 1989). The pituitary gland can enlarge or develop a tumor called prolactinoma in estrogen-using transsexuals (Kovacs, Stefaneanu, Ezzat, & Smyth, 1994; Gooren, Harmsen-Louman, & van Kessel, 1985).

Body and Face Feminization Surgery

With increasing frequency, older individuals are applying for surgery, in particular genital reconstruction surgery. This presents potential for more complications both with anesthesia and the surgical technique. Those who have chronic lung disease and who smoke have added risk. In addition, smoking is the "enemy of good healing," especially when microsurgical techniques are to be employed. Genital reconstructive surgery is a major operation for the MTF transsexual. The possibility always exists of infection, tissue breakdown, and imperfect healing along with loss of vagina length and width because of scarring and stricture formation. Great skill is needed on the part of the surgeon to accomplish good cosmetic and functional results, both at the time of operation and during the convalescence in the weeks that follow.

Of concern is the fact that many MTF transsexuals go to surgeons for all kinds of procedures, particularly genital surgery, who are hundreds and even thousands of miles away. Preoperative preparation and evaluation might be incomplete or inadequate. Even more important, postoperative care once the individual returns home is frequently inadequate and usually provided by caregivers who know very little about the kind of evaluation and care that is needed. Severe problems with infection, poor healing, fistulas, and urinary dysfunction often develop with the operated person who is often considerably out of contact with the operating surgeon.

Sexually Transmitted Infections

Although the entire transgender population has liability to contract sexually transmitted infections, one segment of the community has a very high risk for development of these infections. MTF street or sex workers and those in entertainment are of particular concern (Bockting, Robinson, & Rosser, 1998). Reasons for their high-risk behavior are multiple. Suffice it to say that when one engages in sexual activity to be able to live each day or to accomplish a goal (e.g., drug purchase or genital reassignment surgery), then high-risk behavior will always be in evidence.

The most concerning infection is HIV/AIDS (Chew, Tham, & Ratnam, 1997). The prevalence of HIV-seropositive, transgender sex workers in major cities in the United States ranges from 20 percent to just under 50 percent. We know very little about HIV infection in transgender individuals who are not sex workers.

We know of other sexually transmitted infections in the transpopulation, but prevalence rates are not as well recorded and reported. One of particular concern is human papillomavirus (HPV), and especially certain strains of that organism (Infantolino et al., 2000). These identifiable strains can cause rectal and anal cancer in those who engage in anal sex. We have no information that tells us of this infection and of the cancer potential in transsexuals after having vaginal construction, particularly when a segment of colon is used to create the neovagina. Also, very little is known about gonorrhea

(Haustein, 1995), chlamydia (Kiyan et al., 1993), and syphilis (Baqi, Shah, Baig, Mujeeb, & Memon, 1999) infections in the MTF population.

Other infectious diseases affect the MTF transgender population. Hepatitis A, B, and C (Tsakris, Kyriakis, Chryssou, & Papoutsakis, 1997) and tuberculosis are concerns for those engaging in high-risk behavior. Hepatitis is increasing in the transgender street population. Vaccination against hepatitis A and B is available. We do not know what percentage of the MTF transpopulation have received it and, in fact, how informed they are of its availability.

Substance Use

A number of substances are used in excess by the transgendered community and are considered by them to be pleasures. We will never know to what extent substance use takes place in those who are considered to be just cross-dressers, because they are largely an invisible part of the transgender community. Those who are "out" and live most of the time in an opposite gender role are the only source of research information.

The first substance to be considered is alcohol. Although it is used liberally in the nontransgender population, in the transgender population it may be that it is used at least twice as much and perhaps more. The reasons for its use seem to parallel those known in the general population (e.g., depression, anxiety, low self-esteem, stress, and anger, to name a few). Whatever might be the driving force to drink more than casually or even moderately, it can be postulated that in the transgender population those factors are more evident. The pressures of discrimination and prejudice can contribute to increased alcohol use. Alcohol abuse to relieve these feelings will inevitably lead to physical illness involving the gastrointestinal tract, liver, and central nervous system and will act as a cofactor for a host of other diseases.

Illicit substances and drugs can blunt the fear and pain of rejection and the isolation that MTF transpeople endure. It may be in some instances even more a problem for the transsexual who is post–genital reconstruction.

Another practice that leads the transgendered population into severe health problems and diminished longevity is smoking. It is believed to be higher in transpeople than in the general population. More research needs to be done in this area because we do not know to what extent that increase in smoking leads to increased rates of chronic pulmonary obstructive disease and lung cancer. We also do not know in what way it contributes to cardiac disease in this population.

Another substance should be included in this overview—it is free silicone by injections. Free silicone used to alter the body or face can make its way into the vascular system and then to the lungs, causing death (Hage, Kanhai, Oen, van Diest, & Karim, 2001). In addition, with passage of time, free silicone will follow the dictates of gravity and migrate to more dependant parts of the body. Medical literature has reported cases of individuals being injected to amplify the breasts and buttocks experiencing eventual migration of the silicone to the legs, ankles, and feet.

Tumor Disease

The MTF transsexual on estrogen seems to have a much lower incidence of prostate gland disease than the non-estrogen-using biologic male. Both malignancy (van Haarst, Newling, Gooren, Asscheman, & Prenger, 1998) and benign hypertrophy (Brown & Wilson, 1997) are reported in transsexuals, but those reports are very few. Breast cancer reports are uncommon (Ganly & Taylor, 1995) and it is likely that the incidence in both the transsexual and the nontranssexual, biologic male population is the same. This is a little surprising, since estrogen is such an important factor in the genesis of breast cancer in biologic females. Family history (probably by genetic transmission) does not seem to be as important a factor for MTF transsexuals as it is for biologic females, though we have not looked at this in a well-planned study.

We have already mentioned the pituitary tumor prolactinoma that can develop in estrogen users. Two additional areas of study that must be pursued in MTFs are the incidence of malignancy in the anorectal area because of HPV infection and the incidence of lung cancer in those MTF transsexuals who smoke.

Cardiovascular and Metabolic Disease

The MTF transsexual could be at risk of developing heart disease and stroke while taking estrogen, but it is not clear what other factors are involved in the development of heart and arterial disease and its consequences. The lipid profile is benefited in estrogen-using transsexuals and arterial stiffness is reduced (i.e., arterial wall muscular relaxation and reactivity is enhanced) (McCrohon et al., 1997; New et al., 1997). However, in-depth studies of heart disease and the factors involved in MTF estrogen users have yet to be carried out.

As already mentioned, diabetes can develop or become more of a clinical management problem when using estrogen. However, only a few scattered reports are in the literature. In the monitoring process of MTF individuals on a feminizing regimen, diet regulation, evaluation of glucose tolerance, and close observation of cardiac health are all important.

Street and Domestic Violence

The health and welfare of MTF transsexuals (and cross-dressing individuals) is of great concern when they enter the streets. Reports of violence and mortality hit the newspapers frequently. Members of society are not only prejudiced in their reaction to the transsexual but some can be so violent as to kill. Police indifference is sometimes a part of the problem as well. Another problem seems to be invisible—the occurrence of domestic violence in the MTF transsexual population. We know nothing about the incidence of physical and psychological violence in the relationships of MTF persons.

FEMALE-TO-MALE TRANSSEXUALS

Opposite-Gender Hormone Therapy

For some FTMs, taking testosterone may be the only masculinizing step they will take. But what a step it is! Testosterone is a very powerful hormone, very capable of overcoming estrogen production and erasing many of the physical female changes produced by estrogen at puberty. Along with very successful transformation, using testosterone can produce very serious consequences for some FTMs. Excess body weight leading to obesity can be a considerable problem (van Kesteren et al., 1997). Some preliminary reporting indicates that HDL will be lowered significantly with testosterone (Asscheman et al., 1994). This is the component in the lipid profile that, when in proper range or higher, provides cardio-protective factors. When lower than acceptable, it can lead to coronary artery arteriosclerosis, as is found in biologic males who experience heart attacks. Arterial stiffness and reactivity (the elasticity of the arteries due to muscular wall relaxation) is reduced in FTM persons (McCredie et al., 1998; Giltay et al., 1999). This can result in hypertension, as it does in biologic males. All of these concerns are preludes to heart disease and stroke (Elbers, Asscheman, Seidell, & Gooren, 1997).

We do not know enough about these problems, real or potential, in the FTM population. Many health care providers do not monitor their FTM patients adequately when they are taking testosterone. They do not obtain baseline heart studies before beginning testosterone therapy for comparison in the monitoring stages later on. Monitoring often is cursory and not well oriented to cardiovascular health. Weight management often is ignored.

Breast Removal, Hysterectomy, and Genital Reconstruction

Breast removal is very desired by the FTM transsexual and often the first or only surgical procedure that they will obtain. This very obvious physical marker of femaleness is distasteful to most. The procedures for doing this with the very best cosmetic results, called top surgery, can be very successful for some and very much a failure for others. Extensive scars, poor nipple placement, and retraction and inadequate breast tissue removal are not infrequently the results. Interestingly, many FTMs are so grateful for removal that they will accept unsatisfactory results.

Hysterectomy for the FTM should always be accompanied by removal of both ovaries, and when possible, removal of the vagina, although vaginectomy often is delayed because of the use of vaginal tissue with possibility of genital reconstruction surgery at a later date. Some surgical techniques utilize vaginal wall tissue to create an extension of the urethra to facilitate "stand-up" urination. Although abdominal approaches are common, many FTMs are now aware that vaginal removal with and without laparoscopy is far more desirable. Frequently, FTMs having hysterectomy do not have preoperative ultrasound examinations and consequently undiagnosed disease is found at the time of the operation. Uterine and ovarian tumors are sometimes found inadvertently. Many FTMs do not consider hysterectomy and internal genital removal needed for two reasons. The first is because of expense. Quite often their insurance, if they have it, will not cover the surgery because a disease process is not existent to warrant removal. Second, because ovulation and menstruation have stopped with testosterone use, many believe there is no reason to have this operation.

Genital reconstructive surgery for the FTM is, at best, very difficult to perform (even with very experienced surgeons). The process is fraught with complications in healing and intended outcome and is extremely expensive. Insurance coverage does not exist for these operations. Two basic operations are employed:

1. Metoidioplasty—freeing of the clitoris, which is enlarged with testosterone use. The urethra can be incorporated at the same time to permit "stand-up" urination. Penetrative sexual experience will not generally be possible after this operation.
2. Phalloplasty—a procedure to create a penis using a number of different techniques originated by different surgeons. The forearm graft is now commonly used. Convalescence is difficult, complications with healing are rather common, and although cosmetic results can be quite acceptable, functionality for many in sexual experiences is lack-

ing. The lack of spontaneous erection is problematic and artificial devices to accomplish this are frequently employed and often fail.

With both of these genital surgical operations, a scrotum with silicone ovoid implants is constructed. Phalloplastic surgery is complicated, and although many FTMs are gratified, the costs in time, inconvenience, and money can be extensive. Once more, these operations are out-of-pocket and therefore are not obtainable for many.

Sexually Transmitted Infections

We have been aware for some time that certain sexually transmitted infections can be passed between biologic female, same-sex partners. HIV in FTMs has been reported, but in far lower numbers than in MTFs. The prevalence is 2.5 to 3 percent. It is not always clear if those with STIs, including HIV, are or are not still engaging in sexual activity with biologic males who infect them. There is possibility of infection caused by HPV. Although the possibility of exchanging the virus between biologic females has been proven (Marazzo, Stine, & Koutsky, 2000), it is not always clear if infection took place in a heterosexual relationship months to several years before the current relationship. Certain strains of this infection cause cervical cancer (O'Hanlan & Crum, 1996). Chlamydia, herpes, gonorrhea, and bacterial vaginosis (Marazzo, et al., 2002) are also reported in FTM individuals cohabiting with biologic females.

It is necessary to evaluate much more accurately the potential of STIs or the actual existence of them in FTMs. Many physicians do not diagnose the infections with accuracy or do not carry out follow-up examinations. In addition, they often do not report to public health agencies.

Substance Use

All three types of substances that are misused in the MTF population—alcohol, tobacco, and illicit drugs—are also problems in the FTM community. We have not found much reporting about drug and restricted substance abuse in the FTM community. However, alcohol and tobacco are very much in use. We know that medical caretakers are not much of an influence in altering their usage. Research also has given little insight into their misuse and the consequences that result. Alcohol contributes to excess body weight, which in turn leads to heart disease. Liver disease is also a potential concern. Smoking is also a very large cofactor in the development of heart disease. Logically, both can add to the problems of arterial vessel disease and heart disease that testosterone alone can cause. Last, lung diseases, both benign and malignant, are very much related to smoking, but we do not know to what extent in FTMs.

Tumor Disease

Certain tumor diseases in the FTM population just do not seem to be present—breast cancer is one of these. It is likely that FTMs have breast removal at ages that are young enough to prevent the development of cancer in this site. Ovarian cancer does take place but seems to be uncommon (Hage, Dekker, Karim, Verheijen, & Bloemena, 2000). We know nothing, however, about the incidence of BRCA 1 and BRCA 2 genes in FTMs. This is a genetic inheritance that leads to a very high rate of breast and ovarian cancer development in those who are carriers. Because of the reluctance of FTMs who have kept their uterus and ovaries to have thorough gynecologic evaluations, a notable barrier exists to collecting research information about the potential for pelvic disease.

One condition that could be placed in this tumor category, although it is principally a hematological disorder, is polycythemia, an overabundance of red blood cells. The red-cell volume will be in excess in some FTMs on testosterone. The hormone is a stimulant to red blood cell production in bone and is frequently used to treat certain forms of anemia. In a number of FTMs this positive effect of the hormone works to their disadvantage and becomes a problem, particularly when they apply for surgical procedures. Too many red cells can lead to coagulation problems, which can be problematic and even fatal during surgery and convalescence.

In addition, two other tumor diseases, one benign and the other malignant, should be mentioned. The first, polycystic ovarian disease, is believed to be up to four times more common in FTMs who are pre–testosterone treatment than in nontransgender biologic females (Balen, Schachter, Montgomery, Reid, & Jacobs, 1993). The problems with this tumor are not related to infertility in the FTM, as in nontransgender women. The problems are with the hyperinsulinism that exists in about 40 percent of those with the disease. This will lead to diabetes and heart disease. Most physicians do not know to look for this ovarian disorder in FTMs, particularly before testosterone is started. Many physicians also do not know to look for the possibility of diabetes.

The second is cervical cancer. Certain strains of HPV can and will cause uterine cervical cancer in biologic females (Infantolino et al., 2000). FTMs with a uterus in place must be screened for the earliest signs of this infection and their potential for cancer development because of it. When FTMs resist proper gynecologic evaluation, the problem becomes more difficult to detect and manage.

Cardiovascular and Metabolic Disease

We have already spoken in the hormone therapy section of the potential for heart disease with testosterone use. Studies that identify all the risk factors having to do with development of heart and vessel disease (as well as stroke and hypertension) in the FTM population are lacking. We must consider the research to define these problems more accurately.

As discussed in the tumor section, diabetes can develop in up to 40 percent of those with polycystic ovarian disease. FTMs must be screened for this gynecologic condition and then screened for hyperinsulinism or abnormal glucose tolerance. Early diagnosis for a prediabetes state is such an important part of good health maintenance. To delay the onset of diabetes in a susceptible FTM individual can lessen appreciably the onset of cardiac disease, particularly when other risk factors are identified. Many physicians caring for FTMs do not know of this sequence of events.

Street and Domestic Violence

We have found only scant reports of street violence against FTM individuals. It does take place, but not as frequently as in the MTF population. The movie *Boys Don't Cry* (1999) gave graphic insight into an FTM person who suffered ridicule, beatings, and tragic death because he was transsexual. In addition, information about domestic violence is as lacking in the FTM population as it is in the MTF population.

CONCLUSION

And one last challenge, at least for some of us: How do we maintain a nonjudgmental posture when dealing, for example, with a transwoman who dresses in the sometimes outrageous "femme" style that so many biologic women, informed by the feminist movement, see as regressive or abhorrent? We do not have a simple answer to this. It is a difficult question that many people who work with transpeople grapple with. Some argue that, ultimately, it is simply an issue of personal freedom and choice. Others argue that this challenge reflects the tension between the individual and society and that *society* needs to be changed! For example, if societal "norms" were more fluid, then transpeople could live in whatever ways suited them without having to fit into societal stereotypes, and perhaps without medical interventions. They might not have inadequate or incompetent caretakers or lack of good health because of society's refusal to acknowledge that they deserve the same medical and surgical care offered to others. They would not be tempted to adopt behavior patterns in sexual practice or with substance use that lead to illness and death.

In the meantime, we are faced still with a challenge: How do we help this individual, here and now before us, who does not have time to wait for such monumental changes? Whatever the future brings in terms of society, culture, politics, and the gender binary, if we all can work to answer this question together, the world will soon become a more welcoming place for all transpeople.

SELECTED RESOURCES

Harry Benjamin International Gender Dysphoria Association (HBIGDA)
http://www.hbigda.org
Phone: 612-624-9397

Resources available: Standards of Care, Ethical Guidelines, list of members of the association, links to other organizations

International Foundation for Gender Education (IFGE)
http://www.ifge.org
Phone: 781-899-2212

Resources available: News about current events affecting the transgender community, list of local organizations, information about professionals in your area, bookstore with transgender publications for sale, links to other Web sites and organizations

Intersex Society of North America (ISNA)
http://www.isna.org
Fax: 801-348-5350

Resources available: News of interest to the intersex community, information about intersex ambitions, medical and legal information, recommended readings and bibliography of articles available online

QUESTIONS TO CONSIDER

1. Would a transperson walking into your agency or department feel welcomed? For example:
   - Is your staff well informed about the needs of transpeople?
   - Will the staff person who greets this transperson treat him or her with respect?
   - Do your forms reflect an openness to transpeople? For example, when you ask for a person's sex or gender do you allow for more possibilities than just male or female?
   - How will people in your office respond when an MTF transsexual asks to use the ladies' restroom?
   - How can you make the environment of your workplace more hospitable to transpeople?
2. Would you feel at ease if a transperson walked into your office asking for some kind of help? If not, what would you do? If you feel comfortable but think you do not have the necessary training, what would you do? In either case, how would you find help?
   - Would you be able to recuse yourself and make a good referral?
   - Would you know how to find a good referral for this person?
   - Do you know what resources are available locally, such as professionals working in the field and local trans organizations and social clubs?
   - Do you know how local and state laws affect transpeople?
   - Would you know how to find the training to make you ready and qualified to help?
   - Do you know that you can get help online and/or by phone from HBIGDA and IFGE? (See Selected Resources.)
   - Did you know that although gender identity disorder (GID) is listed in the DSM, most insurance companies will not accept this as a reimbursable diagnosis?
3. You are already working with transpeople. You are already a qualified and caring provider of services to and/or supporter of the trans community.
   - How much gatekeeping do you still do? Why?
   - Do you believe that transpeople who are fully informed about the effects and consequences of medical interventions and transitioning are capable of making their own decisions about proceeding to the various surgeries needed to fully transition—for example, breast reduction/removal, genital reassignment, castration, and so on?

- Are you or your agency advocating for transpeople in your area? Why not?
- Are you on the cutting edge of trans theory and practice—*or are you part of the problem?* As a provider, are you as informed and accepting as you could be?

RECOMMENDED READINGS

Bockting, W. O., & Coleman, E. (1993). *Gender dysphoria: Interdisciplinary approaches in clinical management.* Binghamton, NY: The Haworth Press.

Bornstein, K. (1994). *Gender outlaw: On men, women, and the rest of us.* New York: Routledge.

Brown, M. L., & Rounsley, C. A. (1996). *True selves: Understanding transsexualism: For families, friends, coworkers, and helping professionals.* San Francisco: Jossey-Bass Publishers.

Califia, P. (1997). *Sex changes: The politics of transgenderism.* San Francisco: Cleis Press.

Denny, D. (1991). *Discovering who you are: A guide to self-assessment for persons with gender dysphoria.* Decatur, GA: AEGIS.

Nestle, J., Howell, C., & Wilchins, R. (Eds.). (2002). *Genderqueer.* Los Angeles: Alyson Books.

Stuart, K. E. (1991). *The uninvited dilemma: A question of gender* (Rev. ed.). Portland, OR: Metamorphous Press.

REFERENCES

American Psychiatric Association. (2000). *Diagnostic and statistical manual of mental disorders,* Fourth edition, Text revision. Washington, DC: Author.

Asscheman, H. (1989). *Cross-gender hormone treatment: Some effects and some metabolic aspects.* Amsterdam: Free University Press.

Asscheman, H., Gooren, L. J., Megens, J. A., Nauta, J., Kloosterboer, H. J., & Eikelboom, F. (1994). Serum testosterone level is the major determinant of the male-female differences in serum levels of high-density lipoprotein (HDL) cholesterol and HDL2 cholesterol. *Metabolism: Clinical & Experimental, 43*(8), 935-939.

Balen, A. H., Schachter, M. E., Montgomery, D., Reid, R. W., & Jacobs, H. S. (1993). Polycystic ovaries are a common finding in untreated female to male transsexuals. [See comment.] *Clinical Endocrinology, 38*(3), 325-329.

Baqi, S., Shah, S. A., Baig, M. A., Mujeeb, S. A., & Memon, A. (1999). Seroprevalence of HIV, HBV and syphilis and associated risk behaviours in male transvestites (Hijras) in Karachi, Pakistan. *International Journal of STD & AIDS, 10*(5), 300-304.

Bockting, W. O., Robinson, B. E., & Rosser, B. R. (1998). Transgender HIV prevention: A qualitative needs assessment. *AIDS Care, 10*(4), 505-525.

Brown, J. A., & Wilson, T. M. (1997). Benign prostatic hyperplasia requiring transurethral resection of the prostate in a 60-year-old male-to-female transsexual. *British Journal of Urology, 80*(6), 956-957.

Chew, S., Tham, K. F., & Ratnam, S. S. (1997). Sexual behaviour and prevalence of HIV antibodies in transsexuals. *Journal of Obstetrics & Gynaecology Research, 23*(1), 33-36.

Elbers, J., Asscheman, H., Seidell, J., & Gooren, J. (1997). *Effects of androgens in female to male transsexuals: A shift toward a male cardiovascular risk pattern.* Amsterdam: Free University Hospital, Division of Endocrinology and Andrology.

Ettner, R. (1999). *Gender loving care: A guide to counseling gender-variant clients.* New York: W.W. Norton & Co.

Fausto-Sterling, A. (2000). *Sexing the body: Gender politics and the construction of sexuality.* New York: Basic Books.

Ganly, I., & Taylor, E. W. (1995). Case report: Breast cancer in a trans-sexual man receiving hormone replacement therapy. *British Journal of Surgery, 82*(3), 341.

Giltay, E. J., Lambert, J., Gooren, L. J., Elbers, J. M., Steyn, M., & Stehouwer, C. D. (1999). Sex steroids, insulin, and arterial stiffness in women and men. *Hypertension, 34*(4 Pt 1), 590-597.

Gooren, L. J., Harmsen-Louman, W., & van Kessel, H. (1985). Follow-up of prolactin levels in long-term oestrogen-treated male-to-female transsexuals with regard to prolactinoma induction. *Clinical Endocrinology, 22*(2), 201-207.

Hage, J. J., Dekker, J. J., Karim, R. B., Verheijen, R. H., & Bloemena, E. (2000). Ovarian cancer in female-to-male transsexuals: Report of two cases. *Gynecologic Oncology, 76*(3), 413-415.

Hage, J. J., Kanhai, R. C., Oen, A. L., van Diest, P. J., & Karim, R. B. (2001). The devastating outcome of massive subcutaneous injection of highly viscous fluids in male-to-female transsexuals. *Plastic & Reconstructive Surgery, 107*(3), 734-741.

Haustein, N. F. (1995). Pruritis of the artificial vagina of a transsexual patient caused by gonorrhea infection. *Havtarzt, 46*(12), 858.

Infantolino, C., Fabris, P., Infantolino, D., Biasin, M. R., Venza, E., & Tositti, G. (2000). Usefulness of human papillomavirus testing in the screening of cervical cancer precursor lesions: A retrospective study in 314 cases. *European Journal of Obstetrics, Gynecology, & Reproductive Biology, 93*(1), 71-75.

Intersex Society of North America. (1998). Historian dares to look at the present. *Hermaphrodites with Attitude, Summer,* 1 and 5. Retrieved July 5, 2005, from http://www.isna.org/files/hwa/summer1998.pdf.

Kiyan, M., Cengiz, A. T., Kendi, O., Ugurel, M. S., Bilge, Y., & Tumer, A. R. (1993). [Demonstration of *Chlamydia trachomatis* IgG using ELISA in transsexuals and homosexuals.] *Mikrobiyoloji Bulteni, 27*(3), 233-240.

Kovacs, K., Stefaneanu, L., Ezzat, S., & Smyth, H. S. (1994). Prolactin-producing pituitary adenoma in a male-to-female transsexual patient with protracted estrogen administration: A morphologic study. *Archives of Pathology & Laboratory Medicine, 118,* 562-565.

Marrazzo, J. M., Koutsky, L. A., Eschenbach, D. A., Agnew, K., Stine, K., & Hillier, S. L. (2002). Characterization of vaginal flora and bacterial vaginosis in women who have sex with women. *Journal of Infectious Diseases, 185*(9), 1307-1313.

Marrazzo, J. M., Stine, K., & Koutsky, L. A. (2000). Genital human papillomavirus infection in women who have sex with women: A review. *American Journal of Obstetrics & Gynecology, 183*(3), 770-774.

McCredie, R. J., McCrohon, J. A., Turner, L., Griffiths, K. A., Handelsman, D. J., & Celermajer, D. S. (1998). Vascular reactivity is impaired in genetic females taking high-dose androgens. *Journal of the American College of Cardiology, 32*(5), 1331-1335.

McCrohon, J. A., Walters, W. A., Robinson, J. T., McCredie, R. J., Turner, L., Adams, M. R., Handelsman, D. J., & Celermajer, D. S. (1997). Arterial reactivity is enhanced in genetic males taking high dose estrogens. *Journal of the American College of Cardiology, 29*(7), 1432-1436.

Meyer, W., III, Bockting, W. O., Cohen-Kettenis, P., Coleman, E., DiCeglie, D., Devor, H., Gooren, L., Hage, J. J., Kirk, S., Kuiper, B., et al. (2001). The Harry Benjamin International Gender Dysphoria Association's standards of care for gender identity disorders, Sixth version. HBIGDA. Retrieved July 7, 2005, from http://www.hbigda.org/soc.cfm.

New, G., Timmins, K. L., Duffy, S. J., Tran, B. T., O'Brien, R. C., Harper, R. W., & Meredith, I. T. (1997). Long-term estrogen therapy improves vascular function in male to female transsexuals. [See comment.] *Journal of the American College of Cardiology, 29*(7), 1437-1444.

O'Hanlan, K. A., & Crum, C. P. (1996). Human papillomavirus-associated cervical intraepithelial neoplasia following lesbian sex. *Obstetrics & Gynecology, 88* (4 Pt 2), 702-703.

Stoller, R. J. (1982). Transvestism in women. *Archives of Sexual Behavior, 11*(2), 99-115.

Tsakris, A., Kyriakis, K. P., Chryssou, S., & Papoutsakis, G. (1997). Infection by hepatitis B and C virus in female and transsexual Greek prostitutes with serological evidence of active syphilis. *International Journal of STD & AIDS, 8*(11), 697-699.

van Haarst, D. W., Newling, L. J. G., Gooren, L., Asscheman, H., & Prenger, D. M. (1998). Metastatic prostate carcinoma in a male to female transsexual. *British Journal of Urology, 81*, 776.

van Kesteren, P. J. M., Asscheman, H., Megens, J. A. J., & Gooren, L. J. G. (1997). Mortality and morbidity in transsexual subjects treated with cross-sex hormones. *Clinical Endocrinology, 47*(3), 337-343.

PART IV:
HEALTH CARE DELIVERY SYSTEM

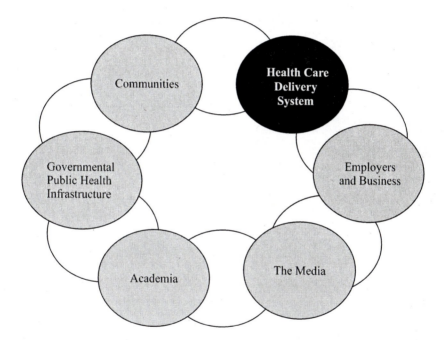

Figure reprinted with permission from *The Future of the Public's Health in the 21st Century.* ©2002 by the National Academy of Sciences, courtesy of the National Academies Press, Washington, DC.

Chapter 8

Barriers to Health Care Access

Manuel Hernandez
Shawn L. Fultz

INTRODUCTION

Health care providers, from bedside clinicians to public health practitioners, researchers, health care executives, and social service specialists, have only recently begun to address the unique health needs of the lesbian, gay, bisexual, and transgender (LGBT) community. As little attention has been given to this topic in formal educational curricula, many practitioners have forged their own paths, gaining the knowledge they need to care for this medically underserved community. Some providers have done so because of their own self-identification as LGBT, while others simply recognize the disparities that presently exist for the LGBT population. Whatever the reason, because health care'clinicians represent the frontline of health care, their commitment to eliminating health care disparities is critical to breaking down the barriers for LGBT patients.

Many barriers impede LGBT patients from gaining access to competent and culturally sensitive health care, yet there remains a dearth of scientific research examining the existence and reinforcement of these barriers. Public health experts have determined, as recently as 2001, that research into the unique medical needs of LGBT patients is still lacking. A 2001 review of MEDLINE articles showed that only 0.1 percent of all articles focused on LGBT-specific topics and, of those, 61 percent were disease-specific, focusing on topics such as HIV, AIDS, sexually transmitted diseases, and "stigma diseases" such as gay bowel disease (Boehmer, 2002). The remaining articles focused on non-disease-specific topics such as identity, sexual behavior, provider and patient attitudes, risk factors, and so forth.

Although some patients and providers see barriers to LGBT-sensitive and culturally competent health care as an isolated issue of external homophobia by providers, the reality is far more complex. Barriers to accessing care can be more accurately discussed by examining three specific levels of the health care continuum: institutional-level barriers, provider-level barriers, and patient-level barriers.

INSTITUTIONAL BARRIERS TO LGBT HEALTH CARE

Third-Party Payer Insurance System

Many working adults under the age of sixty-five who are fortunate enough to have health insurance participate in an employer-sponsored, third-party payer system with coverage ranging from inpatient and emergency care to preventive and health maintenance outpatient care, prescription drug benefits, and mental health care. The third-party health insurance system can afford significant financial security for its enrollees, yet it can also create several potential barriers to accessing care for its LGBT members.

Many employers offering group health insurance do not include coverage for same-sex domestic partners. The reasons for this can be attributed to numerous causes. First, some employers are simply unwilling to provide the benefit. Explanations ranging from the moral to the economic are levied to justify the exclusion of LGBT couples from health insurance. In some states, heath insurers are unwilling or, due to government regulation, unable to write policies for domestic partner coverage.

Although an increasing number of Fortune 500 companies are extending benefits to same-sex domestic partners, many other organizations, especially small and midsized organizations, have yet to jump on the bandwagon. In recent years, some organizations have been embroiled in battles over providing health insurance benefits to same-sex domestic partners. Organizations ranging from commercial airlines to large public universities have been caught up in legal challenges regarding their refusal to offer domestic partner benefits. To date, the courts have ruled both for and against requiring organizations to offer same-sex domestic partner benefits, while the federal government has maintained the position of this being a state's rights issue.

The most obvious consequence of refusing same-sex partners health insurance is that both individuals must continue to maintain gainful employment that provides health insurance coverage, creating a situation whereby same-sex couples are subject to the economic realities of dual health insurance copayments and deductibles. While a married couple may have a $1,500 annual household deductible for out-of-pocket medical expenses, a same-sex couple without domestic partner benefits and similar insurance coverage could see their annual out-of-pocket expenses reach $3,000, in addition to the costs associated with added health insurance premiums. Besides

," both of which

re for sensitive
with their em-
to their health
ation and place
ir sexual orien-
r patients who
providers have

ered from the
gest organiza-
armed forces,
, the military
n in any man-
nts and phy-
ial. Informa-
commanding
he soldier in
orientation
ek help for
o same-sex

a concern
ghteen are
legitimate
ity. Ado-
en them-
ly to dis-
r (Allen,
cted pro-
patients,
smitted
ss indi-
lividual

ients is
along

individuals to maintain gainful
prohibits stay-at-home parent-

ess to health insurance cannot be
he difficult choices of increasing
risking financial or medical catas-
e relationship. Although there are
o help address these economic dis-
significant benefit.

n community resources available to
nples include items as simple as free
d cholesterol to more complex issues
, LGBT-friendly support groups, and
g programs. While clinicians provide
ommunity resources, policy leaders and
orking with government and corporate
p to their responsibility of ensuring every
e coverage.

rds

lity and Accountability Act (HIPAA) es-
tect the confidentiality of patients and their
g the release of specific information without
ient or health care proxy. However, HIPAA
rs to use and disclose specific information re-
ical conditions for the purposes of treatment,
rations without the patient's specific written
lated to payment includes billing for services,
ce companies, utilization reviews, and health
nctions related to the delivery of care and the
ction of the health care organization (West,
the federal level to ensure a patient's medical
dential, holes still remain in this protection.
alth care costs in check, some corporations have
oyees. This creates concern among some employ-
nature of their medical records. When organiza-
es, they cannot guarantee information contained in
ain confidential, even with the protections provided
tives and other organizational members can have un-
loyee medical records and detailed insurance billing

the economic consequences, requiring both individuals to maintain gainful employment with health insurance benefits prohibits stay-at-home parenting for the children of same-sex couples.

The economic impact of restricting access to health insurance cannot be understated. Many LGBT couples face the difficult choices of increasing their medical and child care expenses or risking financial or medical catastrophe by not insuring one member of the relationship. Although there are limits to what clinical providers can do to help address these economic disparities, simple undertakings can yield significant benefit.

Clinicians can provide information on community resources available to LGBT patients and their families. Examples include items as simple as free health screening for blood pressure and cholesterol to more complex issues such as child care, family counseling, LGBT-friendly support groups, and free and discounted prescription drug programs. While clinicians provide LGBT patients and families with community resources, policy leaders and health care executives should be working with government and corporate entities, encouraging each to live up to their responsibility of ensuring every citizen is provided with health care coverage.

Confidentiality of Medical Records

The Health Insurance Portability and Accountability Act (HIPAA) establishes firm guidelines to protect the confidentiality of patients and their medical conditions, prohibiting the release of specific information without the written consent of the patient or health care proxy. However, HIPAA does allow health care providers to use and disclose specific information related to patients and their medical conditions for the purposes of treatment, payment, and health care operations without the patient's specific written authorization. Information related to payment includes billing for services, submitting claims to insurance companies, utilization reviews, and health care operations including functions related to the delivery of care and the general administrative function of the health care organization (West, 2003). Despite attempts on the federal level to ensure a patient's medical information remains confidential, holes still remain in this protection.

As a method to keep health care costs in check, some corporations have elected to self-insure employees. This creates concern among some employees about the confidential nature of their medical records. When organizations self-insure employees, they cannot guarantee information contained in medical records will remain confidential, even with the protections provided by HIPAA. Senior executives and other organizational members can have unrestricted access to employee medical records and detailed insurance billing invoices for the purposes of "billing" and "utilization review," both of which are permissible under HIPAA guidelines.

This situation can prevent employees from seeking care for sensitive medical and psychiatric conditions that may be shared with their employers. Some patients fear disclosing certain information to their health care providers that will draw attention to their sexual orientation and place them at risk of harassment or even termination based on their sexual orientation. As a result, patient satisfaction and quality of care for patients who do not disclose their sexual orientation to their health care providers have declined (Bonvicini & Perlin, 2003).

Examples of how employers can abuse information garnered from the health care setting can be best illustrated by looking at the largest organization to self-insure, the United States Armed Forces. In the armed forces, LGBT soldiers and other enlisted members can be discharged, the military equivalent of termination, for affirming their sexual orientation in any manner. Under current military policy, conversations between patients and physicians or mental health providers are not considered confidential. Information contained within the medical record can be shared with commanding officers, who may then begin discharge procedures against the soldier in question. This encourages LGBT soldiers to hide their sexual orientation from their health care providers, limiting their ability to seek help for mental or physical health concerns they feel may be related to same-sex behaviors.

LGBT Youth

The risk of breaching patient-provider confidentiality is also a concern for LGBT youth and adolescents. Because children under age eighteen are typically covered by their parent's health insurance, there is a legitimate concern that they cannot visit a health care provider with anonymity. Adolescent patients that were made aware of the confidentiality between themselves and their health care providers were three times more likely to discuss their sexual orientation openly with their health care provider (Allen, Glicken, Beach, & Naylor, 1998). Although many states have enacted provisions for limited confidentiality between physicians and minor patients, this is often only related to specific concerns such as sexually transmitted diseases, drug and alcohol use, and mental health conditions, unless individual health care providers establish other parameters in their individual practices.

Another and sometimes more tangible concern for adolescent patients is that information they share with health care providers will be passed along to their parents, yielding disastrous results. A recent survey of Washington, DC, pediatricians demonstrated that many of the physicians surveyed would share information regarding an adolescent patient's sexual orientation with his or her parents. Even more alarming, 5 percent of those surveyed indicated they would do so even if the result were physical violence against the adolescent or expulsion from the home (East & Rayess, 1998). Regrettably, many social service agencies created to assist at-risk adolescents are often ill prepared to manage the complex needs of LGBT youth. The causes of this deficiency are multifactorial, yet the social services literature has failed to provide practitioners with direction in addressing this disparity. Between 1988 and 1997 nearly two-thirds of social work literature focusing on the LGBT community addressed HIV/AIDS, while much of the remaining literature tackled LGBT issues from a problem-oriented approach (Van Voorhis & Wagner, 2002).

LGBT Elders

Older adults also share a fear of the implications of revealing their sexual orientation with their health care providers and family members. Failure of older LGBT patients to share their sexual orientation with their health care providers results in worse clinical outcomes for disease processes such as cancer (Valanis et al., 2000). Other studies focusing on older members of the LGBT community demonstrate higher rates of internalized homophobia, alcohol abuse, and suicidal ideation among those with lower self-esteem and fewer people aware of their sexual orientation (D'Augelli, Grossman, Hershberger, & O'Connell, 2001).

Beyond concerns related to health care disparities and the mental health of LGBT elders, another very real concern relates to how LGBT patients will be received in long-term care facilities. In a study of lesbian and gay elders in Canada, a noted fear was that long-term care facilities, such as personal care and nursing homes, would not provide a supportive and safe environment for older LGBT persons (Brotman, Ryan, & Cormier, 2003). Patients described hiding their sexual orientation from their families and providers. Some older LGBT people reported going so far as to change their last names to match that of their partner in order to appear to be family so they could remain together while living in a long-term care facility.

Although long-term care facilities are often ill prepared to address sexual orientation among their residents, they are not alone in this limitation. Many health care facilities are often unprepared to deal with these very same issues. From heterosexist intake and demographic forms (see Exhibit 8.1) that fail to recognize LGBT relationships and differences in gender

EXHIBIT 8.1. Sample Information for LGBT-Sensitive Intake Forms

Legal name:
_____

Name I prefer to be called: .
_____

Sexual identity

Heterosexual	Bisexual
Gay	Not sure
Lesbian	Don't know
Other _____	

Gender

Male	Male to Female (MTF)
Female	Female to Male (FTM)
Transgender	Other _____

My sexual identity is known to
(circle all that apply)

My spouse/partner/significant
  other
My family
My friends
My co-workers
My children
No one
I am uncertain of my sexual
  identity

Current relationship situation

Single
Legally married
Domestic partner
Multiple partners
Separated from spouse/partner
Divorced/permanently separated
Widowed
Other _____

Are there children living in your home?
(circle all that apply)

No children
My children
My spouse/partner's children
Other children_____

Current living situation

Alone
With spouse/partner
With former spouse/partner
With roommate(s)
With parents
With other relatives
Dormitory/communal housing
Other_____

My current sexual partners are
(circle all that apply)

Men	Other_____
Women	

In the past my sexual partners
have included (circle all that apply)

Men	Other_____
Women	

Do you have any concerns
regarding your sexual identity?

Yes   No

Do you have any concerns
regarding your gender identity?

Yes   No

identity, to visitation policies restricting same-sex partners from visiting their significant others while in the hospital, to failing to address homophobia among clinicians, many hospitals have only begun to address these critical issues.

Issues regarding transgender and intersex patients become even more complex. Anecdotal yet very chilling evidence exists of hospitals being uncertain how to classify the gender of some patients and others not knowing whether to place a transgender or intersex patient in a male or female semiprivate room.

Confidentiality and "Family"

In 2000, Colin Hobbs and Joseph Roth traveled to Maryland to visit Hobbs's sister. During the visit, Roth was admitted to a community hospital with an AIDS-related complication. The hospital, unable to manage Roth's complex medical condition, transferred him to a university medical center.

At the university hospital, Roth was taken to an intensive care unit. When Hobbs arrived, he asked to speak with Roth's physicians and to see his partner. He was advised that the physicians would only speak to "family" members, and he did not meet the definition of family. Hobbs explained that he had a durable power of attorney for health care decisions for Roth and pointed out that they were registered as domestic partners in California.

Hobbs was forced to sit in the waiting room. He was denied access to Roth and was not permitted to speak with Roth's physicians to advise them of his partner's desire to decline life-sustaining interventions such as intubation and artificial ventilation. He never had a voice in Roth's care.

Hobbs was forced to wait four hours in the waiting room until his partner's family arrived. The family was shortly thereafter greeted by a physician, given an update on Roth's condition, and allowed to see him. Hobbs was allowed to visit his partner at this point, only to find him intubated and unconscious. Roth never regained consciousness, and Hobbs was never able to say good-bye before Roth died.

Advanced Health Care Planning

This example illustrates some of the barriers that LGBT patients face in the search for clinically competent health care that is also respectful of the LGBT family unit. Many hospitals and medical centers have difficulty defining and recognizing families beyond the traditional nuclear family. The Joint Commission for the Accreditation of Hospitals has defined family as "The person(s) who plays a significant role in the individual's [patient's] life. This may include a person(s) not legally related to the individual," but many hospitals have not provided their staff with adequate training to help providers better understand the variations on the family unit (Joint Commission Resources JCR, *2001 Hospital Accreditation Standards*, p. 322).

In an article appearing in *American Family Physician* in 2002, many different types of "families" were presented as equally viable definitions of the family unit. One definition, the crisis family, includes any person or persons who are actively involved in the management of a crisis situation (Medalie & Cole-Kelly, 2002). This definition can be interpreted to include biological family, friends, and other loved ones. Another family definition, the functional family, includes all persons in the household and others involved in the everyday affairs of the household (Medalie, 2002). Regardless of the family type or household composition, LGBT patients must make every effort to ensure that their medical affairs are in order and that their wishes will be respected by the health care providers, whether it is related to visitation rights, medical decision making, or withdrawal of care. This is best accomplished though the creation of legal documents outlining the wishes of the individual patient and the designation of a medical decision maker who will maintain sole responsibility for all medical decisions should the patient become incapacitated. This information is typically outlined in documents known as an *advanced directive* and a *durable medical power of attorney.*

An advanced directive, also known as a living will, is a legal document created by a patient outlining his or her wishes regarding resuscitative and life-sustaining care and is executed when a patient is no longer able to make medical decisions on his or her own behalf. Items addressed in an advanced directive may include the initiation of cardiopulmonary resuscitation, the insertion of a breathing tube or a feeding tube to maintain nutrition, or the withholding of life-saving medical interventions such as antibiotics, kidney dialysis, or surgery. A durable medical power of attorney is a legal document designating a person who will act on behalf of a patient to make medical decisions. This document is executed when the patient becomes either physically or mentally incapacitated and is unable to express his or her wishes and make his or her own medical decisions.

These documents have become critical to LGBT patients and their families. Horror stories are common of patients who have not created these documents and have had estranged family members arrive at the hospital and begin making decisions, shutting the patient's partner out of the process, and, at times, even restricting his or her access to visitation. Worse yet, same-sex partners have been denied medical decision-making rights by hospitals because they are not legally married and, as such, are not related and not legally able to make decisions on behalf of an incapacitated patient. Perhaps due to these occurrences, a larger percentage of patients in same-sex relationships have created these documents as compared to their heterosexual counterparts (Stein & Bonuck, 2001).

Information regarding the pervasiveness of LGBT-inclusive visitation policies and guidelines regarding medical decision making remains anecdotal. No large-scale research project or survey has been undertaken to assess how many hospitals and medical centers are taking proactive measures related to LGBT-inclusive policies and what mechanisms are being employed to educate staff about these polices and how they are to be executed.

Many LGBT advocacy groups have begun offering information to assist patients in creating an advanced directive and a durable medical power of attorney. The most comprehensive information can be found on the Web site of the Lambda Legal Defense and Education Fund, a national group based in New York City with regional offices across the country.

The Lambda Legal Defense and Education Fund's Web site (http://www.lambda legal.org) includes important background information on hospital visitation for LGBT patients and families, as well as information on advanced directives and durable medical power of attorney documents. Visitors to the site can find state-specific advanced planning documents that can be downloaded through a link with the Web site of Partnership for Caring (http://www.caringinfo.org), a Washington, DC–based nonprofit organization devoted to educating consumers and providers on end-of-life issues.

Creating a durable medical power of attorney mandates that patients select an individual whom they trust to execute their wishes should they become incapacitated. The designated person is known as the health care proxy. Once this person agrees to the responsibility, the document should be created, signed by the patient, notarized, and copies distributed to the patient, his or her lawyer, the primary health care provider, the designated proxy, and a copy placed in the inpatient medical record when the patient is admitted to the hospital.

Although creating an advanced directive does not require the designation of a health care proxy, this may be included in the document and, like the durable medical power of attorney, a copy should be provided to all parties, including the person designated as health care proxy in the durable medical power of attorney, should one exist. In addition, the advanced directive can be used to designate an approved list of hospital visitors, such that the hospital personnel are aware of who is and, sometimes more important, who is not permitted to visit the patient should the patient be unable to make decisions regarding visitation. Advanced directives can also include important information regarding organ donation and anatomical gifts.

Creating legal documents to protect the decision-making process is critical; however, the example at the beginning of this section illustrated how this might not be enough in every circumstance. In order to ensure that every hospital respects both the information outlined in advanced-planning documents and the LGBT family unit, provider and hospital administrator education must be undertaken to reinforce the diversity of family units and their importance. In addition, hospitals need to enact LGBT-specific policies addressing hospital visitation rights, medical decision making, and guidelines for recognition of LGBT families. The Lambda Legal Defense and Education Fund's Web site includes information on hospital visitation rights for LGBT patients and their loved ones, as well as a sample letter that can be downloaded and mailed to hospital administrators asking them to address hospital visitation policies and definitions of family that are LGBT inclusive. The Web site also includes links to Boston's Beth Israel Deaconess Medical Center's Guide to Childbirth Visitors and the New York State Department of Health's Patients' Bill of Rights, both of which include information that is culturally sensitive to LGBT patients.

Another advanced-planning process that should not be forgotten is planning related to the care of children with same-sex parents. If both parents have not legally adopted the children, it is critical to generate documentation providing both parents with the right to seek medical care for the children in question. Once created, these documents should be provided to both parents, the children's pediatrician, the children's schools or day care centers, and any sporting/recreational organizations in which the children participate.

PROVIDER-BASED BARRIERS TO LGBT HEALTH CARE

Health care providers are people and, as such, carry their own biases and prejudices affecting how they see themselves, their colleagues, and their patients. Providers with negative opinions of LGBT patients or colleagues can carry these views into their interactions with others in the health care arena.

A landmark study released in 1996 showed some disturbing health care trends. More than 50 percent of LGBT physicians surveyed witnessed patients being denied care or receiving substandard care solely based on presumed sexual orientation (Schatz & O'Hanlan, 1994). This is supported by a 1986 San Diego County (California) Medical Association survey indicating that 40 percent of respondents would not refer patients to providers whom they knew to self-identify as LGBT, while 30 percent of respondents would refuse medical school admission to highly qualified LGBT applicants (Matthews, Booth, Turner, & Kessler, 1986). The same study also demonstrated that 23 percent of those surveyed scored within the homophobic range of the heterosexual attitudes toward homosexuality (HATH) scale.

Although the San Diego County study did not explore the reason for this trend, the assumption can be made that this was due in part to the physicians' perceptions of the moral character of LGBT physicians and their prejudices toward the LGBT community. Twelve years later, a New Mexico study showed that although homophobic attitudes were improving, there was much work ahead. This study of academic physicians showed that 11 percent of respondents felt that "out" LGBT obstetrician-gynecologists were at risk of losing referrals due to their sexual orientation. The study also demonstrated that LGBT medical students who were open about their sexual orientation were often discouraged from entering specialties such as pediatrics, psychiatry, and obstetrics and gynecology, and instead were encouraged to pursue training in specialties with limited patient contact, such as radiology and pathology (Ramos, Tellez, Palley, Umland, & Skipper, 1998). Many of the respondents felt that LGBT physicians practicing pediatrics, psychiatry, obstetrics and gynecology, and so on would be in a position to influence patients in vulnerable or compromising situations.

When it comes to health care providers' interactions with LGBT patients, the trend toward negative perceptions of LGBT patients continues. A survey of California health care providers revealed that 40 percent reported they sometimes or often felt uncomfortable treating LGBT patients (Rankow, 1995). This finding was verified by a 2004 study of clinicians which found that, if given the option, 36 percent of clinicians would refrain from caring for LGBT patients (Röndahl, 2004).

Homophobia in health care is not simply a product of "older" providers who come from a different generation. One study looking at medical students found that they were more likely to attribute negative characteristics to homosexual patients, including finding them more offensive, less truthful, less likeable, less attractive, less intelligent, less assertive, more dangerous to others, and more responsible for their own illnesses (Kelly, St. Lawrence, Smith, Hood, & Cook, 1987). Although educating students in the health sciences can decrease homophobic attitudes (Wallick, Cambre, & Townsend, 1995), many health-related professions do not spend enough time educating their students about the nuances of caring for LGBT patients.

A glaring example of the lack of education on LGBT-related issues can be demonstrated by looking at medical education. Medical schools spend very little time educating future providers about the health care issues of LGBT patients. The average time medical schools spend educating their students on LGBT-specific issues was 3.5 hours, with some schools reporting no part of their curriculum devoted to LGBT issues (Wallick, Cambre, & Townsend, 1992). Often, gay men were discussed only in relation to sexually transmitted diseases and HIV. Even less time is spent on educating providers about the health care needs of transgender and intersex patients. Still today, references to homosexuality in some medical specialties only include HIV and conditions such as "gay bowel" disease.

As a result of this lack of appropriate education, even LGBT-sensitive providers are often unaware of the health care issues presented by LGBT patients. For instance, many lesbian women experience delayed diagnosis of life-threatening conditions such as breast and cervical cancer. Reasons for this disparity may include increased periods between mammograms and pap smears for lesbian and bisexual women. In addition, many lesbians are given misinformation and told that they are not at risk for cervical cancer since the HPV virus is transmitted by heterosexual intercourse. Still others have had negative experiences visiting their providers upon revealing their sexual orientation, and over 50 percent of lesbians reported rarely or never going to see their gynecologist (Zeidenstein, 1990).

PATIENT-BASED BARRIERS TO LGBT HEALTH CARE

Many patients coming to terms with their self-identification as an LGBT person may be uncomfortable talking to their health care providers about their sexual orientation or the concerns they have about how their sexual orientation will affect their care. This may be a particular problem in rural areas or for patients who already have long-term existing relationships with their providers. Shame or embarrassment over behaviors can also limit the ability to discuss their health care concerns. Negative past experiences with the health care system can also affect future care. A patient who was ridiculed or lectured at a previous visit will likely feel less comfortable seeking health care or, if they do seek it, will be more likely to remain closeted.

Homophobia is just one reason many LGBT patients have become disenfranchised within the health care delivery system; many other examples of barriers abound. From lack of knowledge about LGBT-specific medical problems, to clinical environments and intake forms that are heterocentric, to the failure to include LGBT patients' life partners in the health care process, many LGBT patients have turned their backs on the health care community.

PROVIDERS' ROLE IN ENSURING HEALTH OF THE LGBT COMMUNITY

In all of the studies addressing health care in the LGBT community one undisputed fact can be unearthed: homophobic attitudes, whether directed at patients or providers, will ultimately serve to construct barriers to the delivery of culturally competent care for LGBT patients. Whether it be by limiting the number of out LGBT practitioners in primary care and specialty settings or by creating an environment that is uncomfortable or inhospitable to LGBT patients and their families, actions such as these have a damaging effect on the well-being of the LGBT community.

Although it would appear that the barriers to access are insurmountable, they are not. The acknowledged existence of these barriers has encouraged innovative approaches to eliminating them. Community organizations, non-profit special interest groups, for-profit commercial and media organizations, academia, clinicians, and even governmental entities have all taken on the task of reducing health care disparities for LGBT patients. They have accomplished this through the creation of community outreach programming, creation and support of LGBT-specific community health centers, education campaigns targeting both health care providers and patients, and promoting policies to support the family units that are unique to the LGBT community.

Importance of Culturally Competent Care

LGBT patients who receive care they perceive to be culturally competent are more likely to seek care and to be compliant with recommended treatment plans (Schilder et al., 2001). Health care providers who are aware of and respectful toward sexual orientation and the differences in cultural and social belief and customs are a large part of why patients are more likely to report a willingness to seek out care and adhere to treatment plans. Programs undertaken to educate providers about how to provide care that is more effective to LGBT patients have been largely successful (Scout, Bradford, & Fields, 2001). In addition, the health care experience is often further improved when providers engage in communication patterns culturally sensitive to the LGBT community (Bakker & Cavender, 2003). These successes have also been extended to the educational process. Evidence demonstrates how the attitudes of students of the health sciences toward LGBT patients are considered less homophobic once LGBT-specific educational programming is introduced into the curriculum (Wallick et al., 1995; McGarry, 2002).

Evolution of LGBT-Specific Health Care
Research and Programming

As the interest in LGBT-related health information grew, providers branched out into many different arenas to provide this information and fill the numerous gaps. Some practitioners began engaging in original research, strictly adhering to scientific method and rigor, while others wrote papers from anecdotal evidence, personal experiences, or feedback from patients. Still other providers forged in entirely different directions, tackling issues related to health policy, while some focused on improving health education. Recognizing the lack of response to LGBT-specific needs by many professional health care organizations, some professionals banded together to create LGBT-specific professional organizations while some mainstream professional organizations created special interest groups or caucuses dedicated to addressing LGBT-specific health issues.

For the health needs of the LGBT community to be addressed in a comprehensive manner, clinical, administrative, academic, and policymaking sectors of health care must work in tandem, ensuring that needs are identified, research is undertaken, and best practice guidelines are developed. The entire process must be shared with providers on all levels, with thoughtful input from representatives of the LGBT community and LGBT-focused health, community, and advocacy organizations.

Community-Based LGBT Health Centers

Many local communities have taken to empowering themselves to meet the growing health care needs of their respective communities. Since the 1980s local community leaders and health care providers have come together to respond to community health needs through the advent of community health centers. Supported by the financial support of the local LGBT communities, billing for services and support of local and national organizations as well as foundation and governmental grants, these centers carry out the unique mission of serving the health care needs of the local LGBT communities. Local health centers have also become a hotbed of LGBT-specific health research. Centers in New York; Boston; Chicago; Washington, DC; and many others have participated in countless research studies that have increased access to care for LGBT patients and improved understanding of many LGBT-specific aspects of common medical illnesses.

One of the best examples of actions to increase access to care for LGBT patients has been the creation of community-based health centers catering to the LGBT community. Callen-Lorde in New York City; Whitman-Walker in Washington, DC; Chicago's Howard Brown Health Center; Boston's Fenway Community Health; and Philadelphia's Mazzoni Center are all local LGBT-focused health centers that have been created to meet the needs of the LGBT communities in which they serve. The health centers offer services as far-ranging as primary care, reproductive services, acupuncture, podiatry, counseling services, and substance-abuse treatment. Many community health centers have partnered with one another, in addition to academic institutions and others in the health care industry, to engage in LGBT-specific medical research, to educate health sciences students, and to initiate various community health and education programs. The underlying goal of all the programming undertaken by community health centers is to improve the overall health care of the LGBT community in a safe and supportive environment.

Community health centers have been met with significant success. In twenty-five years, the patient volume at Fenway Community Health Center has increased ten-fold. Fenway, which provides medical services, mental health programming, and participates in medical education programming, boasts a staff of over 170 individuals and an annual budget that exceeded $10 million in 2001 (Mayer et al., 2001). Fenway and its staff participate in ongoing research projects and are frequent collaborators with local, state, and national agencies. In addition, Fenway has developed programming to educate the general community about the specific health needs of LGBT patients. Fenway has become a model community health center. Its success and depth of programming should serve as a guide for other health centers striving to achieve the same access for their LGBT patients.

Academia and Professional Medical Organizations

While local communities have made great inroads to improving access to care for LGBT patients, academia and professional medical organizations have also taken a lead role in eliminating barriers in the LGBT community. In 2001, the American Public Health Association published a special issue of their journal, *American Journal of Public Health (AJPH),* dedicated solely to health care and public health issues central to the LGBT community. This special edition, the first dedicated to LGBT health in the ninety-one-year history of *AJPH,* was preceded by a resolution highlighting the need for greater research in the relationship among sexual orientation, gender identity, and disease (Meyer, 2001). Through the LGBT Caucus of Public Health Workers, the American Public Health Association continues to remain at the forefront of promoting research in LGBT health issues. In addition to the work of professional organizations, many colleges and universities have established academic centers of excellence that focus solely on LGBT-specific research.

While groups such as the American Public Health Association and the University of Pittsburgh's Center for Research on Health and Sexual Orientation work to promote education through research into LGBT health issues, other professional organizations work to educate health care providers through advocacy and educational programming. The Gay and Lesbian

Medical Association (GLMA), a national organization of health care providers dedicated to improving health care for the LGBT community, works to eliminate barriers to health care through its annual education conference, in addition to extensive work in LGBT health policy and advocacy. In 2002, the GLMA released two articles designed to educate health care consumers about their own health care. The publications, titled "Ten Things Lesbians Should Discuss with Their Health Care Providers" and "Ten Things Gay Men Should Discuss with Their Health Care Providers," detail specific issues that LGBT patients should address with their primary care providers (see Exhibits 8.2 and 8.3). The lists, derived from surveys of GLMA's membership, received wide media coverage and appear on the organization's Web site, in addition to the Web sites of many other organizations.

Governmental Agencies

Some governmental entities have also taken a role in eliminating barriers and increasing access to health care for LGBT patients. In 1997, the Massachusetts Department of Public Health funded the Gay, Lesbian, Bisexual, and Transgender (GLBT) Health Access Project, a five-year public-private partnership dedicated to eliminating barriers to health care for the LGBT community. Through the collaboration of the Department of Public Health, community-based health and human service agencies, and the at-large LGBT community, the project was successful in developing standards for health care and related services for LGBT individuals and provider training programs that included information on making practices more LGBT friendly;

EXHIBIT 8.2. Ten Things Gay Men Should Discuss with Their Health Care Providers

1. HIV/AIDS, Safe Sex
2. Substance Use
3. Depression/Anxiety
4. Hepatitis Immunization
5. STDs
6. Prostate/Testicular/Colon Cancer
7. Alcohol
8. Tobacco
9. Fitness (Diet & Exercise)
10. Anal Papiloma

Source: Gay and Lesbian Medical Association (2002). "Ten Things Gay Men Should Discuss with Their Health Care Providers." San Francisco, CA © (courtesy of GLMA, http://www.glma.org).

**EXHIBIT 8.3. Ten Things Lesbians Should Discuss
with Their Health Care Providers**

1. Breast Cancer
2. Depression/Anxiety
3. Gynecological Cancer
4. Fitness (Diet and Exercise)
5. Substance Use
6. Tobacco
7. Alcohol
8. Domestic Violence
9. Osteoporosis
10. Heart Health

Source: Gay and Lesbian Medical Association (2002). "Ten Things Lesbians Should Discuss with Their Health Care Providers." San Francisco, CA © (courtesy of GLMA, http://www.glma.org).

it also participated in the collection of LGBT-specific health data (Clark, Landers, Linde, & Sperber, 2001).

The GLBT Health Access Project maintains a Web site (http://www.glbthealth.org/) where patients and providers can obtain additional information about the many projects this program undertakes.

Some governmental agencies on the state and national level have acted to promote and fund LGBT-specific research, while other governmental organizations, mostly on the local and regional levels, have engaged in public awareness campaigns to educate the LGBT community and respond to community health threats.

The Public Health Department of King County, Washington, which includes the city of Seattle, maintains a Web site for LGBT health (http://www.metrokc.gov/health/glbt/). The site provides users with information on LGBT-specific resources in King County, including substance abuse counseling centers, HIV testing sites, community health centers, mental health services, and a special section providing resources for the transgender community. The King County Web site also provides educational material to health care providers, giving information about the impact of homophobia in health care and offering tips to provide a treatment environment that is LGBT positive.

Individual Health Care Practitioners

Although organizational and governmental involvement in improving access to care are critical to ensuring that the trend of reducing barriers to care for the LGBT community continues, individual practitioners must also strive to ensure their work environments are LGBT inclusive. Staff must be trained to recognize LGBT-specific concerns and incorporate the entire family unit into the health care process. Steps as simple as using LGBT-sensitive intake forms, providing health education materials that include information for LGBT patients, and making available waiting room reading materials and posters that include LGBT-positive imagery all have the potential to improve the health care experience for LGBT patients. Many of the organizations previously discussed in this section, along with a wide variety of other sources, provide information that can assist health care providers in creating a supportive environment for LGBT patients and their families.

With many health care providers recognizing the *"Will and Grace"* effect of greater acceptance of the LGBT community through increased visibility and exposure, some providers have taken action to help health care come out of the closet. Many providers have made themselves available to LGBT student organizations for mentoring and support while others lend their expertise and services to LGBT issues in professional groups such as the American Medical Association (AMA) and the American Public Health Association (APHA). Another interesting movement to support up-and-coming leaders in LGBT health has been undertaken within the past year. Created in 2004, the LGBT Health, Education, and Research Trust (LGBT HEART) was founded by health care providers representing clinical care, public health, and academia who are committed to providing need- and merit-based scholarships to out LGBT students pursuing careers in the health sciences.

PITFALLS TO PROGRESS

In assuring that the needs of the community are addressed, it is important that members of the health care delivery system look not only to the present but also to the future. As the LGBT community continues to grow and evolve, it also continues to age. The LGBT community has begun to realize that a growing population of LGBT people heading into their "golden years" will increasingly utilize health care services. Unfortunately, many older members of the LGBT community perceive significant marginalization in their social and political lives (Brotman et al., 2003). From this extends a concern about the implications this feeling of marginalization will have on the delivery of long-term care and social support for older LGBT persons and their families. As such, the health care system will need to adapt, ensuring that the health care and long-term care needs of the LGBT community are met.

Unintended Consequences

Despite improvements in programming, research, and policy related to LGBT health care, providers, researchers, and academicians must ensure that their actions, although often well intentioned, do not cause further harm or isolation for LGBT patients. Many gay and bisexual men who engage in anal intercourse saw their self-expression and decision-making capacity limited as a result of attempts to educate them about the risks of HIV transmission. Many primary care providers and public health workers provided HIV education that recommended restrictions on anal intercourse that were often interpreted as sex-phobic (Odets, 1996). Members of the transgender community expressed concern when transgender health issues were not included in the final draft of the *Healthy People 2010 Companion Document for LGBT Health* (Gay and Lesbian Medical Association & LGBT Health Experts, 2001), a collaborative effort involving nearly 200 individuals, organizations, and agencies spearheaded by the GLMA (Dean et al., 2000).

In addition to ensuring that the actions of health care providers are perceived in the manner in which they are intended, providers must also be mindful of the role of sexual orientation as it relates to the self-awareness of LGBT patients. This self-awareness varies widely and is influenced by various socioeconomic, cultural, gender-related, religious, and geographic factors (Meyer, 2001; Mills et al., 2001). Perceptions of personal sexual orientation of a white, gay man living in South Beach may be significantly different from that of a Chinese lesbian living in San Francisco's Chinatown. Gay men who reside in urbanized "gay ghettos" tend to be more involved with the larger LGBT community than those who reside in suburban, rural, and non-LGBT-concentrated urban areas (Mills et al., 2001). An anal-receptive Latino man may perceive himself as gay, while his anal-insertive partner may perceive himself as straight. Some patients may see their sexual orientation as central to their emotional well-being, while others see it as peripheral and instead focus on other issues such as religion, culture, profession, or family.

CONCLUSION

In order for the interests of the LGBT community to be represented in the delivery of health care, all aspects of the delivery system must work in tandem to recognize potential barriers to assess to quality care and work to eliminate the barrier. Clinical health care practitioners, health educators, public health workers, researchers, and administrators must all play a role in this process. Students of the health sciences should receive education that is inclusive of LGBT health issues. Researchers should be encouraged to pursue further study on disparities in health care for the LGBT community. They should also continue to assess the unique health care needs of the LGBT community. Practitioners should continue to promote open and honest communication with their patients. They should also include the family in the care process when possible and remain open to learning as much as possible about their LGBT patients and families. Health care advocates should continue to hold all parties accountable and push for increased education. Health policy analysts should lobby for legislation to protect the needs of the community. Finally, and probably most important, LGBT patients must take an active role in their own health care.

SELECTED LGBT RESOURCES FOR STUDENTS IN THE HEALTH SCIENCES

The following groups provide information, links, or resources for LGBT students enrolled in health science education programs. This list is by no means exhaustive and changes regularly.

- Association of Gay and Lesbian Psychiatrists
  www.aglp.org
- Gay and Lesbian Medical Association
  www.glma.org
- Gay Nurses' Alliance
  214 Market Street
  Wilmington, DE 19801
- Healthy Lesbian, Gay, and Bisexual Students Project of the American Psychological Association
  www.apa.org/ed/hlgb/
- Iranian Gay and Lesbian Healthcare Providers Association
  www.iraniangaydoctors.com

- Lesbian, Gay and Bisexual Health Concerns Office of the American Psychological Association
  www.apa.org/pi/lgbc/homepage.html
- Lesbian, Gay, Bisexual and Transgender Caucus of Public Health Workers
  www.stophiv.com/lgbtc/
- Lesbian, Gay, Bisexual and Transgendered Health Science Librarians Special Interest Group of the Medical Library Association
  www.lgbtsig.org/
- Lesbian, Gay, Bisexual and Transgender People in Medicine (LGBTPM) of the American Medical Student Association
  www.amsa.org/adv/lgbtpm/
- National Association of Lesbian and Gay Addiction Professionals
  www.nalgap.org
- National Association of Social Workers Committee on Lesbian and Gay Issues
  www.naswdc.org/Diversity/default.asp

QUESTIONS TO CONSIDER

1. Recalling ten things gay men and lesbians should discuss with their health care providers (see Exhibits 8.2 and 8.3), how are the items listed for gay men and lesbians similar? How are they different? What challenges could be expected in tailoring the messages for similar items to each group? What challenges can be expected for delivering messages within each group?
2. Recalling Exibit 8.1, outlining the information essential to developing an LGBT-sensitive intake form, think of the variety of responses that can be expected from patients responding to the questionnaire. Discuss what type of techniques can be undertaken to help LGBT and questioning patients feel more comfortable with providing such detailed and often sensitive information. How would you justify the need to obtain this information, if asked, to your heterosexual patients or to patients with very strong moral and/or religious convictions who look unfavorably upon such information?
3. It has been recommended that LGBT patients in long-term committed relationships establish a durable medical power of attorney, an advanced directive, and documents related to medical care of children. Given the myriad laws governing same-sex relationships across the nation, how would you advise your patients and their families regarding these documents? What are the advantages and limitations of advanced-planning documents?

4. Reference has been made to the "unintended consequences" of trying to provide an LGBT-sensitive approach to health care. Examples abound of "what she said isn't what she meant" in everyday communications. Think of examples in your experience of attempts to provide culturally sensitive health care that only resulted in offending or alienating a patient. Given the diverse nature of the LGBT community, how can you as a health care provider tailor the appropriate message to such a multifaceted audience?

5. Experts and laypersons from university academia to the media have argued that everyone has prejudices and stereotypes regarding other groups. As a health care provider, what types of prejudices and stereotypes do you have regarding different subcultures within the LGBT community? How do these preconceived beliefs affect how you approach your patients and deliver care? What specific steps can be taken on individual, institutional, academic, and governmental levels to help minimize the effects of prejudice and stereotyping?

REFERENCES

Allen, L., Glicken, A., Beach, R., & Naylor, K. (1998). Adolescent health care experiences of gay, lesbian and bisexual young adults. *Journal of Adolescent Health, 23*(4), 212-220.

Bakker, L. J., & Cavender, A. (2003). Promoting culturally compentent care for gay youth. *Journal of School Nursing, 19*(2), 65-72.

Boehmer, U. (2002). Twenty years of public health research: Inclusion of lesbian, gay, bisexual and transgender populations. *American Journal of Public Health, 92*(7), 1125-1130.

Bonvicini, K., & Perlin, M. (2003). The same but different: Clinician-patient communication with gay and lesbian patients. *Patient Education and Counseling, 51*(2), 115-122.

Brotman, S., Ryan, B., & Cormier, R. (2003). The health and social service needs of gay and lesbian elders and their families in Canada. *The Gerontologist, 43*(2), 192-202.

Clark, M., Landers, S., Linde, R., & Sperber, J. (2001). The GLBT Health Access Project: A state-funded effort to improve access to care. *American Journal of Public Health, 91*(6), 895-896.

D'Augelli, A., Grossman, A., Hershberger, S., & O'Connell, T. (2001). Aspects of mental health among older lesbian, gay and bisexual adults. *Aging and Mental Health, 5,* 149-158.

Dean, L., Meyer, I. H., Robinson, K., Sell, R. L., Sember, R., Silenzio, V. M. B, Bowen, D. J., Bradford, J., Rothblum, E., White, J., Dunn, P., Lawrence, A., Wolfe, D., & Xavier, J. (2000). Lesbian, gay, bisexual and transgender health:

Findings and concerns. *Journal of the Gay and Lesbian Medical Association, 3,* 101-151.

East, J., & Rayess, F. (1998). Pediatricians' approach to the health care of lesbian, gay and bisexual youth. *Journal of Adolescent Health, 23*(4), 191-193.

Gay and Lesbian Medical Association & LGBT Health Experts. (2001). *Healthy people 2010 companion document for lesbian, gay, bisexual, and transgender (LGBT) health.* San Francisco, CA: Gay and Lesbian Medical Association.

Joint Commission Resources. (2001). Hospital accreditation standards. Available at www.jcrinc.com.

Kelly, J. A., St. Lawrence, J. S., Smith, S., Jr., Hood, H. V., & Cook, D. J. (1987). Medical students' attitudes toward AIDS and homosexual patients. *Journal of Medical Education, 62,* 549-556.

Matthews, W., Booth, M., Turner, J., & Kessler, L. (1986). Physicians' attitudes toward homosexuality—Survey of a California county medical society. *The Western Journal of Medicine, 144,* 106-110.

Mayer, K., Appelbaum, J., Rogers, T., Lo, W., Bradford, J., & Boswell, S. (2001). The evolution of the Fenway Community Health model. *American Journal of Public Health, 91*(6), 892-895.

McGarry, K. (2002). Evaluating a lesbian and gay health care curriculum. *Teach and Learn Medicine, 14*(4), 244-248.

Medalie, J. H., & Cole-Kelly, K. (2002). The clinical importance of defining family. *American Family Physician, 65*(7), 1277-1279.

Meyer, I. (2001). Why lesbian, gay, bisexual and transgender health? *American Journal of Public Health, 9*(6), 856-859.

Mills, T., Stall, R., Pollack, L., Paul, J., Binson, D., Canchola, J., & Catania, J. (2001). Health-related characteristics of men who have sex with men: A comparison of those living in "gay ghettos" with those living elsewhere. *American Journal of Public Health, 91*(6), 980-983.

Odets, W. (1996). Why we stopped doing primary prevention for gay men in 1985. In Dangerous Bedfellows (E. G. Coulter, W. Hoffman, E. Pendleton, A. Redick, & D. Serlin) (Eds.), *Policing public sex: Queer politics and the future of AIDS activism* (pp. 115-140). Boston, MA: South End Press.

Ramos, M. M., Tellez, C. M., Palley, T. B., Umland, B. E., & Skipper, B. J. (1998). Attitudes of physicians practicing in New Mexico toward gay men and lesbians in the profession. *Academic Medicine, 73,* 436-438.

Rankow, E. J. (1995). Lesbian health issues for the primary care provider. *Journal of Family Practice, 40,* 486-496.

Röndahl, G. (2004). Nursing staff and nursing students' emotions toward homosexual patients and their wish to refrain from nursing, if the option existed. *Scandinavian Journal of Caring Sciences, 18*(1), 19-26.

Schatz, B., & O'Hanlan, K. A. (1994). *Anti-gay discrimination in medicine: Results of a national survey of lesbian, gay and bisexual physicians.* San Francisco, CA: American Association of Physicians for Human Rights.

Schilder, A. J., Kennedy, C., Goldstone, I. L., Ogden, R. D., Hogg, R. S., & O'Shaughnessy, M. V. (2001). "Being dealt with as a whole person"—Care seeking and adherence: The benefits of culturally competent care. *Social Science & Medicine, 52*(11), 1643-1659.

Scout, Bradford, J., & Fields, C. (2001). Removing the barriers: Improving practitioners' skills in providing health care to lesbians and women who partner with women. *American Journal of Public Health, 91*(6), 989.

Stein, G. L., & Bonuck, K. A. (2001). Attitudes on end-of-life care and advance care planning in the lesbian and gay community. *Journal of Palliative Medicine, 4*(2), 173-190.

Valanis, B. G., Bowen, D. J., Bassford, T., Whitlock, E., Charney, P., Carter, R. A. (2000). Sexual orientation and health: Comparsions in the Women's Health Initiative sample. *Archives of Family Medicine, 9*(9), 843-853.

Van Voorhis, R., & Wagner, M. (2002). Among the missing: Content on lesbian and gay people in social work journals. *Social Work, 47*(4), 345-354.

Wallick, M., Cambre, K., & Townsend, M. (1992). How the topic of homosexuality is taught at U.S. medical schools. *Academic Medicine, 67,* 601-603.

Wallick, M., Cambre, K., & Townsend, M. (1995). Influence of a freshman-year panel presentation on medical students' attitudes toward homosexuality. *Academic Medicine, 70*(9), 839-841.

West, J. (2003). Medical-legal issues: The patient relationship and risk management. *Clinics in Family Practice, 5*(4), 905.

Zeidenstein, L. (1990). Gynecological and childbearing needs to lesbians. *Journal of Nurse Midwifery, 35,* 10-18.

Chapter 9

Lesbian, Gay, Bisexual, and Transgender Substance Abuse

Rodger L. Beatty
Rosemary Madl-Young
Wendy B. Bostwick

INTRODUCTION

This chapter highlights the special concerns of substance use (alcohol, tobacco, and other drugs) in the LGBT community. The goal is to help those individuals who treat persons with substance use to better understand the unique issues and needs within the LGBT community. Practitioners will be more effective if they understand how the contemporary LGBT community is defined, the distinctive patterns and unique risk factors of LGBT substance abuse, and treatment options and resources.

Various ways of defining lesbian, gay, bisexual, and transgender (LGBT) include behavior, identity, and attraction. Although there is some overlap, most lesbians and gays acknowledge that their sexual identity, behavior, and attraction are not consistently same-gender. Sexuality is often fluid rather than static (Finnegan & McNally, 2002). Researchers have not agreed on definitions of sexual orientation, sexual identity, or sexual attraction. It is often left up to research subjects to define these words for themselves. In addition, these words have different meanings in different cultures. Researchers rarely collect information on individuals that do not conform to societal perceptions of male or female. Finnegan and McNally (2002) further stress that it is extremely important to understand that any of these labels—homosexual, heterosexual, bisexual, asexual—can be misleading because they do not account for the subtleties and intricacies of human emotions and behavior or changes in the human condition.

Epidemiological data and information related to alcohol, tobacco, and other drug (ATOD) use and abuse among LGBT persons are, for the most part, limited to regional or local studies of specific populations (e.g., lesbians, men living with or at risk for HIV). No studies to date have utilized a national sample of LGBT individuals. Few studies have included sufficient numbers of bisexual women to permit separate analyses, and no studies to date have focused exclusively on this subset of the population. Data from bisexual women are usually combined with data from lesbians, reflecting an unexplored assumption that bisexual women have more in common with lesbians than with heterosexual women. Therefore, many of the results reported in studies of lesbian women likely include some proportion of bisexual women. However, bisexual men are included in studies of gay men in much greater numbers. One reason for this variance is the disproportionately large number of studies that focus on behavior rather than identity to better understand risk factors associated with STDs, including HIV/AIDS, among men who have sex with men (Hughes & Eliason, 2002).

In one of the earliest and most frequently cited studies, Fifield, DeCresenzo, & Latham (1975) surveyed 98 bartenders and 200 bar patrons. Based upon their subjects' alcohol consumption, these investigators concluded that alcohol abuse occurred with approximately 32 percent of the gay population in Los Angeles County, California. Methodological limitations, such as small, nonrepresentative samples that often included bar patrons and a lack of appropriate comparison groups, certainly raises questions about the validity of these findings. An additional concern with this seminal work is that the term "gay" was utilized when it reflected both lesbians and gay men. In even more recent research it is often challenging to separate the data by categories and subpopulations.

LESBIANS AND BISEXUAL WOMEN

In another large study, Skinner reported findings from lesbians and gay men in Lexington and Louisville, Kentucky (Skinner, 1994; Skinner & Otis, 1996). To compare the lesbians in their study to the general population, Skinner and Otis geographically matched a subsample of women from the 1988 National Household Survey on Drug Abuse (NHSDA). More lesbians (87 percent) than women in the NHSDA (64 percent) reported alcohol consumption in the past year (lesbians are likely included within the NHSDA, but the telephone surveys do not distinguish that category). Lesbians in this study also reported more drinking days and more binge drinking (five or more drinks on one occasion) than did the NHSDA women. Past-year use of marijuana was also significantly higher for lesbians (36 percent) than for women in the NHSDA (8 percent). In fact, lesbians' rates of marijuana use were comparable to those of the gay men (37 percent) in this study. Overall prevalence rates for past-year cocaine use was relatively low for both lesbian women (7 percent) and NHSDA women (3 percent), none-theless, still more than twice as much.

In one of the few studies of lesbians' alcohol use to employ probability sampling and include a heterosexual comparison group, Bloomfield (1993) discovered findings that differ somewhat from studies using convenience samples. In this study, fifty-two lesbians and six bisexual women were com-pared with 397 heterosexual women in a household sample of San Fran-cisco residents eighteen to fifty years old. No significant differences were found between lesbians' and bisexual women's levels of drinking and those of heterosexual women. Only the number of recovering alcoholics signifi-cantly differed for the two groups: 13 percent of the lesbian and bisexual women and 3 percent of the heterosexual women reported being in recovery.

Similarly, in a multisite study conducted by Hughes, Hass, Razzano, Cassidy, & Matthews (2000), significantly more lesbians (14 percent) than heterosexual women (6 percent) indicated that they had gotten help for al-cohol and other drug problems at least once in the past ($p < .001$). Of the nondrinking lesbians, 68 percent reported that they had gotten help for an alcohol or drug problem. This finding suggests that the majority of lesbian abstainers were likely in recovery from substance-related problems. Re-searchers (Cochran and Mays, 2000; Gilman et al., 2001; Sanfort, de Graaf, Bijl, & Schnabel, 2001) used data from large national population-based da-tabases to compare women who reported any same-sex partners with those who reported only male partners. Each study found a substantially higher rate of alcohol or drug dependency among women who reported same-sex partners. Because questions about self-identity were not included, it cannot be assumed that these women are lesbian or bisexual. However, findings suggest that same-sex sexual behavior and alcohol dependence are strongly associated and emphasize the need for including a measure of sexual iden-tity, in addition to measures of sexual behavior, in all large-scale popula-tion-based studies.

GAY AND BISEXUAL MEN

In the only population-based study (Stall & Wiley, 1988), investigators of the San Francisco Men's Health Study conducted a random household study of 748 gay men and a comparison group of 286 nongay men. The prevalence of frequent/heavy drinking for gay men (19 percent) was higher than the rate for nongay men (11 percent), but about twice as many gay men (6 percent) as nongay men (3 percent) reported that they did not drink at all in the previous twelve months. Gay men younger than thirty-five were much more likely than their age-matched counterparts to report use of poppers, ecstasy, barbiturates, and amphetamines. Differences between gay and nongay men in use of marijuana and psychedelics were not nearly as large, though the young gay men were also more likely to report use of both of these drugs. Among men older than thirty-five, only use of poppers and amphetamines differed significantly from older nongay men.

Stall et al. (2001) conducted a telephone survey of a stratified probability sample of men who identified as gay, bisexual, or reported having sex with another man in the past five years (men who have sex with men) drawn from selected zip codes in the city limits of San Francisco, New York, Chicago, and Los Angeles ($n = 2172$). Both recreational drug use (52 percent) and alcohol use (85 percent) were highly prevalent among these urban men, while current levels of multiple drug use (18 percent), three or more alcohol-related problems (12 percent), frequent drug use (19 percent), and heavy-to-frequent alcohol use (8 percent) were not uncommon. The associations of heavy and/or problematic substance use are complex, with independent associations found at the level of demographics, adverse early life circumstance, current mental health status, social and sexual practices, and connection to gay male culture. In addition, this study further indicated substances used by these men as marijuana (42.4 percent), poppers (19.8 percent), cocaine (15.2 percent), crack cocaine (3.0 percent), ecstasy (11.7 percent), speed (9.5 percent), downers (8.8 percent), and opiates (3.2 percent). These data support the view that drug and alcohol use is highly prevalent among urban men who have sex with men. In addition, current problems attributed to drug or alcohol use were not uncommon.

TRANSGENDER MEN AND WOMEN

Scarce research has been carried out concerning substance use among transgender persons. The few studies that do involve transgender individuals have been conducted as part of HIV-related research. Studies have typically employed convenience samples from large urban areas. Although results of these studies cannot be generalized to transgender persons as a whole, they provide evidence of the extent of substance abuse problems in some urban transgender groups. One study examining the past-month alcohol and other drug (AOD) use of 209 transgender women found that 37 percent used alcohol, 13 percent marijuana, 11 percent methamphetamine, 11 percent crack, 7 percent powdered cocaine, and 2 percent heroin (Reback & Lombardi, 1999). In comparison, the most recent National Survey on Drug Use & Health (2002), an annual survey of the noninstitutionalized United States population aged twelve years or older, 8.3 percent of the population were current illicit drug users (i.e., use of an illicit drug during the month prior to the survey). Marijuana is the most commonly used illicit drug for men and women, with a rate of 6.2 percent, half of the rate cited by Reback and Lombardi for transsexuals. The 1999 Clements study done in San Francisco by the Department of Public Health found that, in the preceding six months, the drugs most commonly used by male-to-female (MTF) transgender persons were marijuana (64 percent), speed (30 percent), and crack cocaine (21 percent); female-to-male (FTM) transgender persons reported using only marijuana frequently (43 percent). Another study reported that alcohol, cocaine/crack, and methamphetamines were the drugs most commonly used by MTF transgender persons in Los Angeles (Reback & Lombardi, 1999).

Valentine's study (1998) of intake records from 1989 to 1997 at the Gender Identity Project in New York City showed high rates of substance abuse in the transgender population: 27.1 percent reported alcohol abuse and 23.6 percent reported drug abuse. Three hundred ninety-two transgender people participated in San Francisco's Transgender Community Health Project (Clements, 1999). Twenty-one percent (eighty-two individuals) identified as bisexual; 16 percent of the total number revealed they had received treatment for alcohol problems and 23 percent for drug problems. In addition, among this group of transgender persons it was shown that lifetime use of marijuana was 90 percent, cocaine 66 percent, crack 48 percent, and heroin 24 percent. Of the injection drug users, 84 percent used speed, 58 percent heroin, and 54 percent cocaine. Of the 252 participants in Xavier's Washington, DC, study (2000), 13.1 percent self-identified as bisexual. Thirty-four percent of all the participants stated that alcohol was a problem and 36 percent reported drugs to be a problem.

LESBIANS AND GAY MEN

Cochran and Mays (2000) examined alcohol-use patterns among adults interviewed in the 1996 National Household Survey on Drug Abuse. Sexually active respondents were classified into two groups: those with at least one same-gender sexual partner ($n = 194$) in the year prior to the interview and those with only opposite-gender sexual partners ($n = 9,174$). The authors compared these two groups separately by gender. For men, normative alcohol-use patterns or morbidity did not differ significantly between the two groups. However, women with same-gender sexual preference reported using alcohol more frequently and in greater amounts and experienced greater alcohol-related morbidity than exclusively heterosexual women (see Exhibit 9.1).

EXHIBIT 9.1. April 2000 Millennium March in Washington, DC

730 self-identified gay males surveyed:

- 26.3 percent reported that party drugs such as ecstasy, special K, and GHB are used once a month
- 13.4 percent reported party drugs are used one or more times a week
- 21.9 percent reported one or two times per year
- 34.8 percent reported that party drugs are never used in their circle of friends
- 45.1 percent reported that they consume alcohol once a week or less
- 28.4 percent reported using alcohol two or three times a week
- 14.6 percent reported using alcohol four times a week.

307 self-identified lesbians surveyed:

- 61.9 percent reported that party drugs are never used in their group of friends
- 11.4 percent reported once a month
- 5.9 percent one or more times a week
- 20.8 percent one or two times a year
- 57.4 percent reported using alcohol once a week or less
- 20.5 percent reported consuming alcohol two or three times a week
- 14.6 percent reported using alcohol four times a week

Nearly 12 percent of gay males and nearly 6 percent of lesbians who participated in the survey reported that they never use alcohol. Lesbians ranked alcohol abuse as the second highest health concern for the community and more than 30 percent of gay men reported the same concern.

Source: K-Y Liquid Community Health Survey, 2000.

LGBT YOUTH AND SENIORS

LGBT youth use alcohol and other drugs for many of the same reasons as their heterosexual peers: to experiment and to assert independence, to relieve tension, to increase feelings of self-esteem and self-adequacy, and to self-medicate for underlying depression or other mental health problems (Ryan & Hunter, 2001). Adolescents grow up in an environment that assumes heterosexuality. Little acceptance is available to LGBT youth within most sectors of their world (e.g., families, peers, schools, and churches). Youth of color face additional stresses and challenges in integrating multiple sexual, gender, racial, and ethnic identities (Wisconsin Survey Research Laboratory, 2000), which may contribute to their use of alcohol and other drugs.

Available data suggest that the risk of alcohol and drug abuse is greater for youth who identify as lesbian, gay, or bisexual and those who report same-sex experiences, as well as for youth who have been harassed by their peers because they are perceived to be lesbian, gay, or bisexual. In the 1997 Massachusetts Youth Risk Behavior Survey (1998), 46 percent of youth who identified as lesbian or gay or who reported having same-gender sex reported ever having used hallucinogens, 77 percent reported ever having used marijuana, and 33 percent reported ever having used cocaine (Garofalo et al., 1998).

Similarly, the 1997 Vermont Youth Risk Behavior Survey found that youth with same-sex sexual experience were significantly more likely than other youth to use alcohol and other drugs in the past thirty days. Specifically, of those youth with same-sex sexual experiences, 64 percent smoked cigarettes; 16 percent drank alcohol daily; 22 percent reported smoking marijuana ten or more times; 29 percent reported using cocaine; and 19 percent had injected illegal drugs two or more times in their lifetimes.

The 1997 Wisconsin Youth Risk Behavior Study compared ninth through twelfth graders who reported having been threatened or hurt because someone thought they were lesbian, gay, or bisexual with youth who reported no such harassment. Among harassed youth, 53 percent had smoked cigarettes and 52 percent had used marijuana in the past thirty days. In addition, 38 percent had sniffed inhalants (glue, aerosol cans, paints), 25 percent had used LSD ("acid"), and 23 percent had used cocaine (powder, freebase, or crack) at least once in the past (Wisconsin Survey Research Laboratory, 2000).

One of the largest studies of older LGBT persons (416 individuals) found 9 percent of respondents could be classified as "problem drinkers," using the Alcohol Use Disorders Identification Test (AUDIT). Within this cohort men were likely to report more alcohol use than women and more men could be classified as problem drinkers. The studies found no relationship between alcohol use and living status, number of people in the respondents' support network, age, household income, or victimization experiences (Grossman, D'Augelli, & O'Connel, 2001). Shankle, Maxwell, Katzman, & Landers (2003) reveal that the lack of research on substance abuse among older LGBT persons is a huge gap that needs to be addressed.

TOBACCO USE

   Studies of tobacco use among lesbians and gay men, like research on alcohol use, have generally used nonrandom samples. *Healthy People 2010*
designates sexual orientation as one of six demographic categories in which
health disparities exist, and states that some evidence suggests that lesbian
and gay individuals have higher rates of smoking than women and men in
the heterosexual community (USDHHS, 2000). Despite the substantial increase in research on smoking conducted during the past several decades,
the lesbian, gay, bisexual, and transgender population has been largely ignored. The Institute of Medicine's (IOM) report on the status of lesbian
health research concludes that large gaps exist in the current body of knowledge regarding lesbian health, citing substance abuse, including tobacco
use, as one of the primary health problems about which more research is
needed (Solarz, 1999). Although reports of current smoking among lesbian
and gay persons vary widely, the majority of studies report rates that are
substantially higher than those for women and men in the general population
(Hughes, Johnson, & Wilsnack, 2001; Ryan, Wortley, Easton, Pederson, &
Greenwood, 2001).

   Some of the differences in alcohol and tobacco use between lesbians and
their heterosexual counterparts seem to diminish with age. One study found
that lesbians under age fifty smoked at higher rates than their heterosexual
peers. However, lesbian and bisexual women age fifty and older were found
to smoke cigarettes at a similar rate (12.1 percent, 11.3 percent) as their
nonlesbian peers (Gruskin, Hart, Gordon, & Ackerson, 2001).

   Almost no data exist on smoking among LGBT people of color. Heather,
Wortley, Easton, Pederson, & Greenwood (2001) searched studies from
1987 through 2000 on tobacco use among lesbians, gays, and bisexuals.
Smoking rates in these studies of lesbians, gays, and bisexuals ranged from
38 percent to 59 percent among youth and from 11 percent to 50 percent
among adults. National smoking rates during comparable periods ranged
from 28 percent to 35 percent for adolescents and were approximately 28
percent for adults. However, results from a recent study (Hughes, Haas,
Razzano, Cassidy, & Matthews, 2000) of lesbian and heterosexual women
in Chicago, New York City, and St. Paul (Minnesota) suggest that racial/
ethnic minority lesbians may be at greater risk for smoking than their white
counterparts. In this study, racial/ethnic minority lesbians with a high
school education or less were most likely to be current and lifetime smokers.
These investigators conclude that multiple marginalized statuses appear to
compound the risks for smoking.

   In addition to stress, race, age, education, and socioeconomic status,
other important influences include cultural gender-role norms, tobacco ad-

vertising, perceptions of risks and benefits of smoking, peer-group norms and behaviors, and other health behaviors such as alcohol and other drug use (Skinner & Otis, 1996). Sexual orientation may interact with some or all of these factors in ways that influence risk for smoking. For example, lesbians are less likely than heterosexual women to adhere to traditional female gender-role norms and more likely to drink alcohol—factors that may increase risk for smoking. Conversely, lesbians as a group tend to be more highly educated, in part because of fewer family roles and responsibilities (Gonzales et al., 1999). Lesbians also appear to be less influenced by societal pressures to be thin, a factor associated with lower risk of smoking among women (Arday, Edlin, Giovino, & Nelson, 1993). Although interesting and potentially important, until population-based studies that include large samples of lesbians are more feasible, the previously mentioned relationships will remain an untested hypothesis and the question of whether lesbians are more likely than heterosexual women to smoke will remain unanswered (Stall, Greenwood, Acree, Paul, & Coates, 1999).

To date, no empirical data on tobacco use among transgender persons exist. However, given risk factors identified in this population, including poverty, low educational attainment, a high prevalence of injection and noninjection substance use and abuse, stressful living and work environments (e.g., unstable housing, violence), incarceration, HIV seropositivity, and risky sexual behaviors (Clements, 1999), the risk for smoking is likely high.

MEDIA/ADVERTISING INFLUENCES

Media portrayals directly and indirectly influence how people, especially youth and young adults, perceive smoking and the use of alcohol and other drugs. Advertising affects how youth perceive substance use by influencing their perception of people who drink, smoke, or use other substances. Evidence suggests that the tobacco industry aggressively targets the LGBT community (Engardio, 2000). In a survey of the perceptions of more than 300 gay men and lesbians in Los Angeles, 59 percent of respondents either "disagree" that tobacco companies target the LGBT community or were "not aware" that they were being targeted. Nearly one-half (44 percent) of respondents reported that they recalled seeing tobacco companies sponsor bar and nightclub events to promote their products and 50 percent reported using cigarettes during the seven days prior to completing the survey. More than half (53 percent) agreed that tobacco use is an acceptable norm among their peers (Clements, 1999).

Tobacco companies have been successful in adopting the strategies of the alcoholic beverage industry—positioning the tobacco industry as a valuable "friend" to the LGBT community. A spokesperson for Philip Morris Companies, Inc., noted that in 1990 the company contributed more than $800,000 to AIDS-related charities and the following year donated $10,000 to the Gay and Lesbian Alliance (Brucker, 1997). At the same time, LGBT community leaders, organizers, health professionals, advocates, and HIV/AIDS service organizations appear unaware of or unwilling to discuss the implications of accepting tobacco money.

If the media or advertising is used to promote drinking and/or smoking, then media can be effective in discouraging its use. Media messages that overtly include LGBT youth in general are rare, yet media messages represent an untapped resource in conveying positive messages about self-esteem and in decreasing substance use. Federal, state, and local agencies should join forces with LGBT national and community organizations to sponsor counteradvertising that promotes health-positive messages and discourages substance use. Developing partnerships with key individuals in large advertising and marketing firms could facilitate the development of appropriate media messages that both serve the advertisers' function (e.g., selling a product) and the LGBT community (e.g., increasing positive LGBT images, reducing health-negative behaviors, reducing homophobia, and addressing other issues of concern to the LGBT community). Assisting LGBT youth and adult service organizations to reduce dependency on tobacco-industry funding and identifying and cultivating alternative funding to meet their financial needs would loosen the tobacco industry's grip on the LGBT community.

INFERENCES

Too few studies of substance use or abuse in LGBT populations have included sufficient numbers of racial/ethnic minority persons to permit separate analyses. However, the interaction of gender and race/ethnicity also is apparent in LGBT populations, though not always in the same form as is often reported in other non–LGBT-specific research. Gays who are also members of racial/ethnic minority groups are subjected to both antigay and racist attitudes and treatment. Moreover, they are stigmatized, in turn, by their own racial/ethnic and sexual minority communities. Thus, they find themselves occupying a peripheral position in the sexual minority community and within the dominant/mainstream culture (Icard & Traunstein, 1987). This may mean that those of other ethnic cultures may not experience this process in the same manner. It may also suggest that those of nonwhite backgrounds are viewed as "selling out" (Chan, 1995) to the values of another culture. Some evidence suggests that African-American men are more likely than white men to trade sex for drugs (Peterson, 1995). Because heavy drinking is prevalent in the Latino heterosexual and gay male culture, Latino gay men may have higher rates of drinking than either group alone (Tori, 1989).

Bux (1996) drew four conclusions comparing previous and recent research through 1995 relative to gay and lesbian use of alcohol. First, gay men and lesbians appear to be less likely than heterosexuals to abstain from alcohol consumption. Second, gay men appear to exhibit little or no elevated risk for alcohol abuse or heavy drinking (using categories defined by the National Institute of Alcohol Abuse and Alcoholism [NIAAA] as sixty or more drinks per month) relative to heterosexual men. Third, lesbians appear to be at higher risk for heavy drinking and for drinking-related problems than heterosexual women are. At times, lesbians have been found to match gay and heterosexual men in rates of heavy and/or problem drinking. Fourth, studies examining trends in drinking have reported recent decreases in drinking and alcohol-related problems among gay men.

In addition, it is clear that alcohol-free and drug-free alternatives for coming-out or questioning youth, as well as the LGBT adult population, are lacking. Youth who are coming out have few options for socializing other than clubs and bars. In these settings, they are susceptible to exposure to the use of tobacco, alcohol, and illicit drugs. Without question, the LGBT community shares the responsibility for establishing safer and healthier opportunities for LGBT individuals to gather and to socialize. At the same time, the LGBT community is among the groups targeted by the alcohol industry (Drabble, 2000).

RISK FACTORS

Frequently identified as risk factors for increased substance use in the LGBT community, heterosexism and homophobia increase internalized homophobia, shame, and a negative self-concept (Niesen, 1993). Older LGBT individuals, who grew up at a time when societal attitudes toward them were very negative, are likely to be at high risk for alcohol and other substance use.

Likewise with transgender populations, Lombardi and van Servellen (2000) note, "transgendered individuals must navigate through a health care system that is unable to comprehend let alone support transgendered individuals" (p. 293). Bockting, Robinson, & Rosser (1998) and Kammerer, Mason, & Connors (2001) report that in Boston there are no alcohol or drug treatment groups or facilities specifically for transgender people. In addition, when transgender individuals went to lesbian and/or gay twelve-step meetings, friction often came from the lesbian and gay Alcoholics Anonymous (AA) members about their presence. Mental health and substance abuse treatment providers need additional cultural sensitivity training in order to work with transgender clients to identify when gender issues are or are not relevant. Sometimes gender issues are central to mental health or substance abuse treatment, sometimes they are peripheral, and sometimes they are unrelated (JSI Research and Training Institute, 2000).

IMPLICATIONS

In late 1993, the Substance Abuse and Mental Health Services Administration (SAMHSA) Center for Substance Abuse Treatment (CSAT) convened a national multiracial and multiethnic work group of lesbian and gay policy experts, community leaders, and substance abuse treatment providers. Their task was to develop recommendations for increasing access to substance abuse services for lesbian, gay, bisexual, and transgender individuals. The work group believed that their personal and work experience showed that societal bias against homosexual expression and gender role conflicts were the leading causes of the lack of or inappropriate substance use treatment service. Higher rates of substance abuse and addiction put LGBT individuals at higher risk for HIV disease, breast cancer, and other health problems. They concluded that LGBT individuals have historically been underserved or have had to seek substance abuse treatment services that were culturally incompetent, homophobic, and frequently hostile to them regarding their sexual orientation (Craft & Mulvey, 2001).

Craft and Mulvey further shared that in 1997, following requests from the National Association of Alcohol and Drug Abuse Counselors and the six largest HIV/AIDS care providers in the United States, CSAT began to develop, with multiple experts from the LGBT communities, the first primer on LGBT substance abuse. In January 2001, the resulting document—*A Providers Introduction to Substance Abuse Treatment for LGBT Individuals* (Substance Abuse and Mental Health Services Administration, 2001)—CSAT published and disseminated to nearly 20,000 treatment providers and other constituents.

The *Healthy People 2010 Companion Document on Lesbian, Gay, Bisexual, and Transgender (LGBT) Health* (Gay and Lesbian Medical Association & LGBT Health Experts, 2001) illustrates that most health care providers need additional education and training to offer culturally appropriate and linguistically accessible services. The CSAT work group realized that, in the interests of enhancing the likelihood of effective treatment outcomes, mainstream substance abuse treatment providers (i.e., providers who have not recognized or provided specific services to LGBT individuals) were, for the most part, ready to accept guidance that would help them initiate or strengthen culturally competent services for LGBT individuals.

As it is in the general population in the United States, substance abuse in the LGBT community is associated with a myriad of public health challenges, including HIV/AIDS, sexually transmitted infections, violence, and chronic disease conditions such as cirrhosis of the liver. LGBT people may be at high risk for problems that are not directly related to sexual orientation or gender identity (e.g., smoking, obesity, alcohol and drug use). Although such problems are not unique to LGBT people, to the extent that they have a higher prevalence in LGBT populations these problems require special public health attention and unique approaches for investigation, prevention, and treatment (Meyer, 2001). Social conditions that are characterized by rejection and discrimination distinguish the public health of LGBT populations from the general population. Those concerns affect a wide range of issues, including the selection of research priorities, the design of public health prevention and intervention programs, the development of standards of care, access to care, and the provision of culturally sensitive care. Meyer (2001) further explains that the most often addressed area under the public health category is risk related to sexual behavior. Just as important, however, are risks related to social conditions characterized by prejudice, discrimination, and rejection (e.g., antigay violence or racial stress). Such risks may have direct impacts on the incidence of mental and somatic disorders, as well as access to care, health care utilization, and quality of care. Prejudice about same-sex sexuality or gender roles can also lead to the design of insensitive and alienating public health interventions and prevention programs that fail to respect the values and needs of the LGBT community. Finally, a specialized focus may still be required in all public health areas, even those in which LGBT populations do not have a unique or increased risk for disease. For example, provision of adequate care requires that care providers be sensitive to the needs of these populations. Insensitive or hostile care may lead to inappropriate interventions, fail to effect change, and further add to alienation and mistrust of public health recommendations.

The National Institute on Drug Abuse (NIDA) director, Nora Volkow, MD, postulates that "the best approach to reducing the tremendous toll substance abuse exacts from individuals, families, and communities is to prevent the damage before it occurs" (Volkow, 2003, p. 3). The science of drug and alcohol prevention is still in its early stages of developing. What many experts believe is that tomorrow's prevention programs will more closely reflect the people who will take part in them. Beatty et al. (2003) point out that "methods needed to adapt research-based interventions to local community needs or to tailor them to different populations are rarely discussed in journal articles" (p. 235).

Nationally, health care and alcohol and drug treatment organizations are struggling with the challenges to respond to the needs of the LGBT population in all areas of service delivery. Alcohol and drug services to the LGBT population must identify and incorporate cultural factors that are specific to the community. They include an understanding of

- Beliefs, values, traditions, and practices within the LGBT community, which are often dictated by geography, ethnicity, and age
- Identification of the LGBT culturally defined AOD service needs
- Belief systems regarding the etiology of the addiction/abuse and those related to approaching treatment and recovery
- Attitudes toward seeking help from the treatment provider whose staff may exhibit institutional or personal homophobia

Why are alcohol and drug treatment services and prevention efforts different for the LGBT population? The answer is clearly echoed by the LGBT population: because of the need to reveal or hide their LGBT identity with providers they do not know and who are the vital link to treatment. Being honest about one's sexual orientation is a crucial factor in determining health care needs. Knowledge of the beliefs that shape the LGBT person's approach to health and treatment often stem from a direct, negative interaction with his or her primary health care provider. More often than not, the primary health care provider who is vital for the triaging of the LGBT's treatment is unaware of the degree of discrimination a LGBT person has already experienced in the health care/treatment setting. Likewise, they are also unaware of the LGBT individual's resulting fear, discomfort, and mistrust in seeking and getting information. These fears are reasonable and well grounded. A Kings County (Seattle, Washington) 1998 survey of nursing students showed 8 to 12 percent despised lesbian, gay, and bisexual people; 5 to 12 percent found LGB people disgusting, and 40 to 43 percent believed that LGB people should keep their sexuality private. In 1996, 20 percent of 1,027 New Mexico general practitioners, 9.3 percent of family practice physicians, and 4 percent of pediatricians reported that they would discontinue patient referrals to gay or lesbian surgeons.

LGBT individuals are not afforded the same protections in many areas of the country. Disclosure of one's sexual orientation can lead to employment problems or the denial of housing and social services. LGBT individuals may lose custody of their children if their sexual orientation becomes known during a custody dispute. LGBT individuals regard protecting information about their sexual orientation and substance abuse histories as critically important. Programs that treat this population must be particularly sensitive about maintaining clients' confidentiality, because the consequences of an inappropriate disclosure can be devastating.

In order for the LGBT population to trust treatment providers and prevention programs, an atmosphere of openness and affirmation is vital to being successful. Many different components go into creating a prevention approach that is viewed by the LGBT population as inclusive and safe. Few prevention efforts target the LGBT population with marketing and outreach for alcohol and other drugs. Most emphasis has been placed on HIV. Prevention efforts will require that

- experts speak at meetings of LGBT organizations;
- advertisements be placed in LGBT periodicals (do not forget the local service directories and "underground" newsletters);
- information be posted on LGBT Web pages;
- information is tailored to be culturally specific to the geographic area; many times different linguistics exist based on the town or city;
- promotional information specifically states what services are provided without discrimination based on sexual orientation or gender identity;
- a system for maintaining confidentiality of contacts and records is designed, enforced, and publicized;
- health workers have a familiarity with appropriate LGBT health service providers and LGBT groups or organizations are in the area to provide information on specific treatment services, prevention, and medical contacts that are LGBT safe;
- research protocols that are combinations of qualitative and quantitative methods are initiated; and
- key LGBT community figures who are willing to be educated in the area of disseminating alcohol and drug abuse prevention information are identified and educated.

A Washington State family practice physician summarizes the difficulty in eliminating disparities across geographical, ethnic, racial, and sexual orientation lines. "I think it has been hard to get a handle on this . . . we're talking about a culture that was underground 30 years ago" (Pownall, 2001).

RESOURCES

Aftercare and support are critical to full recovery from substance use. Bittle suggested in 1982 that those participating in Alcoholics Anonymous

(AA) meetings should secure a sponsor who is either LGBT or who is comfortable with and knowledgeable about the LGBT community. In addition, he suggests that it must be assumed that a majority of LGBTs coming into AA will require more than an AA group for continued sobriety. Many of the problems will not be considered in standard AA meetings, so it is essential that they maintain contact with a supportive LGBT community. The concepts of "higher power" and "spirituality" are core to traditional AA; however, many religious organizations have been extremely judgmental and condemning of LGBTs. Therefore, these terms may become barriers for many who associate them with organized religion. Many alternative support groups have been developed, such as Women for Sobriety or those exclusive to LGBTs, such as "Gidget Gets Sober" in Pittsburgh, Pennsylvania.

Two of the oldest substance abuse inpatient/outpatient treatment programs exclusively serving the LGBT community are Alternatives, Inc. (www.alternativesinc.org), for more than twenty-five years, and Pride Institute (www.pride-institute.com), for more than seventeen years. The National Association of Lesbian and Gay Addiction Professionals—Serving the LGBT Communities Since 1979 (www.nalgap.org), has a listing of local and national resources (NALGAP, 901 North Washington Street, Suite 600, Alexandria, VA 22314-1535, 703-465-0539). Many local programs also offer separate tracks for LGBT clients or have developed good reputations for working with LGBT communities despite their overall focus on all substance abusers. *A Provider's Introduction to Substance Abuse Treatment for Lesbian, Gay, Bisexual, and Transgender Individuals* (Substance Abuse and Mental Health Services Administration, 2001) is a free government publication. This document serves as both a reference tool and program guide by providing statistical and demographic information, prevalence data, case examples and suggested interventions, treatment guidelines and approaches, and organizational policies and procedures.

Effective treatment for LGBT substance abusers must address the primary symptoms of substance abuse with sensitivity to society and interpersonal concerns that make this community unique. Effective therapists *are* knowledgeable about, skillful in, and comfortable with certain topical areas above and beyond standard clinical substance abuse treatment.

QUESTIONS TO CONSIDER

1. Should drug and alcohol treatment administrators check and edit the mission philosophy or service statement to ensure it includes a commitment to serve LGBT communities?

2. Should drug and alcohol treatment administrators include sexual orientation and gender identity in their nondiscriminatory employment policy?
3. Should drug and alcohol treatment administrators establish firm guidelines regarding client behavior and consistently enforce these guidelines to ensure a treatment atmosphere of safety for LGBT clients?
4. Does establishing the proper ethic of care for LGBT clients require that counselors be aware of and work through their own feelings about these clients?
5. Should providers consult with experts in LGBT issues, such as clients, staff, advocacy groups, or organizations, to provide assistance in developing an LGBT program that is sensitive, supportive, and effective?

REFERENCES

Arday, D. A., Edlin, B. R., Giovino, G. A., & Nelson, D. E. (1993). Smoking, HIV infection and gay men in the United States. *Tobacco Control, 2,* 156-158.

Beatty, R. L., Gruskin, E., His, A., Jillson, I. A., Neisen, J., & Ross, M. (2003). Bridging science and practice in LGBT health. *Clinical Research and Regulatory Affairs, 20,* 229-246.

Bittle, W. E. (1982). Alcoholics Anonymous and the gay alcoholic. In T. O. Ziebold & J. E. Mongeson (Eds.), *Alcoholism and homosexuality* (pp. 81-88). Binghamton, NY: The Haworth Press.

Bloomfield, K. A. (1993). A comparison of alcohol consumption between lesbians and heterosexual women in an urban population. *Drug and Alcohol Dependence, 33,* 257-269.

Bockting, W. O., Robinson, B. E., & Rosser, B. R. S. (1998). Transgender HIV prevention: A qualitative needs assessment. *AIDS Care, 10,* 505-526.

Brucker, E. L. (1997). *Out and free: Sexual minorities and tobacco addiction.* Seattle, WA: King County Health Department.

Bux, D. A. (1996). The epidemiology of drinking in gay men and lesbians: A critical review. *Clinical Psychology Review, 16,* 277-298.

Chan, C. S. (1995). Issues of sexual identity in an ethnic minority: The case of Chinese American lesbians, gay men, and bisexual people. In A. R. D'Augelli & C. J. Peterson (Eds.), *Lesbian, gay and bisexual identities over the lifespan: Psychological perspectives* (pp. 87-101). New York: Oxford University Press.

Clements, N. K. (1999). *The transgender community health project: Descriptive results.* San Francisco: San Francisco Department of Public Health.

Cochran, S. D. & Mays, V. M. (2000). Relation between psychiatric syndromes and behaviorally defined sexual orientation in a sample of the U.S. population. *Journal of Epidemiology, 151*(5), 516-523.

Craft, E. M. & Mulvey, K. P. (2001). Addressing lesbian, gay, bisexual and transgender issues from the inside: One federal agency's approach. *American Journal of Public Health, 91*(6), 163-165.

Drabble, L. (2000). Alcohol, tobacco and pharmaceutical industry funding: Considerations for organizations serving lesbian, gay, bisexual and transgender communities. *Journal of Gay and Lesbian Social Services, 11,* 2.

Engardio, J. P. (2000). Outgoing Marlboro man: Document reveals new details on how tobacco companies target gays. *San Francisco Weekly* (February), 16-22.

Fifield, L., DeCresenzo, T. A., & Latham, J. D. (1975). *On my way to nowhere: Alienated, isolated, drunk.* Los Angeles: Gay and Lesbian Community Services Center.

Finnegan, D. G. & McNally, E. B. (2002). *Counseling lesbian, gay, bisexual and transgender substance abusers: Dual identities.* Binghamton, NY: The Haworth Press.

Garofalo, R., Wolf, R., Cameron, M. S., Kessel, S., Palfrey, J., & DuRant, R. H. (1998). The association between health behaviors and sexual orientation among a school-based sample of adolescents. *Pediatrics, 101,* 895-902.

Gay and Lesbian Medical Association & LGBT Health Experts. (2001). *Healthy people 2010 companion document for lesbian, gay, bisexual, and transgender (LGBT) health.* San Francisco, CA: Gay and Lesbian Medical Association.

Gilman, S. E., Cochran, S. D., Mays, V. M., Hughes, M., Ostrow, D., & Kessler, R. C. (2001). Risks of psychiatric disorders among individuals reporting.same-sex sexual partners in the National Comorbidity Survey. *American Journal of Public Health, 91*(6), 933-939.

Gonzales, C., Washienko, K. M., Krone, M. R., Chapman, L. I., Arredondo, E. M., Huckeba, H. J., & Downder, A. (1999). Sexual and drug-use risk factors for HIV and STDs: A comparison of women with and without bisexual experiences. *American Journal of Public Health, 89*(12), 1841-1846.

Grossman, A. H., D'Augelli, A. R., & O'Connel, T. S. (2001). Being lesbian, gay, bisexual and 60 or older in North America. *Journal of Gay and Lesbian Social Services, 13*(4), 171-179.

Gruskin, E. P., Hart, S., Gordon, N., & Ackerson, L. (2001). Patterns of cigarette smoking and alcohol use among lesbians and bisexual women enrolled in a large health maintenance organization. *American Journal of Public Health, 91*(6), 976-979.

Heather, R., Wortley, P., Easton, A., Pederson, L., & Greenwood, G. (2001). Smoking among lesbians, gays, and bisexuals: A review of the literature. *American Journal of Preventive Medicine, 21*(2), 142-149.

Hughes, T. L. & Eliason, M. (2002). Substance use and abuse in lesbian, gay, bisexual and transgender populations. *Journal of Primary Prevention, 22*(3), 263-298.

Hughes, T. L., Hass, A. P., Razzano, L., Cassidy, R., & Matthews, A. K. (2000). Comparing lesbian and heterosexual women's mental health: Findings from a multi-site study. *Journal of Gay and Lesbian Social Services, 11*(1), 57-76.

Hughes, T. L., Johnson, T. P., & Wilsnack, S. C. (2001). Sexual assault and alcohol abuse: A comparison of lesbian and heterosexual women. *Journal of Substance Abuse, 13,* 515-532.

Icard, L. & Traunstein, D. M. (1987). Black, gay, alcoholic men: Their character and treatment. *Social Casework, 68*(5), 267-272.

JSI Research and Training Institute. (2000). Access to health care for transgendered persons in greater Boston. Retrieved July 9, 2005, from http://www.glbthealth.org/documents/transaccessstudy.pdf.

Kammerer, N., Mason, T., & Connors, M. (2001). Transgender health and social service needs in the context of HIV risk. In W. O. Bockting & S. Kirk (Eds.), *Transender and HIV: Risks, prevention and care* (pp. 13-38). Binghamton, NY: The Haworth Press.

K-Y Liquid Community Health Survey. (2000). Conducted at the LGBT Millennium March, Washington, DC, April 29-30.

Lombardi, E. L., van Servellen, G. (2000). Building culturally sensitive substance use prevention and treatment programs for transgendered populations. *Journal of Substance Abuse Treatment 19*(3): 291-296.

Massachusetts Youth Risk Behavior Survey. (1998). 1997 Massachusetts Youth Risk Behavior Survey Results. Retrieved September 13, 2005, from http://www.doe.mass.edu/hssss/yrbs97/97yrbsexec.html.

Matthews, A. K., Hughes, T. L., Johnson, T., Razzano, L. A., & Cassidy, R. (2002). Prediction of depressive distress in a community sample of women: The role of sexual orientation. *American Journal of Public Health, 92*(7), 1131-1139.

Meyer, I. H. (2001). Why lesbian, gay, bisexual and transgender public health? *American Journal of Public Health, 91*(6), 14-17.

National Survey on Drug Use and Health. (2002). Results from the 2002 National Survey on Drug Use and Health: National findings. Rockville, MD: DHHS, SAMHSA. Retrieved April 12, 2004, from http://www.osa.samhsa.gov/NHSDA/2k2NSDUH/Results/2k2results.htm.

Niesen, J. H. (1993). Healing from cultural victimization: Recovery from shame due to heterosexism. *Journal of Gay and Lesbian Psychotherapy, 2,* 49-63.

Peterson, J. L. (1995). AIDS-related risks and same-sex behaviors among African American men. In G. Herek & B. Green (Eds.), *AIDS, identity and community* (pp. 85-104). Thousand Oaks, CA: Sage Publications.

Pownall, E. (2001). Removing the barriers: Subtle and not-so-subtle forms of discrimination create obstacles in lesbian health care. *Eugene Weekly,* Online edition, *20*(18). Retrieved July 11, 2005, from http://www2.eugeneweekly.com/2001/05_03_01/coverstory.html.

Rebac, C. & Lombardi, E. L. (2001). A community-based harm reduction program for male-to female transgenders at risk for HIV infection. In W. Bocking & S. Kirk (Eds.), *Transgender and HIV* (pp. 59-68). Binghamton, NY: The Haworth Press.

Ryan, C. & Hunter, J. (2001). Clinical issues with youth. In *A provider's introduction to substance abuse treatment for lesbian, gay, bisexual and transgender individuals* (pp. 99-104). UDHHS/SAMHSA/CSAT publication number (SMA) 03-3819. Washington, DC: U.S. Department of Health and Human Services.

Ryan, H., Wortley, P. M., Easton, A., Pederson, L., & Greenwood, G. (2001). Smoking among lesbians, gays, and bisexuals. *American Journal of Preventive Medicine, 21,* 142-149.

SAMHSA Office of Applied Science. (1989). *National Household Survey on Drug Abuse.* Rockville, MD: SAMHSA.

Sanfort, T. G. M., de Graaf, R., Bijl, R. V., & Schnabel, P. (2001). Same-sex sexual behavior and psychiatric disorders: Findings from the Netherlands Mental Health Survey and Incidence Study (NEMESIS). *Archives of General Psychiatry, 58*(1), 85-91.

Shankle, M. D., Maxwell, C. A., Katzman, E. S., & Landers, S. (2003). An invisible population: Older lesbians, gay, bisexual and transgender individuals. *Clinical Research and Regulatory Affairs, 20,* 159-182.

Skinner, W. F. (1994). The prevalence and demographic predictors of illicit and licit drug use among lesbians and gay men. *American Journal of Public Health, 89,* 1307-1310.

Skinner, W. F. & Otis, M. D. (1996). Drug and alcohol use among lesbian and gay people in a southern U.S. sample: Epidemiological, comparative, and methodological findings from the Trilogy Project. *Journal of Homosexuality, 30*(3), 59-92.

Solarz, A. L. (Ed.). (1999). *Lesbian health: Current assessment and directions for the future Institute of Medicine Committee on Lesbian Health Research Priorities.* Washington, DC: National Academy Press, Institutes of Medicine.

Stall, R. D., Greenwood, G. L., Acree, M., Paul, J., & Coates, T. J. (1999). Cigarette smoking among gay and bisexual men. *American Journal of Public Health, 89*(12), 1875-1878.

Stall, R. D., Paul, J. P., Greenwood, G., Pollack, L. M., Bein, E., Crosby, G. M., Mills, T. C., Binson, D., Coates, T. J., & Catania, J. A. (2001). Alcohol use, drug use and alcohol-related problems among men who have sex with men: The urban men's health study. *Addiction, 96,* 1589-1601.

Stall, R. D. & Wiley, J. (1988). A comparison of alcohol and drug use patterns of homosexual and heterosexual men: The San Francisco Men's Health Study. *Drug and Alcohol Dependence, 22,* 63-73.

Substance Abuse and Mental Health Services Administration. (2001). *A provider's introduction to substance abuse treatment for lesbian, gay, bisexual, and transgender individuals.* Rockville, MD: U.S. Department of Health and Human Services.

Tori, D. C. (1989). Homosexuality and illegal residency status in relation to substance abuse and personality traits among Mexican nations. *Journal of Clinical Psychology, 45*(5), 814-821.

U.S. Department of Health & Human Services. (2000). *Healthy people 2010* (2nd ed.) (Volumes1 & 2). Washington, DC: GPO.

Valentine, E. (1998). *Gender identity project: Report on intake statistics, 1989-April.* New York: The Lesbian and Gay Community Center.

Vermont Department of Health. (1997). The 1997 Youth Risk Behavior Survey. Retrieved July 11, 2005, from http://www.state.vt.us/adap/yrbs97a.htm.

Volkow, N. D. (2003). Bringing research and practice together to improve drug abuse prevention. *NIDA Notes, 18,* 3.

Wisconsin Survey Research Laboratory. (1997). Wisconsin Youth Risk Behavior Survey. Madison: University of Wisconsin—Extension of Public Instruction. Retrieved December 14, 2000, from www.dpi.state.wi.us/dpi/dlsea/sspw/yrbsindex97.html.

Xavier, J. M. (2000). *The Washington transgender needs assessment survey.* Washington, DC: Department of Health of the District of Columbia.

Chapter 10

Health Care Delivery and Public Health Related to LGBT Youth and Young Adults

Joyce Hunter
Alwyn T. Cohall
Gerald P. Mallon
Matthew B. Moyer
James P. Riddel Jr.

INTRODUCTION

Many lesbian, gay, bisexual, and transgender (LGBT) youth are resilient, live at home, and are not seen in social services agencies or community health clinics. Others have very different accounts of their lives. Homosexual and transgender youth are stigmatized within their communities and schools. This stigmatization plays a role in increasing vulnerability to and risk for negative mental, emotional, and physical health outcomes. In a heterosexist culture, many youth hide their sexual orientation, creating stressful situations that contribute to increased mental health problems, including depression and suicide ideation (Hunter & Mallon, 2000; Havens, Mellins, & Hunter, 2002). Although coming out to others is often a positive step in their personal identity development, it greatly increases their risk for harassment and violence (D'Augelli, 1996). This stigmatization also results in harassment and violence toward those who cannot hide their sexual orientation or gender identity (Hunter & Schaecher, 1992; Human Rights Watch, 2001). Many LGBT youth suffer from a lack of adult and/or peer support once they have disclosed their sexual identities, creating barriers to accessing care (Cohall et al., 2004; East & El Rayess, 1998; Ginsburg et al., 2002). Risk behaviors, including early sexual activities; sexually transmitted infections (STIs), including HIV; and substance use are higher in the LGBT populations than in the heterosexual adolescent population (Garofalo, Wolf, Kessel, Falfrey, & DuRant, 1998).

When addressing the health concerns and needs of LGBT youth, we must look at the myriad influences on their health. Parent and family support and supervision may have an impact on a young person's comfort with his or her sexual and/or gender identity (Li, Stanton, & Feigelman, 2000; U.S. Surgeon General, 2001). Many parents or guardians, however, do not have accurate knowledge of their young people's sexual activities or health risks, as many young people do not disclose their sexual or drug behaviors to their families. Parents may not be effective as teachers of knowledge and attitudes regarding sexual health, including HIV (Sigelman, Mukai, Woods, & Alfeld, 1995). As youth reach adolescence, a time of significant physical, psychosocial, and sexual development, many heterosexual adolescents confide in their peers and rely on them for information and support (Ryan & Hunter, 2001). LGBT adolescents have issues and needs in relation to their emerging sexual orientation and are not always able to confide in either their families or peers.

Youth who identify as transgender are many times included in programs serving LGB youth. They face a multitude of additional challenges, trying to find a sense of themselves in terms of their gender and sexual identities in a hostile society. Youth who identify as transgender (gender identities/expressions different from birth sex) have often been rejected by family, peers, and social institutions, including health care providers, and as a result experience high levels of homelessness and denial of employment and education, creating mental-health- and stress-related risk behaviors. As a result of this "transphobia," they often underutilize medical and social services (Israel & Tarver, 1997).

Communities and cultures, including schools, social service agencies, religious institutions, and faith-based social services, teach and influence youth. Cultures vary greatly in their attitudes toward and treatment of LGBT youth. State and federal laws for funding influence and in many cases restrict the curriculum for sexual health and HIV prevention in the schools (e.g., funding for an abstinence-only or abstinence-based curriculum in recent years). Supportive role models for LGBT youth, both adult and peer, are often lacking in the school and community.

Thus, many young LGBT individuals are without the traditional resources of family, peers, and community. In addition to the alienation and isolation, many others experience high levels of harassment and violence, often in middle and high school settings. These experiences result in high drop-out rates among the most vulnerable (Garofalo & Katz, 2001). In extreme cases, young people find themselves homeless or in the foster care system.

Lack of access to needed health care can be a result of both the alienation from society and the hiding of one's sexual activities. Youth who are not living at home or do not have the family and community support they need for other reasons find health care difficult to access and are at increased risk for health problems. Often these young people do not trust health care providers and will not disclose sexual activities that may put them at risk for diseases such as HIV or STIs (Hunter, Cohall, Castrucci, & Ellis, 2001).

Young men and women in disadvantaged urban communities, communities of color, those who are homeless, and young men who have sex with men (YMSM) are the tragic new face of AIDS in communities across the United States (Centers for Disease Control & Prevention [CDC], 2002a; Kates & Wilson Leggoe, 2005). Their partners and others in neighborhoods or venues already impacted by HIV are also at high risk.

Health care professionals have important roles to play as they interact with youth at regular checkups or in times of health crisis—developing rapport, asking questions, gathering assessment data, giving information, and providing services and referrals. These opportunities are often missed because of provider discomfort in discussing sexual behaviors, sexuality, and homosexuality; a lack of training on the part of the health care professional in general to care for LGBT youth; and/or a lack of knowledge or confusion about the youth's legal rights to information and privacy in the health care setting (Ryan & Futterman, 1998; Allen, Glicken, Beach, & Naylor, 1998).

This chapter will focus on LGBT youth and young adults' general health care, STI and HIV issues, and the health needs of at-risk youth in and out of the foster care system. Recommendations and resources for health care professionals in schools, community-based organizations (CBOs), hospitals, and clinics are included to effectively enable health care professionals to provide service to LGBT youth.

PROVIDING OPTIMAL HEALTH SERVICES
FOR LGBT YOUNG PEOPLE IN MEDICAL SETTINGS

Why a Special Focus on Health Needs of LGBT Young People?

Adolescence represents a time period marked by experimentation—a necessary prerequisite for cognitive growth and maturation. In some cases, significant risk-taking and health-compromising behaviors may be initiated during adolescence with resultant morbidity and mortality. Steps have been made to improve the general well-being of adolescents. In recognition of the need for health providers to improve their ability to identify, address, and prevent risk-taking behaviors, the American Medical Association (Elster & Kuznets, 1997), the Society for Adolescent Medicine (Rosen, Elster, Hedberg, Paperny, 1997), and other professional organizations have developed several guidelines and protocols that are broadly applicable to all youth, including LGBT youth.

LGBT youth deserve special care and attention, with a higher prevalence of voluntary and involuntary involvement in risk-taking behaviors than their heterosexual peers (Rosario, Meyer-Bahlburg, Hunter, & Gwadz, 1999). Levels of risk taking are higher, begin earlier, and are frequently clustered together. Examples of risk-taking behaviors include school avoidance, substance use, alcohol use, multiple sexual partners, suicidal attempts, carrying a weapon, and fighting (Garofalo et al., 1998). Although care must be taken to balance this "deficit" model with an appreciation of the strengths and assets of LGBT youth, it is important for providers to pay special attention to the health issues that may compromise the well-being of LGBT young adults.

In addition to the heightened risks for physical and emotional health problems, these youth also have to cope with other health concerns such as asthma, obesity, and diabetes. Thus, the importance of comprehensive medical evaluation and management is underscored with appropriate linkages to community resources for mental health, substance-abuse counseling, and concrete services to address vocational, educational, housing, and recreational needs.

Barriers to Accessing Care

Close supervision and support by health care professionals of these populations are frequently lacking (Hunter, Cohall, Castrucci, & Ellis, 2001). LGBT youth have had previous negative encounters with health professionals, which may affect their subsequent interactions with medical providers (Cohall et al., 2004; East & El Rayess, 1998; Garofalo, 2001; Ginsberg et al., 2002; Ryan & Futterman, 1998). LGBT young people are reluctant to seek services of health care professionals for fear of further stigmatization, rejection, and embarrassment. This reluctance, combined with concomitant depression, may undermine help-seeking behavior. They may also harbor concerns about whether health providers can truly keep their interactions confidential. Thus LGBT youth will often either avoid services altogether or keep their sexual identity hidden from the provider (East & El Rayess, 1998; Ginsberg et al., 2002). Extrinsically, they may not know where to go to receive appropriate care, or the services in their communities may be inadequate or inconvenient. Those who run away, are displaced, homeless, or have recently entered the United States often lack adequate health insurance, which often precludes acquisition of comprehensive health services in a consistent medical setting.

Effective Interventions with LGBT Youth in Primary Care Settings

LGBT youth can be found in any practice setting in any community. Thus, "finding" LGBT youth is not difficult. However, as noted previously, unless providers create a welcoming atmosphere and demonstrate a nonjudgmental attitude, LGBT youth may be reluctant to disclose personal information, thus limiting opportunities for prevention, early identification and intervention, and appropriate follow-up (see Exhibit 10.1).

In general, providers should adopt a "client-centered" approach to patient care that strives to identify the specific strengths as well as concerns of the individual client. Careful attention to establishing privacy, confidentiality, and rapport will facilitate communication between adolescent and provider, leading to subsequent disclosure of information that will ultimately form the basis of developing a tailored treatment plan. The provider may become a critical link in providing support and arranging for additional services as needed for the young LGBT clients and their families. Thus, a higher premium should be placed on the provider's ability to successfully engage LGBT youth in care. Establishing this connection may be a critical step in the successful transition for LGBT youth into healthy adulthood.

The following is an approach to working with LGBT youth in general primary care settings, such as private practice, outpatient, hospital, or community health centers. Modifications may be necessary in working with youth in other clinical settings such as the emergency room, runaway shelter, or juvenile detention facilities.

EXHIBIT 10.1. Effective Medical Interventions with LGBT Youth

Effective medical interventions with LGBT youth should focus on, but not be limited to

1. *prevention* (immunizations to protect against hepatitis and counseling on safer sex practices to reduce HIV exposure);
2. *early identification of health issues* (screening and detection of STIs, depression, and substance use, including tobacco);
3. *treatment* (antibiotics for gonorrhea and other STIs; counseling and careful use of antidepressants);
4. *health promotion counseling* (importance of diet, exercise, stress management, tobacco cessation, etc.); and
5. *referral for additional services* (individual, couples, family psychosocial counseling; educational, vocational, legal, and recreational services).

Creating a Welcoming Atmosphere

1. *Sensitivity and cultural competency training of frontline and ancillary staff (receptionists, medical assistants, etc.) is essential.* The adage "you may never get a second chance to make a first impression" is very important, as youth may be turned off (or, alternatively, comforted) by the comments or behavior of other staff. For example, male-to-female transgender youth may welcome the opportunity to be addressed by their female name by the receptionist. Conversely, failure to acknowledge and respect the client's wishes in this regard sets the stage for confrontation and alienation.

2. *Providers should have an array of health information materials in their waiting rooms that include topics of interest to LGBT young people.* These materials (e.g., LGBT newsletters, magazines, comic books), are available from CBOs serving this population. They are educational and also alert youth that the practice setting is comfortable addressing their needs.

3. *As standard practice, providers need to escort patients to a private area and explain, with appropriate written and/or audiovisual materials, the practice's approach to providing confidentiality.* Although Health Insurance Portability and Accountability Act (HIPAA) regulations underscore the overall importance of protecting patient confidentiality, specific language should be added to patient materials that let adolescents know that their discussions with providers will be protected from parental intrusion unless the provider becomes concerned about suicide, homicide, or the adolescent's inability to make concerted efforts to safeguard his or her health. Providers should clearly articulate to youth that in the event that they will need to break confidentiality, youth must be given the courtesy of an explanation.

4. *The assessment/evaluation process begins with the provider asking the young person to fill out a brief questionnaire to elicit responses to questions in order to assess health-promoting and health-compromising behaviors* (Elster & Kuznets, 1997). Audio or computerized questionnaires have been well received (Boekeloo et al., 1994). Adolescents report they answer queries honestly and in many instances prefer the computer to live interviewers (Paperny, 1997).

The Initial Interview: Recommendations

1. If the adolescent is accompanied by a parent, guardian, or friend, *it is critically important to conduct the interview in private* after a suitable time period has passed for introductions, establishing the reason for the visit, and

obtaining specific pieces of information the adolescent may not know (e.g., birth and early childhood history, family medical history, etc.).

2. *Establishing clear ground rules for privacy and confidentiality* become key cornerstones prior to initiating the evaluation of any young patient, particularly LGBT young people who may understandably be sensitive to these issues.

3. *The provider must establish rapport with the adolescent patient,* such as with a few minutes of "small talk," allowing the adolescent to relax and begin to trust the provider. Sample strategies for putting the adolescent at ease include

    A. minimizing distractions from telephones, pagers, and beepers;
    B. looking directly at the patient and avoiding initially taking notes;
    C. asking the young person for his or her preferred name or nickname; and/or
    D. initiating an innocuous inquiry about jewelry, clothing, tattoos, or piercings.

Providers must not presume heterosexuality in evaluating and treating adolescent patients. This implies that heterosexuality is the norm and may further inhibit the LGBT young person from honest disclosure of his or her sexual behaviors.

4. *After responding to any urgent presenting health problems, a comprehensive assessment of health-promoting and health-compromising behaviors may begin.* If written or computerized questionnaires have been utilized, the responses should be reviewed with the client. If not, the provider may consider using the "HEADSS" acronym (home, education, activities, drugs, suicide, and sex) as a guide for the types of subject areas to investigate (Goldenring & Rosen, 2004) (see selected sample questions in Table 10.1). The structure of the conversation can contribute to making the patient feel comfortable enough to answer honestly.

    A. *Providers need to start the interview by asking about relatively nonthreatening areas such as hobbies or activities before pursuing potentially sensitive areas such as sexuality or substance use.* Providers may initially feel reluctant to ask sensitive questions because of a lack of training in these areas, or providers are not sure how to address affirmative responses regarding these areas. Despite outward appearances to the contrary, adolescents want and need support and advice from adults, particularly health professionals. As long as they perceive the provider to be genuine and empathetic, they will generally be open and honest in their responses—even if the provider fumbles a bit in the delivery of the question.

    B. *Normalize the exploration of these sensitive areas.* Sample questions are provided only as a starting point to initiate conversation.

"In my practice, many of the young people who come in have begun to date. Can you tell me a bit about your feelings about dating? Are you attracted to anyone? How about right now? If so, is that person male or female?"

C. *Further questions about sexual experimentation, along with an exploration of attitudes toward and use of condoms and contraceptive devices, potential or actual exposure to infectious diseases, experience with pregnancy, and involvement in coercive relationships, are essential.*

Inquiry into aspects of a youth's general health, e.g., activities, environment, safety, abuse, depression, drug use, and sexual behaviors, are important. Following are rationale and sample questions for these areas from the HEADSS Questionnaire (Goldenring & Rosen, 2004). These give providers direction in the assessment interview.

5. *The Examination*

A. *Exam may be complete or focused on a particular concern,* depending on the nature of the presenting complaint and time constraints.

B. *Pay particular attention to scars and healed wounds and note how the adolescent acquired them.* In some cases, this may lead to provision of information requiring further evaluation, such as about trauma, abuse, victimization, or self-mutilation.

C. *Examination should also include anal-genital inspection and evaluation for signs of infection or trauma.* Regardless of sexual orientation, adolescents may experiment with sexual activities with either sex. All females should be encouraged to obtain regular pelvic exams and pap smears. Even those female adolescents who currently state that they have only same-sex partners may have had a history of voluntary or involuntary sexual experiences with males. It is important to determine potential exposure to human papillomavirus (HPV) or herpes simplex virus (HSV) infections for both sexes.

6. *Lab Tests and Immunizations.* Obtaining and/or ordering lab tests and immunizations should be geared to findings from the medical history and physical exam, as well as an understanding of pertinent health concerns of adolescents and LGBT youth.

7. *Youth who report sexual activity should receive HIV counseling and testing during the office visit.* The availability of effective treatment underscores the need for early detection. Providers may delay testing temporarily until the youth has obtained additional evaluation and needed resources.

8. *Health Promotion*

A. Provide young people with information and guidance about health promotion (e.g., diet, handling peer pressure, safer sex, substance abuse, tobacco cessation, coping with stress).

B. Specific issues of focused importance to LGBT youth include disclosure of orientation to parents and friends and dealing with stigma, violence, and victimization as a result of their sexual orientation.
C. Providers may need to focus on one or two main issues for discussion at the initial visit and reserve others for review at subsequent visits.
D. Have print and/or audiovisual materials on hand to disseminate to adolescents and their significant others.
E. Young people can be referred to additional health information and engage in interactive health communication through the additional Internet resources listed in Prevention Programs.

9. *Referrals*. After identifying a need to further evaluate or treat the adolescent, the provider may address other issues not covered during subsequent visits or may refer certain concerns to other professionals or agencies. Providers should have a listing of community resources in their offices in order to facilitate appropriate referrals.

10. *"Oh by the way . . ."* Not infrequently, as the visit draws to a close and the adolescent is preparing to leave, he or she will reveal another concern or may correct information that was previously presented to the provider. The provider should quickly assess the parameters of the concern and make a plan with the adolescent for further evaluation (Boggio & Cohall, 1990).

TABLE 10.1. Sample Questions from the HEADSS Questionnaire

Topic	Sample Questions
Activities: Can provide a glimpse into potential strengths/talents of the client in addition to their support network. This may also indicate potential areas of concern, particularly for youth who appear isolated.	What kinds of things do you like to do with your friends? What are some things that your friends are involved with that might be considered dangerous? What is the most dangerous thing you have ever done? How much time do you spend on the Internet? How do you use the Internet? Do you ever visit chat rooms? Have you ever used the Internet to meet someone?
Environment and Safety: May provide an indication of potential or actual stressors that can influence risk-taking behaviors.	Tell me a bit about your neighborhood. Any concerns about the safety of yourself or your friends? Any specific incidents? Have you felt threatened by anyone or by a group of youths who threatened you, either verbally or physically? Have you ever been involved in a fight? If so, what were the circumstances? Do you ever carry a weapon? Have you ever been arrested for loitering?

TABLE 10.1 *(continued)*

Topic	Sample Questions
Abuse: May provide an indication of potential or actual stressors that can influence risk-taking behaviors.	Has there ever been a time in your life when you were verbally, physically, and/or sexually assaulted or victimized?
Depression:	Do you ever feel down or sad? In an average week, how often do you cry? Do you feel like you just cannot get out of bed in the morning? Do you ever feel as if life is not worth living? Have you ever had any thoughts of hurting yourself? Have you actually made any attempts to hurt yourself? If so, what did you do and did anyone find out? When was the last time you felt like this?
Drugs: May provide an indication of potential maladaptive coping strategies that can ultimately exacerbate other risk-taking behaviors.	During adolescence, some young people will experiment with alcohol, tobacco, or other drugs (ATOD). Are any of your friends involved with any of these activities? How about you? If so, which ones and how often do you participate in these activities? Do you ever get high by yourself? Do you find that using ATOD helps you cope with stress? Do you have concerns about your involvement with ATOD?
Sex: Can be either source of support or tension, and thus can either mitigate or accentuate problems in other areas.	Have you started to date? Do you find yourself attracted to males, females, or both sexes? Are you currently involved in a relationship? If so, how are things going? What makes your current partner special? How physically intimate has this relationship gotten? Have you had sex with your current partner? If so, what kinds of sexual experiences have you tried with your current partner? How do you stay safe during sex? How old were you when you began to have sex? From then until now, how many different partners have you had? How many partners were male? How many partners were female? (If male and history of same-sex experiences: Generally are you a "top" or "bottom"? Have you ever had any experiences with unprotected oral or anal sex?) Any concerns about sexual performance? Have you ever been tested for any STIs? If so, how did the tests come out? Have you ever been tested for HIV? When and where were you tested? How did your test results come out? Have you ever been involved in a pregnancy? If so, what happened?

Source: Adapted from Goldenring & Rosen, 2004.

SEXUAL HEALTH: RISK FACTORS AND PREVENTION RELATED TO HIV AND STIs

Risk Factors

HIV/AIDS and other STIs among LGBT young people are a major concern of public health researchers and service providers. Public-health-related programs and services targeting these populations continue to be needed in response to unacceptably high rates of new cases of HIV and STIs, reports of depression, suicide ideation, violence, and other health-related conditions.

It is estimated that at least 40,000 new cases of HIV infection occur each year in the United States. As many as 50 percent of these are among young people under the age of twenty-five, and as many as 25 percent of those cases are among young people under age twenty-two (CDC, 2002b). HIV testing centers continue to report new infections among young men and women in their early twenties and a relative decline in young adults tested.

Most individuals who are infected with HIV have not been tested and do not know their HIV status, which denies them opportunities for treatment or for taking precautions to protect themselves and their partners (CDC, 1999). The long incubation period of the HIV virus, the steady increase in cases every year, and the continued seroconversion of previously negative men in high-risk groups strongly indicate that young people are continuing to become infected at unacceptable rates. Many young people, including young gay men, underestimate how likely they are to be exposed to STIs, including HIV (Crosby & DeCarlo, 2000).

Young gay males and ethnic minority men are particularly vulnerable to STIs (CDC, 2001). The MSM population (men who have sex with men), including men of color, is still the largest exposure group (Valleroy et al., 2000). In some metropolitan areas 3 to 4 percent of young men who have sex with men (YMSM) from the ages of fifteen to twenty-five contract HIV each year, surpassing the rate of men over the age of twenty-five. Depending on the geographic region, rates of syphilis and gonorrhea continue to increase among young gay male populations.

Sexual identity development is a normal process of exploration and adolescent development. Not all young men who have sex with men identify as gay or bisexual. Some also have sex with women. The use of "MSM," and for young men "YMSM," describe the behaviors rather than the self-identification as gay or bisexual.

Transgender youth are a largely hidden population. Therefore few data are available on prevalence of HIV incidence in this population. Many of them are homeless and/or street youth with accompanying health risks. One risk behavior in particular is injection of hormones. Many obtain the hormones illegally and often share needles to inject the hormones, creating a high risk for spreading HIV. Most HIV-prevention and safer sex messages do not reach these youth, or the messages may be ignored by them as not applicable (Dugan, 1998).

Young women have high rates of infections such as chlamydia, gonorrhea, and pelvic inflammatory disease (CDC, 2001). Although woman-to-woman transmission of HIV has rarely been documented, the virus can be transmitted through vaginal secretions and menstrual blood. Some bisexual women and lesbians, especially during exploration of personal and sexual identity, have unsafe sex with men, inject drugs, or practice unsafe sex. STIs are just as common for lesbians as for women who have sex with men (CDC, 2001a).

The advent of HIV drug therapies and medications that reduce morbidity and mortality offer false hope and seem to encourage unsafe behaviors (CDC, 2002b). Many reasons are put forward for these attitudes: now that drugs are available, young people are not as afraid of the disease (e.g., they see posters of muscle-bound men with messages such as "life goes on, take your meds"); they are tired of hearing about what they should not do; they desire to be part of a group of people who are getting attention, such as the young HIV-positive adults receiving services in the community; or they lack hope for the future (Hogarth, 2003).

These increased risk-taking behaviors (e.g., increased sexual risk taking, high rates of drug and alcohol use), apparent complacency, and lack of information continue to place young people at even greater risk of HIV infection (CDC, 2001b).

Young people who are sexually active need to get tested at least annually for HIV and STIs. Testing is not a substitute for safer sex behaviors. Young women also need annual gynecological checkups and pap smears. Youth with evidence of STIs or abnormal pap smears may need semiannual evaluations. Sexually active youth should receive hepatitis A and B immunizations prophylactically.

Prevention and the Roles of Health Care Professionals

Community-level interventions are needed to fight the epidemic in America's youth. Due to the increasing prevalence of HIV, other STIs, and the reported increases in risk behaviors by many LGBT young people, prevention efforts must be increased. Health care professionals and organizations, singly and through links among social service agencies, medical institutions, and local and state health departments, must reach out to both

HIV-negative and HIV-positive young people. A range of comprehensive prevention and treatment services—outreach; medical counseling, testing, and referral (CTR) for social and mental health issues; individual and group counseling; and follow-up support—are essential services for these populations (HRSA, 1997).

HIV-positive young people are themselves at risk for reinfection (secondary infection). They are also at high risk for emotional and behavioral problems, including unsafe sexual and drug behaviors, that put themselves and their partners at risk (Hunter & Haymes, 1997; Rotheram-Borus, Mann, & Chabon, 1999). These young people need extensive intervention for adherence to medications and for the development of coping skills to deal with the physical and emotional issues that arise with having a seropositive status.

Strategies for Providing Competency-Based Health Services for LGBT Youth and Young Adults

1. *Acknowledge that LGBT young people are your clients.* In making an assessment, do not assume that your client is heterosexual. The only way that you will know someone's sexual orientation is if they tell you. Clients will tell you who they are when and if they feel ready. They will also come out when they feel that a safe environment has been created for them to disclose.
2. *Educate yourself and your co-workers about LGBT-youth issues.* Familiarize yourself with the literature, bring in speakers, or ask an openly gay or lesbian professional to discuss gay and lesbian issues with colleagues.
3. *Use gender-neutral language.* If you use language that assumes a person is heterosexual (e.g., inquiring about a woman's boyfriend or husband), gay or lesbian clients may not feel that you are knowledgeable about their orientation and may not share valuable information with you. The use of words and terms such as "partner" or "someone special in your life" are appropriate to use.
4. *Use the words "gay," "lesbian," "bisexual," and "transsexual" in an appropriate context.* As health care professionals, we often refer to groups of people (i.e., Latino, African American, Asian American, etc.). Be inclusive and also mention LGBT people.
5. *Have literature and other visible signs in the waiting room or office that help to create an LGBT-affirming environment.* Magazines, pamphlets, and posters with the words "lesbian" or "gay" printed on them

let clients know that you are sensitive and that your office is a safe place.

6. *If clients disclose to you that they are LGBT—Talk about it!* Do not just move on; talk about what it means for this client to be LGBT and process those feelings with the client.

7. *Do not confuse gender-identity issues* (i.e., transsexuality or transvestism) *with sexual-orientation issues.* Be aware that young people with gender-identity issues are also members of sexual minority communities and will require services to meet their needs.

8. *Research resources in the gay and lesbian community.* Find out about and go visit the resources that exist for people from the gay and lesbian community.

PREVENTION PROGRAMS

Several things need to occur for HIV-prevention efforts to be successful (CDC, 1999; Harper & DiCarlo, 1999). Information is essential, but information alone is not sufficient for stopping the continuing spread of the virus. Effective HIV-prevention programs may need to be targeted to high-risk young people (particularly those who use drugs and are sexually active) in order to reach these often-hidden populations.

Sex Education in Our Schools

Comprehensive sex education and HIV-prevention education does not increase sexual activity among young people. In fact, the United States still has much higher rates of teen pregnancy and HIV than European countries, where the age of first intercourse is similar, but where sexuality education is taught in the schools from early ages (Ehrhardt, 1993). Young people continue to report that sexual health education in schools lacks needed information and skills building for healthy and safe sexual development (SIECUS, 2001).

Abstinence-only or abstinence-based curricula, currently funded by public (i.e., CDC, state and city departments of health) and private sources and implemented widely in schools and faith-based organizations, has not been shown to be effective in providing young people with the skills to protect themselves from sexual risks (Jemmott, Jemmott, & Fong, 1998). Furthermore, "abstinence only until marriage" alleviates discussing sensitive issues such as gay, lesbian, or transgender identities, which marginalizes LGBT young people even more (SIECUS, 2001).

Recommendations—Comprehensive Sex Education

1. Appropriate and comprehensive sex education needs to begin early, before young people have become sexually active (Bachanas et al., 2002).
2. Quality sex-education curricula must include sexual development, sex- and drug-related risk-taking behaviors, development of negotiation skills, and discussion of social and cultural norms as well as feelings and values.
3. Comprehensive health and sexuality education must target both those who identify as LGBT and those who do not (Hunter & Mallon, 1998). Young LGBT people who face homophobia, hatred, racism, poverty, and isolation are very much struggling day to day, finding the means to live while avoiding violence. Youth struggling with sexual identity issues need reassurance that sexual identity development is a process.
4. Sustained interventions as well as more intense interventions are more likely to lead to sustained behavior change or risk reduction (Collins, 1997; IOM, 2000; CDC, 1999). Skills building, information, and modification of the group's social norms taken together are more likely to enhance behavior change (St. Lawrence et al., 1995). Young people need to personalize general knowledge into behavior change and to develop skills in order to negotiate safer sex and change their risky behaviors (Hunter & Schaecher, 1992).

According to the American Academy of Pediatrics, children and adolescents need accurate and comprehensive sex education in order to practice healthy, less risky sexual behavior. Early exploitive or risky sexual activity may lead to health and social problems, such as unintended pregnancy and sexually transmitted diseases, including HIV/AIDS.

Group Interventions for LGBT Youth in Community-Based Clinics, Social Service Agencies, and Other Community-Based Settings

Frontline workers doing outreach and prevention work with at-risk populations report the need to target young LGBT people with messages that address issues that are important to their own ethnic, racial, religious, and cultural frameworks and peer-group norms. Collaborations among community, research, and government have identified essential components of prevention programs and developed effective interventions that help young people develop coping strategies to deal with stressful life events and reduce risky behaviors (Pratt, 2002).

Recommendations—Group Interventions for LGBT Youth

1. HIV-prevention messages targeted to LGBT youth must be delivered in various ways, targeted to at-risk populations (i.e., by age, gender, sexual experience, ethnicity, behavioral risk, or neighborhood) (AIDS Action Council, 2001; Hunter & Mallon, 1998; Pratt, 2002).
2. HIV prevention should be carried out within the context of other issues important to young LGBT people. Barriers keeping youth from being safe, such as dealing with stress, coming out, or self-esteem and identity issues, must be addressed creatively (Hunter & McKay, 2003; Miller et al., 1996). Relationships, intimacy, and sexual health should also be addressed (see Recommendations—Comprehensive Sex Education).
3. Use positive and trustworthy LGBT adult and peer role models as group facilitators. Establish peer-based educational programs as an effective strategy in reaching hard-to-reach youth (UNAIDS, 1997; Kegeles, Hays, Pollack, & Coates, 1999).
4. HIV-prevention programs themselves should be fun and comfortable. Provide "safe zones" where young people can meet one another socially and develop social skills.
5. Prevention programs for young people deserve support from community-based agencies, funders, families, the LGBT community, and the society at large (Forum for Collaborative HIV Research, 2001).
6. Services need to be available, including counseling and testing, either on-site or by referral, for HIV and STIs (Bachanas et al., 2002).

These community-level interventions with proven effectiveness use a variety of approaches and are aimed at changing attitudes and personal norms about sex, health, and responsibility that will then influence risk behavior. Several sources, including the CDC's *Compendium of HIV Prevention Interventions with Evidence of Effectiveness* (1999), describe successful, science-based behavioral programs targeting youth and MSMs. Although not all are LGBT-specific, many intervention designs can be adapted to the LGBT population.

The Internet

Popular Internet Web sites provide a forum where LGBT young people can find resources, interact with others, ask questions, make friends, and share stories. Although the Internet does not provide socialization experiences for young, isolated teens, it does provide resources and information that they might not otherwise have access to. Doing so over the Internet gives youth some privacy while exploring their sexuality and doing it safely. (A word of caution: Among young people, ages ten to seventeen, who use the Internet on a regular basis, one-fifth had been exposed to unwanted sexual solicitations or approaches through the Internet [Finkelhor, Mitchell, & Wolak, 2000].)

The following are popular Web sites for LGBT youth:

> www.advocatesforyouth.org
> www.apa.org/pi/reslgbc.html
> www.ashastd.org
> www.avert.org
> www.centeryes.org/SIGNS/
> www.glsen.org
> www.nyacyouth.org
> www.sxetc.org
> www.youthresource.com

GAY AND LESBIAN YOUTH IN FOSTER CARE

"Self-identified LGBT youth who are in state custody are a little-known, not well-recognized, and generally invisible population in child welfare" (Mallon, Aledort, & Ferrera, 2002, p. 407).

As with their nongay peers, approximately one-third of LGBT youth are placed in out-of-home care before early adolescence (Aldgate, Maluccio, & Reeves, 1989). The majority of these youth came into placement for many of the same reasons that other children are placed: family disintegration, divorce, death or illness of a parent, substance abuse, alcoholism, physical abuse, and neglect. Mallon (1998) found that less than one-third of the young people he studied reported that they came into care for reasons that were directly related to their sexual orientation. Although most gay and lesbian youth in care are not thrown out of their homes when they come out or are found out, those that are face marginalization and oppression in the child welfare system.

Reflecting widely held taboos against homosexuality, families and child welfare systems indirectly encourage these young people to suppress their sexual orientation (Mallon, 1997). The misconceptions, stereotypes, and fears that lead to parents' reluctance to acknowledge the possibility that their children may be lesbian, gay, bisexual, or transgender is mirrored in the attitudes of child welfare professionals (Mallon, 1997). LGBT youth in out-of-home care settings receive fewer services than do their heterosexual peers (Mallon, 1998). They need equal access to the same quality of care afforded to other children in child welfare settings.

The Lambda Legal Defense and Education Fund (Sullivan, Sommer, & Moff, 2001) found that none of the foster care agencies in the United States had policies prohibiting discrimination against foster care youth on the basis of sexual orientation. Further, these agencies did not require training for foster parents or foster care staff on issues related to LGBT youth. Child welfare professionals often label those youth in foster care who are known to be LGBT as "difficult." Youth who are perceived as difficult may receive less responsive care than they require. The emergence of several out-of-home programs to serve this population in New York and Los Angeles reflects changing standards in the child welfare and legal systems (Mallon et al., 2002). For youth who cannot access LGBT-focused youth homes, local crisis service hotlines are important resources. Other resources are recommended by the Child Welfare League of America on their Web site, www.cwla.org.

The most significant challenges identified by LGBT youth in the child welfare system include fear for personal safety, rejection at intake, verbal harassment, and physical violence (Mallon, 1998; Ryan & Futterman, 1998).

Lesbian and gay youth "often are not reunified with their families" (Sullivan, 1994, p. 291). They have a difficult time attending community-based educational programs and accessing appropriate physical or mental health services. These young people often experience very long lengths of stay and multiple placements (Mallon, 1999; Mallon et al., 2002). The prevalence of a history of child welfare involvement for street-involved and homeless youth is significant (Holdway & Ray, 1992). Some LGBT youth would prefer to live on the streets rather than face the threats or experience of personal violence in their out-of-home care setting (Mallon, 1998).

Following are experiences of two young people.

Vinette is a thirteen-year-old self-identified transgender Latina. She lives with her mother, a single parent, and her nine-year-old brother. Vinette, who has identified as transgender since age nine, has had significant difficulty in school placements and has experienced conflict with her mother, who cannot accept Vinette's identity. Vinette and her mother, accompanied by a family friend, came to Green Chimneys LGBT programs in New York City to explore placement in their group home for youths ages twelve to fifteen years.

Vinette was accepted into the Green Chimneys program after an interview and was placed in an LGBT-affirming school in the community. Very soon her school difficulties seemed to be resolved, but other interpersonal issues with peers and adults required some other intervention. Vinette and her mom engaged in weekly sessions with an experienced bilingual therapist. Initial ground rules about use of gender pronouns, dress, and mutual respect were agreed upon and written into a contract, which all parties signed. After five sessions, Vinette and her mom agreed to try bimonthly visits to facilitate reunification. Home visits occurred once a month. After eight months, visits were increased to weekly weekend visits. She was reunited with her mom after one year. Her case was followed by her social worker while she remained in her family home.

Joshua is a sixteen-year-old, self-identified gay, Jamaican youth. Joshua comes from a very traditional, conservative Christian family, including his mother, his father, and three older brothers. Joshua has done very well in school and has been the pride of his family. His family has no idea that he is gay. He is very concerned that if they knew, they would never be able to accept his sexual orientation.

One day while talking on the phone to a boy from his school, Joshua heard a click at the other end of the phone—he had not realized that his father had come home early from work and had listened to the last few minutes of his conversation. After Joshua hung up the phone he walked into the kitchen where his father sat, clearly upset. Joshua asked him what was wrong and he stood up and slapped him across the face. Joshua was caught completely off guard and was even more stunned when his father screamed at him to get all of his things and get out of the house. Scared, upset, and worried about where he was going to go, Joshua left the house and spent the night at a friend's. When he called home, his mother told him not to call again. Joshua finally went to an emergency shelter.

Youth Leaving Foster Care or "Aging Out"

Each year almost 20,000 young people aged sixteen years or older leave the foster care system and are expected to live independently. Once discharged from the foster care system, depending on the state from which they are placed, a youth may receive some transitional services from the foster care caseworker or no services at all (English, Morreale, & Larsen, 2003).

Several studies have documented the high rates of physical and mental health problems among children and youth as they enter foster care and while they are in care. No nationally representative sample of adolescents in foster care has been studied (English et al., 2003).

Recommendations—Youth in Foster Care

1. LGBT youth need appropriate, least-restrictive out-of-home place-ment. Whenever possible, family and relatives are the preferred place-ment/permanency option, keeping youth within their community and culture whenever it is safe to do so, due to the deleterious effects of a hostile environment on LGBT youth in foster care (Mallon, 1998, 1999).
2. When they must be separated from their families, gay-affirming placements with trained staff are safer places than regular foster care placements (Mallon et al., 2002).
3. LGBT youth are subject to discrimination and are often difficult to place. They need, as do all youth in these circumstances, comprehen-sive family and child assessment, written case plans, goal-oriented practice, frequent case reviews, and concurrent permanency plans.
4. These youth need reasonable efforts, where safety can be assured, to reunify families and to maintain family connections and continuity in these relationships (Mallon et al., 2002).

QUESTIONS TO CONSIDER

1. How do we better identify and address the needs of our young LGBT clients?
2. Do our services get input directly from young people? Are LGBT youth involved in the agency's planning process? Do we evaluate our services with young LGBT people in mind?
3. What resources are available in my community for LGBT youth?
4. Are LGBT youth-friendly resources available in my community to which I may refer youth?
5. How does my agency address adolescent sexuality?
6. How is my agency creating a safe and accepting environment for LGBT youth accessing our services?
7. As youth-serving agencies are we equipped to address such issues as teen suicide, HIV/STI, pregnancy, homelessness, mental health, and substance abuse? If not, what are ways agencies can prepare to ad-dress these youth issues successfully?

REFERENCES

AIDS Action Council. (2001). *What works in prevention for youth.* The Body: An AIDS and HIV Information Resource. Retrieved September 6, 2005, from www.thebody.com.

Aldgate, J., Maluccio, A. N., & Reeves, C. (1989). *Adolescents in foster homes.* London: B.T. Batsford; Chicago: Lyceum Books.

Allen, L. B., Glicken, A. D., Beach, R.K., & Naylor, K. (1998). Adolescent health care experiences of gay, lesbian, and bisexual young adults. *Journal of Adolescent Health, 23,* 212-20.

Bachanas, P. J., Morris, M. K., Lewis-Gess, J. K., Sarrett-Cuassay, E. J., Sirl, K., Ries, J. K., & Sawyer, M. K. (2002). Psychological adjustment, substance use, HIV knowledge, and risky sexual behavior in at-risk minority females: Development differences during adolescence. *Journal of Pediatric Psychology, 27,* 373-384.

Boekeloo, B. O., Schaivo, L., Rabin, D. L., Conlon, R. T., Jordan, C. S., & Mundt, D. J. (1994). Self reports of HIV risk factors by patients at a sexually-transmitted disease clinic: Audio vs. written questionnaires. *American Journal of Public Health, 84*(5), 754-760.

Boggio, N., & Cohall, A. (1990). Evaluating the adolescent patient: The search for the hidden agenda. *Emergency Medicine, 22*(2), 18-34.

Centers for Disease Control and Prevention (CDC), USDHHS. (1999). *Compendium of HIV prevention interventions with evidence of effectiveness.*

Centers for Disease Control and Prevention (CDC), USDHHS. (2001a). *HIV/AIDS and U.S. women who have sex with women (WSW).* Atlanta: U.S. Department of Health Services. Available at www.cdc.gov/hiv/pubs/facts/wsw.htm.

Centers for Disease Control and Prevention (CDC), USDHHS. (2001b). *Youth risk behavior. Surveillance-United States 2001.* Atlanta, GA: U.S. Government Printing Office.

Centers for Disease Control and Prevention (CDC), USDHHS. (2002a). *HIV/AIDS surveillance reports, 2000-2002.* Atlanta, GA: U.S. Government Printing Office.

Centers for Disease Control and Prevention (CDC), USDHHS. (2002b). *Young people at risk: HIV/AIDS among America's youth.* Atlanta, GA: U.S. Government Printing Office.

Cohall, A. T., Cohall, R., Ellis, J. A., Vaughan, R. D., Northridge, M. E., Watkins-Bryant, G., & Butcher, J. (2004). More than heights and weights: What parents of urban adolescents want from health care providers. *Journal of Adolescent Health, 34*(4), 258-261.

Collins, C. (1997). *Dangerous inhibitions: How America is letting AIDS become an epidemic of the young.* Monograph Series Occasional Paper #3. Center for AIDS Prevention Studies (CAPS). San Francisco, CA: University of San Francisco.

Crosby, M., & DeCarlo, P. (2000). *What are men who have sex with men (MSM)'s HIV prevention needs?* Center for AIDS Prevention Studies (CAPS). San Francisco, CA: University of San Francisco.

D'Augelli, A. R. (1996). Lesbian, gay, and bisexual development during adolescence and young adulthood. In R. P. Cabaj & T. S. Stein (Eds.), *Textbook of homosexuality and mental health* (pp. 267-288). Washington, DC: American Psychiatric Press.

Dugan, T. (1998). Transgendered people. In R. A. Smith (Ed.), *Encyclopedia of AIDS: A social, political, and scientific record of the HIV epidemic* (pp. 492-494). Chicago, IL, and London, U.K.: Fitzroy Dearborn Publishers.

East, J. A., & El Rayess, F. (1998). Pediatricians' approach to the health care of lesbian, gay and bisexual youth. *Journal of Adolescent Health, 23*, 191-193.

Ehrhardt, A. (1993). Sex education for young people. *National AIDS Bulletin, 32*, 32-35.

Elster, A. B., & Kuznets, N. J. (1997). *Guidelines for adolescent preventive services (GAPS)*. Baltimore, MD: Williams and Wilkens.

English, A., Morreale, M. C., & Larsen, J. (2003). Access to health care for youth leaving foster care: Medicaid and SCHIP. *Journal of Adolescent Health, 32*(S), 6S.

Finkelhor, D., Mitchell, K. J., & Wolak, J. (2000). *Online victimization: A report on the nation's youth*. Washington, DC: National Center for Missing and Exploited Children.

Forum for Collaborative HIV Research. (2001). *Linkage and integration of HIV testing, prevention, and care services*. Project of CDC, HRSA, and the Forum for Collaborative Research. Retrieved September 6, 2005, from www.hivforum.org.

Garofalo, R., & Katz, K. E. (2001). Health care issues of gay and lesbian youth. *Current Opinions in Pediatrics, 13*, 298-302.

Garofalo, R., Wolf, R. C., Kessel, S., Falfrey, J., & DuRant, R. H. (1998). The association between health risk behaviors and sexual orientation among a school-based sample of adolescents. *Pediatrics, 101*, 895-902.

Ginsburg, K. R., Winn, R., Rudy, B. J., Crawford, J., Zhao, H., & Schwarz, D. F. (2002). How to reach sexual minority youth in the health care setting: The teens offer guidance. *Journal of Adolescent Health, 31*, 407-416.

Goldenring, J., & Rosen, D. (2004). Getting into adolescent HEADSS: An essential update. *Contemporary Pediatrics, 21*, 64.

Harper, G. W., & DiCarlo, P. (1999). *What are adolescents' HIV prevention needs?* Fact sheet, Center for AIDS Prevention (CAPS), University of California at San Francisco, April.

Havens, J., Mellins, C. A., & Hunter, J. (2002). Psychiatric aspects of HIV/AIDS in childhood and adolescence. In M. Rutter & E. Taylor (Eds.), *Child and adolescent psychiatry* (4th ed.) (pp. 828-841). Oxford, U.K.: Blackwell Science.

Hogarth, L. (2003). *The Gift*, a documentary film. Los Angeles, CA: Dream Out Loud Productions.

Holdway, D. M., & Ray, J. (1992). Attitudes of street kids toward foster care. *Child and Adolescent Social Work, 9*(4), 307-317.

Human Resources and Services Administration (HRSA), USDHHS. (2003). *Needs assessment and self-assessment module*. Document HAB00322. Rockville, MD: Government Printing Office.

Human Rights Watch. (2001). Hatred in the hallways: Violence and discrimination against lesbian, gay, bisexual and transgender students in U.S. schools. New York/Washington: Human Rights Watch. Retrieved September 6, 2005, from http://www.hrw.org/reports/2001/uslgbt/.

Hunter, J., Cohall, R., Castrucci, B., & Ellis, J. (2001). Lesbian, gay, bisexual and transgender adolescent perceptions of medical providers. Presentation at the American Public Health Association Annual Meeting, Atlanta, GA, October 24.

Hunter, J., & Haymes, R. (1997). It's beginning to rain: Gay/lesbian/bisexual adolescents and AIDS. In M. S. Schneider (Ed.), *Pride and prejudice: Working with lesbian, gay, and bisexual youth* (pp. 137-163). Toronto, Canada: Central Toronto Youth Services.

Hunter, J., & Mallon, G. (1998). Adolescents. In R. A. Smith (Ed.), *Encyclopedia of AIDS: A social, political, and scientific record of the HIV epidemic* (pp. 41-43). Chicago, IL, and London, U.K.: Fitzroy Dearborn Publishers.

Hunter, J., & Mallon, G. (2000). Lesbian, gay, and bisexual adolescent development: Dancing with your feet tied together. In B. Green & G. L. Croom (Eds.), *Education, research, and practice in lesbian, gay, bisexual, transgendered psychology: A resource manual* (pp. 226-243). Thousand Oaks, CA: Sage Publications.

Hunter, J., & McKay, M. (2003). Research-community collaborative partnerships: CHAMP and Working It Out. Presentation at the 15th National Conference on Social Work and HIV/AIDS, HIV/AIDS and Families: Special Needs for Families of Orgin, Families of Choice, Albuquerque, New Mexico, May 30.

Hunter, J., & Schaecher, R. (1992). Adolescents and AIDS: Coping issues. In P. I. Ahmed (Ed.), *Living and dying with AIDS* (pp. 35-45). New York: Plenum Press.

Institute of Medicine (IOM). (2000). *No time to lose: Getting more from HIV prevention.* Report to Congress. Washington, DC: National Academy Press.

Israel, G. E., & Tarver, D. E. (1997). *Transgender care: Recommended guidelines, practical information, and personal accounts.* Philadelphia, PA: Temple University Press.

Jemmott, J. B., Jemmott, L. S., & Fong, G. T. (1998). Abstinence and safer sex HIV risk-reduction interventions for African American adolescents: A randomized controlled trial. *Journal of the American Medical Association, 279,* 1529-1536.

Kates, J., & Wilson Leggoe, A. (2005). *HIV testing in the United States,* HIV/AIDS policy fact sheet. Washington, DC: The Henry J. Kaiser Foundation. Retrieved September 8, 2005, from http://www.kff.org/hivaids/6094=04.cfm.

Kegeles, S. M., Hays, R. B., Pollack, L. M., & Coates, T. J. (1999). Mobilizing young gay and bisexual men for HIV prevention: A two-community study. *AIDS, 12,* 1753-1762.

Li, X., Stanton, B., & Feigelman, S. (2000). Impact of perceived parental monitoring on adolescent risk behavior over 4 years. *Journal of Adolescent Health, 27*(1), 49-56.

Mallon, G. P. (1997). Toward a competent child welfare service delivery system for gay and lesbian adolescents and their families. *Journal of Multicultural Social Work, 5*(3/4), 177-194.

Mallon, G. P. (1998). *We don't exactly get the welcome wagon: The experiences of gay and lesbian adolescents in the child welfare system.* New York: Columbia University Press.

Mallon, G. P. (1999). Gay and lesbian adolescents and their families. *Journal of Gay and Lesbian Social Services, 11*(1/2), 23-33.

Mallon, G. P., Aledort, N., & Ferrera, M. (2002). There's no place like home: Achieving safety, permanency, and well-being for lesbian and gay adolescents in out-of-home care settings. *Child Welfare, 81*(2), 407-437.

Miller, S., Hunter, J., Haymes, R., Hughes, B., Kilmnick, D., Scarella, J., Schreibman, J., & Baer, J. (1996). *Working It Out: An intervention manual for lesbian, gay, and bisexual youth.* HIV Center for Clinical & Behavioral Studies/NYSPI, New York. Retrieved September 6, 2005, from www.hivcenternyc.org.

Paperny, D. M. (1997). Computerized health assessment and education for adolescent HIV and STD prevention in health care settings and schools. *Health, Education, & Behavior, 24,* 54-70.

Pratt, D. (2002). Working It Out: Scenes from the lives of lesbian and gay youth. *Body Positive Magazine, 15*(6), 7-12.

Rosario, M., Meyer-Bahlburg, H. F. L., Hunter, J., & Gwadz, M. (1999). Sexual risk behaviors of gay, lesbian, and bisexual youths in New York City: Prevalence and correlates. *AIDS Education and Prevention, 11,* 475-496.

Rosen, D. S., Elster, A., Hedberg, V., Paperny, D. (1997). Clinical preventive services for adolescents: Position paper of the Society for Adolescent Medicine. *Journal of Adolescent Health, 21,* 203-214.

Rotheram-Borus, M. J., Mann, T., & Chabon, B. (1999). Amphetamine use and its correlates among youths living with HIV. *AIDS Education and Prevention, 11*(3), 232-242.

Ryan, C., & Futterman, D. (1998). *Lesbian and gay youth: Care and counseling.* New York: Columbia University Press.

Ryan, C., & Hunter, J. (2001). Clinical issues with youth. In *A provider's guide to substance abuse treatment for lesbian, gay, bisexual, and transgender individuals* (pp. 99-103). Washington, DC: Center for Substance Abuse Treatment (CSAT)/ SAMHSA.

Sexuality Information and Education Council of the United States (SIECUS). (2001). Lesbian, gay, bisexual, and transgendered youth issues. SIECUS fact sheet. *SIECUS Report, 29*(4), 37-41.

Sigelman, C. K., Mukai, T., Woods, T., & Alfeld, C. (1995). Parents' contributions to children's knowledge and attitudes regarding AIDS: Another look. *Journal of Pediatric Psychiatry, 20,* 61-77.

St. Lawrence, J. S., Brasfield, T. L., Jefferson, K. W., Alleyne, E., O'Bannon, R. E., & Shirley, A. (1995). Cognitive-behavioral intervention to reduce African American adolescents' risk for HIV infection. *Journal of Consulting Clinical Psychology, 63*(2), 221-237.

Sullivan, C., Sommer, S., & Moff, J. (2001). Youth in the margins: A report on the unmet needs of lesbian, gay, bisexual, and transgender adolescents in foster care. New York: Lambda Legal Defense and Education Fund. Available at www.lambdalegal.org.

Sullivan, T. (1994). Obstacles to effective child welfare service with gay and lesbian youths. *Child Welfare, 73*(4), 291-304.

UNAIDS. (1997). *Impact of HIV and sexual health education on the sexual behaviour of young people: A review update.* Geneva: Joint United Nations Programme on HIV/AIDS.

U.S. Surgeon General. (2001). The Surgeon General's call to action to promote sexual health and responsible sexual behavior. Retrieved September 6, 2005, from http://www.surgeongeneral.gov/library/sexualhealth/default.htm.

Valleroy, L. A., MacKellar, D. A., Karon, J. M., Rosen, D. H., McFarland, W., Shehan, D. A., Stoyanoff, S. R., LaLota, M., Celentano, D. D., Koblin, B. A., et al., for the Young Men's Survey Study. (2000). HIV prevalence and associated risks in young men who have sex with men. *Journal of the American Medical Association, 284*(2), 198-204.

Chapter 11

As Time Goes By: An Introduction to the Needs of Lesbian, Gay, Bisexual, and Transgender Elders

Jodi B. Sperber

INTRODUCTION

Lesbian, gay, bisexual, and transgender (LGBT) elders have many things in common with their peers. All elders—who, for the purposes of this chapter, are those over the age of sixty-five—are affected by increased health care needs as they grow older and encounter ageism, increasing isolation, challenges associated with day-to-day living, and living on a fixed income while the cost of living climbs. At the same time, unique challenges remain for LGBT seniors that the aging, health care, and LGBT networks must address.

Ageism is defined as prejudice or negative stereotypes about people based on chronological age. This marginalization can result in a damaging impact on one's ability to thrive socially, economically, and physically.

In 2001, the United States Department of Health and Human Services Administration on Aging publicly recognized and acknowledged that discrimination based upon sexual orientation can be a barrier to receiving high-quality services (Administration on Aging, 2001). This discrimination is due to a host of factors, including the assumption by most service providers that all seniors are heterosexual and no senior identifies as transgender. These assumptions can lead to an incomplete and inaccurate picture of the lives, support systems, and priorities of LGBT elders.

Many thanks to Holly Hartman, Megan Bower, and Eliza Shulman for generous feedback and editorial suggestions.

In recent years, increased attention has been paid to LGBT communities. From popular television shows (such as *Ellen, Will & Grace,* and *Queer Eye for the Straight Guy,* among others) to the popular press, the lives of gay and lesbian (and less frequently bisexual and transgender) people are a more common part of conversation. Great strides have been made in securing civil rights and equal treatment for these populations, including the repeal of all sodomy laws, increased access to health benefits for domestic partners in the workplace, and the presence of antidiscrimination legislation in various state municipalities (*Lawrence v. Texas,* 2003; Human Rights Campaign, 2003).

The mainstream idea of LGBT individuals' physical appearance has not changed over the years; the individuals' physical appearance comprising the LGBT community, however, have changed. Like every other member of society, LGBT individuals age. Unfortunately, the mainstream image of the LGBT community has not expanded to include older people. The sterotype is a young person, who is also typically white, urban, and financially comfortable. In reality, LGBT individuals come in all shapes, sizes, colors, and ages.

Some choose to identify as LGBT, while others do not. This and other decisions made by LGBT elders have been mitigated by surrounding cultural and sociopolitical factors experienced by each individual. This chapter explores the lives of the aging population in an attempt to shed light on an often hidden, commonly ignored, and rarely honored segment of the community.

DEMOGRAPHICS OF THE AGING POPULATION

Although some aspects of the lives of LGBT elders are unique, they also face concerns and questions regarding aging that are similar to those faced by their non-LGBT peers. To better understand the lives of LGBT elders, it is useful to review demographic trends characteristic of the elder population in the United States on the whole. In this way, LGBT elders can be understood as both a unique subpopulation and part of a greater whole.

The overall size of the aging population in the United States is growing rapidly. In 1997, one in eight Americans was elderly; by 2030, one in five will be sixty-five years of age or older. From 1900 to 1997, the number of persons aged sixty-five and older has increased elevenfold, from 3.1 million to 35 million, while the total population has tripled. By 2050, projections show that elderly populations will more than double to about 79 million.

Despite many decades of civil rights activism, racial disparities still exist among older Americans. The average life expectancy in the United States is almost 76 years: 79 years for women and 72 for men (Shapiro, 1997). In addition, persons who reach the age of 65 have a life expectancy of 82.4 years (Administration on Aging, 2001). Differences are seen, however, along racial lines: white men who reach 65 can expect to live 15.7 more years, while black men can expect to live 13.6 more years; life expectancy for white women is 19.4 additional years but 17.6 for black women (Shapiro, 1997).

Today's older Americans enjoy a higher standard of living than any preceding generation of elderly. The median income of the elderly has more than doubled since 1957. However, of the 35.6 million Americans living below the poverty level in 1997, 9.4 percent were age sixty-five or older. Gender disparities remain when examining income levels. In 1996, elderly men had a median income of $17,768, compared with $10,062 for elderly women. Here again, racial disparities exist. Rates of poverty for minority elderly are two to three times higher than for the white population. As of 1997, 9 percent of white elders lived in poverty, compared with 26 percent of black elders and 23.8 percent of Hispanic elders (Social Security Administration, 2000).

Due to the paucity of research on LGBT elders, little information exists concerning the economic status of this subpopulation, and thus it is challenging to make similar comparisons. Some speculation can be made, however, by reviewing research studies demonstrating the relationship between marriage and income (Cahill, South, & Spade, 2001). Marriage often contributes to many positive effects in old age: incomes are typically higher among couples; spouses may provide care during illness; and many elderly couples derive benefits from companionship. In 1994, 78 percent of men and 52 percent of women aged sixty-five to sixty-nine were married. Among those eighty-five and older, 57 percent of men and 13 percent of women were married (U.S. Census Bureau, 2000).

Legal recognition of same-sex partnership would significantly affect access to critical services and supports. Many policies and benefits—including Social Security, hospital visitation rights, and tax laws—are structured around marriage. Same-sex couples face insecurity and unequal treatment when these benefits cannot be accessed. At a time when such benefits are most frequently relied upon, they are often unattainable for LGBT elders.

At this point in time, it is unclear how many LGBT elders are in relationships akin to legally sanctioned marriage. The 2000 Census included information on unmarried partner households, but due to the way the information is compiled and reported, it is difficult to decipher an accurate picture of households actually representing LGBT couples or those in which one or more partners are over the age of sixty-five (U.S. Census Bureau, 2000;

Badgett & Rogers, 2003). Therefore, it is a more challenging task to find these individuals and make reasonable comparisons to their legally married peers.

Although further research is needed to confirm this, it is possible that significant numbers of LGBT elders live in poverty (Cahill et al., 2001). It is often thought that gays and lesbians are wealthier than their heterosexual counterparts, a contention that has been used by more socially and politically conservative individuals as an argument against granting "special rights" (i.e., legal rights and protections afforded others) to this community (Haber, 2003). Others have challenged this analysis, concluding that, on average, gay men earn less than heterosexual men (even if they have attained a higher level of formal education), while lesbians have similar earnings when compared to heterosexual women (Badgett, 1998).

LGBT AGING RESEARCH

At present, little demographic knowledge of LGBT seniors exists. This stems from the fact that limited research has been done on LGBT populations in general. Research that has been conducted generally focuses on individuals under age sixty-five. Boehmer illustrated the scarcity of empirical research in a 2002 article: the results of a comprehensive MEDLINE search (a wide-ranging database from the National Library of Medicine containing over 3.8 million articles published in English) showed that 0.1 percent of all articles therein focused on LGBT populations. Of these, 61 percent of the articles were disease specific, and 85 percent omitted reference to race/ethnicity (Boehmer, 2002).

As data on sexual orientation and gender identity are not requested on the U.S. Census or other large-scale data-collection instruments, no true count has been taken of the number of LGBT elders in this country. Previous studies regarding the prevalence of homosexuality estimate that approximately 8 percent of the overall population identifies as homosexual. Using these studies as a basis for estimation, about 2.8 million lesbian and gay elders over the age of sixty-five are currently living in the United States. Far less is empirically known regarding bisexual and transgender populations, thus similar estimates cannot be drawn. If population projections are correct, the number of gay and lesbian elders will increase to between 2 and 6 million by the year 2050. Little, if any, data exist on the racial profile of this population; research involving random studies has documented profiles as diverse as the general population (Cahill et al., 2001).

LGBT elders are everywhere. They live in cities, rural areas, and everywhere in between. They are diverse in their gender, ethnic and racial backgrounds, and experiences. Sexual orientation and gender identity are just pieces of one's identity, and individuals identifying as LGBT come from every race, ethnicity, economic background, and religious denomination.

Research among LGBT elders is a nascent but growing field. Many articles written on LGBT elders are not scientific research, but rather literature simply telling the stories of the lives of these elders (Clunis & Greene, 1988; Kehoe, 1989). Still, these books and essays give insight into the lives of a once-hidden population. Over the past fifteen years, an increasing amount of qualitative and quantitative research has been conducted with LGBT elders. These studies focus largely on lesbians and gay men, although some studies do include bisexual and transgender individuals. As one might speculate, the concerns of LGBT elders are often similar to those of their non-LGBT peers: fears of poor health, physical limitations, mortality, and adequate finances (Berger, 1984; Kehoe, 1989; Quam & Whitford, 1992). LGBT elders have also been found to hold additional concerns.

Several investigations have found that gay and lesbian people of all ages have reported a range of negative reactions from health and social service providers, including rejection as a patient, provider exhibition of hostility, harassment, excessive curiosity, pity, condescension, ostracism, refusal of treatment, avoidance of physical contact, or breach of confidentiality. These studies document the health care experiences of gay men and lesbians regardless of age, but discrimination in health care has particular impact on elders, because with aging comes an increased level of interaction with health care systems. Among today's LGBT seniors, discrimination has been recognized and documented (Cahill et al., 2001; Boxer, 1997). Indeed, aging services have often been found to be discriminatory environments in which seniors come into contact with much of the same discrimination faced by LGBT individuals of all ages within the health care system (Brotman, Cormier, & Ryan, 2001). In addition, in environments where elders live alongside one another (such as an assisted living facility), LGBT elders may be more vulnerable to further marginalization from peers who hold homophobic and heterosexist attitudes. This can be of particular concern for those who have less choice in their living arrangements due to financial constraints.

Transgender elders face unique challenges. Transgender individuals face additional barriers from service providers and peers due to misunderstanding, discomfort, and lack of experience or comfort with individuals whose self-expression of gender falls outside of rigid norms. Little is known about this population, including answers to concerns surrounding long-term hormone use. Targeted inquiry is needed to assess the barriers faced and to create successful strategies to address them.

Some forms of discrimination are reported not as overt, but rather as "an atmosphere of silence" (Brotman, Ryan, & Cormier, 2002). This can be viewed as an important component of discrimination. Older LGBT individuals are rarely visible in mainstream senior networks, in health care institutions, and in society generally. This oversight may further marginalize LGBT seniors and their care providers. When the needs of gay and lesbian seniors are raised, the most prominent reaction is one of discomfort (Brotman, Ryan, & Cormier, 2003).

Available research expresses differing health outcomes among older lesbians and gay men. Some of this work has documented greater health and mental health problems among gay and lesbian seniors due to discrimination (Cabaj & Stein, 1996; Rothblum, 1994; Robertson, 1998). Research has also argued that managing stigma over long periods of time results in higher risks of depression and suicide, addictions, and substance abuse (Hughes & Wilsnack, 1997; O'Hanlan, Cabaj, Schatz, Lock, & Nemrow, 1997).

Other research has pointed to coping mechanisms developed by LGBT individuals as a successful result of managing stigma and discrimination. Many contend that older lesbian and gay individuals may have advantages over heterosexuals in adapting to old age and may experience more "successful aging." In fact, some research suggests that older lesbians and gays may be more able to adjust to aging and deal with ageism than their heterosexual counterparts. Developing resilience in the face of discrimination has helped some gay and lesbian seniors become experts in dealing with adversity, facing change, and learning how to take care of themselves. For those who have shown such resiliency, the capacity to adapt may follow them into old age such that, if they perceive that they are unable to rely on public services, these LGBT elders have developed a unique capacity to do for themselves and for one another (Humphreys & Quam, 1998; Friend, 1999). Transforming the experiences, concerns, and strategies used by LGBT elders into informed programming or service decisions is beginning, although it remains a task that has been only marginally undertaken (Greater Boston LGBT Aging Project, 2002).

One theory of adaptive coping argues that, for some, the process of "coming out" and the associated stigma earlier in life may cause an individual to better deal with the later stigma of "old age" (Berger, 1996; Francher & Henkin, 1973). Gender-role flexibility may also add to more successful aging, as some individuals may have developed skills not developed by their heterosexual peers (Friend, 1980; Francher & Henkin, 1973). Similar research on bisexual and transgender populations has not yet been documented.

Gender role flexibility—the decreased rigidity of expectations and norms of roles and responsibilities within a relationship, due to the absence of one man and one woman comprising a couple. In many heterosexual couples, men and women have distinct roles determined by expectations placed upon them due to their gender identity (i.e., men are the primary breadwinners, women are the primary homemakers). For same-sex couples, such roles are often negotiated differently.

As they may be estranged from their families of origin, lesbian and gay individuals may learn self-reliance at an earlier age (Berger & Kelly, 1986). This has required many elder lesbian and gay individuals to find and create familial structures among their friends (e.g., a family of choice) (Ramirez-Barranti & Cohen, 2000; Berger, 1996). Investigations have suggested that some older lesbian and gay individuals have more friends than their heterosexual counterparts (Lipman, 1986).

Family of choice appears to be a strong source of support for many older lesbians and gays. In a 1999 study of 160 gay men and lesbians ages forty-five to ninety, almost 70 percent reported having a family of choice with whom they could socialize and spend holidays. Close friends are often noted as sources of support, followed by partners, and then family of birth (Beeler, Rawls, Herdt, & Cohler, 1999; Perlmutter & Sperber, 2002). Interestingly, in the Beeler study, the most important contributor to the respondents' satisfaction with the support they received was the degree to which support persons knew about their sexual orientation.

Informal support networks, regardless of their strength, often need to be augmented by more formal services. The use of health care services by LGBT elders has not been widely studied in any formal manner, although some research has touched on this topic. In one qualitative study, focus-group participants expressed fear over having providers entering their homes and wondered if they would feel the need to alter its appearance in order to hide their sexual orientation (Perlmutter & Sperber, 2002).

The empirical evidence and informal information paints a seemingly contradictory picture of LGBT elders. The mixed conclusions that can be drawn from the research to date indicate a population that has often successfully navigated a personal life but remains reasonably wary of formal services and programs. At a time in their lives when LGBT individuals should be reaping the benefits of years of work and citizenship, many are often placed into systems that are uneducated about or blind to their experiences and concerns.

As times have changed, so have expectations and identities. The current cohort of individuals over age sixty-five grew up in an era where silence about sexuality was the norm; the next generation (i.e., the "baby boomers") is less likely to be willing to go back "into the closet."

We need to ensure that local, regional, and national systems are equipped to respond to LGBT elders in a caring, educated, and welcoming manner. The first step in achieving this goal involves information gathering and education. Increasingly, materials and services are being created to help elder-service providers better serve their LGBT clients. Organizations such as Senior Action in a Gay Environment (SAGE) have created targeted programming for LGBT elders and at the same time educated mainstream providers and the general public regarding the concerns of this population. Mainstream organizations such as the American Society on Aging have also begun to recognize the importance of acknowledging LGBT elders and creating opportunities to learn more about this growing population.

Ongoing training and educational opportunities are crucial and should be sought out or requested within elder-serving agencies. As laid out in this chapter, the root of many of the concerns of LGBT elders is the fear of a negative reaction from providers and peers. This fear can lead an individual to delay or avoid seeking needed care and assistance, thus leading to a lower quality of life. Given this, perhaps the single most important factor in providing good services to all elders is creating an atmosphere in which all people are welcomed to be who they are, regardless of their sexual orientation or gender identity.

Simple actions, such as the posting of LGBT-positive materials, the inclusion of sexual orientation and gender identity in an agency's nondiscrimination policy, or the availability of LGBT magazines and newsletters in the waiting area, can make all the difference to an LGBT elder. In addition, avoiding assumptions about relationships and support networks, and using open-ended, gender-neutral questions that allow the clients to describe their lives can help establish a trusting and constructive relationship between provider and client. The Gay and Lesbian Medical Association has made clear and reasonable guidelines freely available on their Web site (see Selected Resources for more information) to assist providers in making their programs and services accessible to all.

We live in a remarkable and exciting era in regard to LGBT populations. Using the 1969 Stonewall riots in New York City as a chronological marker, we now live among individuals who came of age "pre-Stonewall" (born 1930 to 1949), those that are of the Stonewall generation (born 1950 to 1969), and those who were born "post-Stonewall" (born 1970 and beyond). Each of these three generational cohorts has had a distinct experience of managing relationships and self-identity (see Table 11.1 for examples).

Although individual experiences and expressions of sexuality and gender identity are unique and affected by a variety of factors, including race, education, socioeconomic background, and religious upbringing, among others, it is reasonable to expect that in the coming years many more self-identified LGBT individuals will be entering into the networks constructed to serve and honor our elder citizens. By continuing to educate ourselves and our peers, we will be ready to meet this challenge with confidence.

SELECTED RESOURCES

The following is a list of organizations of interest to LGBT elders and those who work with them. They provide a starting point for those interested in learning more about LGBT elders, as well as an idea of what programs and services are available.

American Society on Aging: Lesbian and Gay Aging Issues Network (LGAIN)
www.asaging.org/networks/lgain/index.html
800-537-9728

LGAIN works to raise awareness about the concerns of LGBT elders and about the unique barriers they encounter in gaining access to housing, health care, long-term care, and other needed services. LGAIN seeks to foster professional development, multidisciplinary research, and wide-ranging dialogue on LGBT issues in the field of aging through publications, conferences, and cosponsored events.

GLBT Health Access Project
www.glbthealth.org
617-988-2605

The Gay, Lesbian, Bisexual, and Transgender Health Access Project exists to foster the development of comprehensive, culturally appropriate health promotion policies and health care services for LGBT people through a variety of venues, including community awareness, policy development, advocacy, direct service, and prevention strategies.

TABLE 11.1. Looking at Events in Recent History Through the Eyes of an LGBT Elder

If, in 2004, you were age	65	85	Event
You would have been age . . .	—	15	when gay and bisexual men were forced to wear pink triangles, and lesbians and bisexual women were forced to wear black triangles, in Nazi Germany (1934)
	12	32	when the Mattachine Society, the first known gay group, was formed (1951)
	14	34	when Christine Jorgenson made headlines for being the first American to undergo sexual re-assignment surgery (1953)
	16	36	when Daughters of Bilitis, the first lesbian group, was formed (1955)
	22	42	when Illinois became the first state to decriminalize homosexual acts (1961)
	30	50	when the Stonewall Riots, considered by many to be the beginning of the LGBT rights movement, took place (1969)
	34	54	when homosexuality was removed from the *Diagnostic and Statistical Manual of Mental Disorders* (DSM-III) as a diagnosable mental disorder (1973)
	38	58	when Harvey Milk, the first openly gay elected official, was elected to office (1977)
	39	59	when Harvey Milk, the first openly gay elected official, was assassinated (1978)
	42	62	when Wisconsin passed the first gay rights bill in the country (1981)
	58	78	when Ellen DeGeneres became the first major character in a sitcom to "come out" on television (1997)
	61	81	when civil unions were created in Vermont (2000)
	64	84	when the United States Supreme Court struck down discriminatory sodomy laws (2003)

LGBT Aging Project
www.lgbtagingproject.org
617-522-6700 ext. 307

The Massachusetts-based LGBT Aging Project works to ensure that LGBT elders and their caregivers have equal access to the same benefits, protections, aging programs, services, and institutions on which their non-LGBT neighbors rely.

Pride Senior Network
www.pridesenior.org
212-675-1936

Pride Senior Network's mission is to encourage and promote services that foster maximum health, well-being, and quality of life for the aging LGBT community through advocacy, education, and research.

Senior Action in a Gay Environment (SAGE)
www.sageusa.org
212-741-2247

SAGE was founded in 1977 and is the nation's oldest and largest social service and advocacy organization dedicated to LGBT elders.

Transgender Aging Network (TAN)
www.forge-forward.org/TAN/
414-540-6456

TAN exists to improve the lives of current and future transgender elders and their significant others, friends, family, and allies.

QUESTIONS TO CONSIDER

1. Do you know if your program or agency currently serves any LGBT elders? How do you know?
2. Upon first meeting a new elder in your program or agency, do you assume the person is heterosexual? Why or why not?
3. Do images or materials in public areas of your program or agency create a welcoming atmosphere for LGBT elders?
4. Are staff and clients within your program or agency aware of the difference between sexual orientation (i.e., gay, lesbian, bisexual, heterosexual) and gender identity (i.e., transgender)?

5. Do staff members intervene when homophobic or transphobic comments are made by clients or other staff? How is this situation handled?
6. Are you aware of local resources of particular interest to LGBT elders and those who work with them?
7. Are your program's or agency's policies inclusive of LGBT individuals?
8. Do all staff within your program or agency participate in trainings involving LGBT populations? If no such trainings exist locally, can they be created or requested?
9. Are you aware of local, state, and national laws and policies that may affect same-sex couples and heterosexual couples differently (such as Social Security, Medicare and Medicaid, 401[k] and pension regulations, and so on)?

REFERENCES

Administration on Aging. (2001). *Fact sheet for older Americans month.* May 2001. Retrieved January 5, 2002, from www.aoa.gov/press/fact/alpha/fact_lgbt.asp.

Administration on Aging. (2002). *A profile of older Americans: 2002.* Retrieved September 9, 2005, from http://www.aoa.gov/prof/statistics/profile/profiles2002.asp.

Badgett, M. V. L. (1998). *Income inflation: The myth of affluence among gay, lesbian, and bisexual Americans.* Retrieved September 9, 2005, from http://www.ngltf.org/downloads/income.pdf.

Badgett, M. V. L., & Rogers, M. (2003). *Left out of the count: Missing same-sex couples in Census 2000.* Institute for Gay and Lesbian Strategic Studies. Retrieved September 9, 2005, from http://www.thetaskforce.org/downloads/income.pdf.

Beeler, J. A., Rawls, T. W., Herdt, G., & Cohler, B. J. (1999). The needs of older lesbians and gay men in Chicago. *Journal of Gay and Lesbian Social Services, 9*(1), 31-49.

Berger, R. M. (1984). Realities of gay and lesbian aging. *Social Work, 29*(1), 57-62.

Berger, R. M. (1996). *Gay and gray: The older homosexual man* (2nd ed.). Binghamton, NY: The Haworth Press.

Berger, R. M., & Kelly, J. J. (1986). Working with homosexuals of the older population. *Social Casework, 67*(4), 203-210.

Boehmer, U. (2002). Twenty years of public health research: Inclusion of lesbian, gay, bisexual, and transgender populations. *American Journal of Public Health, 92*(7), 1125-1130.

Boxer, A. (1997). Gay, lesbian and bisexual aging into the twenty-first century: An overview and introduction. *Journal of Gay, Lesbian and Bisexual Identity, 2*(3/4), 187-196.

Brotman, S., Cormier, R., & Ryan, B. (2001). The marginalization of gay and lesbian seniors in eldercare services. *Vital Aging, 7*(3), 2.

Brotman, S., Ryan, B., & Cormier, R. (2002). Mental health issues of particular groups: Gay and lesbian seniors. In *Writings in gerontology, National Advisory Council on Aging, Canada.* Retrieved September 9, 2005, from http://www. naca-ccnta.ca/writings_gerontology/writ18/writ18_5_e.htm.

Brotman, S., Ryan, B., & Cormier, R. (2003). The health and social service needs of gay and lesbian elders and their families: An exploration in four Canadian cities. *The Gerontologist, 43,* 192-202.

Cabaj, R. P., & Stein, T. S. (1996). *Textbook of homosexuality and mental health.* Washington, DC: American Psychiatric Press.

Cahill, S., South, K., & Spade, J. (2001). *"Outing age": Public policy issues affecting gay, lesbian, bisexual and transgender elders.* New York: National Gay and Lesbian Task Force Foundation. Retrieved September 9, 2005, from http://www.thetaskforce.org/downloads/outingage.pdf.

Clunis, D. M., & Greene, G. D. (1988). Growing older together. In D. M. Clunis & G. D. Greene, *Lesbian couples* (pp. 219-231). Seattle: Seal Press.

Francher, J. S., & Henkin, J. (1973). The menopausal queen: Adjustment to aging and the male homosexual. *American Journal of Orthopsychiatry, 43*(4), 670-674.

Friend, R. A. (1980). Gayging: Adjustment and the older gay male. *Alternative Life-styles, 3*(2), 231-248.

Friend, R. A. (1999) Older lesbian and gay people: A theory of successful aging. *Journal of Homosexuality, 20*(3/4), 99-117.

Greater Boston LGBT Aging Project. (2002). *The LGBT Aging Project: A call to action.* Retrieved September 9, 2005, from http://www.lgbtagingproject.org/plan.php.

Haber, P. (2003). *The gay affluence debate: Myth or marketing hype?* The Gay Financial Network, October 3, 2003. Retrieved September 9, 2005, from http://www.gfn.com/archives/story.phtml?sid=10532.

Hughes, T. L., & Wilsnack, S. C. (1997). Use of alcohol among lesbians: Research and clinical implications. *American Journal of Orthopsychiatry, 66*(1), 20-36.

Human Rights Campaign. (2003). *Corporate equality index 2003.* Retrieved September 9, 2005, from http://www.hrc.org.

Humphreys, N., & Quam, J. (1998). Middle-aged and old gay, lesbian, and bisexual adults. In G. A. Appleby and J. W. Anastas (Eds.), *Not just a passing phase: Social work with gay, lesbian, and bisexual people* (pp. 245-267). New York: Columbia University Press.

Kehoe, M. (1989). *Lesbians over 60 speak for themselves.* Binghamton, NY: The Haworth Press.

Lawrence et al. v. Texas, 539 U.S. (2003). Retrieved July 14, 2005, from http://www.supremecourtus.gov.

Lipman, A. (1986). Homosexual relationships. *Generations, 10*(4), 51-54.

O'Hanlan, K., Cabaj, R. B., Schatz, B., Lock, J., & Nemrow, P. (1997). A review of the medical consequences of homophobia with suggestions for resolution. *Journal of the Gay and Lesbian Medical Association, 1*(1), 25-40.

0

Perlmutter, D., & Sperber, J. (2002). *Addressing the needs of LGBT seniors.* Boston: JSI Research and Training Institute, Inc.

Quam, J., & Whitford, G. (1992). Adaptation and age-related expectations of older gay and lesbian adults. *The Gerontologist, 32*(3), 367-374.

Ramirez-Barranti, C. C., & Cohen, H. L. (2000). Lesbian and gay elders: An invisible minority. In R. L. Shneider, N. P. Kropf, & A. J. Kisor (Eds.), *Gerontological social work: Knowledge, service settings and special populations* (2nd ed.) (pp. 343-367). Belmont, CA: Wadsworth Press.

Robertson, A. E. (1998). The mental health experiences of gay men: A research study exploring gay men's health needs. *Journal of Psychiatric and Mental Health Nursing, 5*(1), 33-40.

Rothblum, E. D. (1994). Introduction to the special section: Mental health of lesbians and gay men. *Journal of Consulting and Clinical Psychology, 62*(2), 211-212.

Shapiro, R. (1997). *The demographics of aging in America.* Population resource center. Retrieved September 9, 2005, from http://www.prcdc.org/summaries/aging/aging.html.

Social Security Administration. (2000). *Income of the population 55 or older, 1998.* Tables VIII.4 and VIII.11. Washington, DC: U.S. Government Printing Office.

United States Census Bureau. (2000). *QT-P18. Marital status by sex, unmarried-partner households, and grandparents as caregivers: 2000.* Retrieved September 9, 2005, from factfinder.census.gov.

PART V:
GOVERNMENT AND PUBLIC HEALTH INFRASTRUCTURE

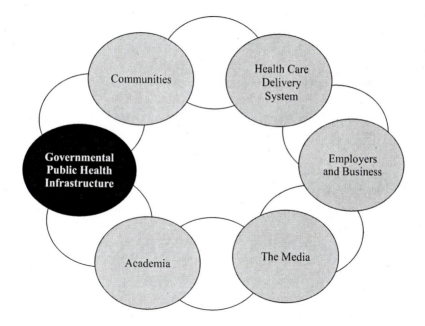

Figure reprinted with permission from *The Future of the Public's Health in the 21st Century.* ©2002 by the National Academy of Sciences, courtesy of the National Academies Press, Washington, DC.

Chapter 12

Strategies for Improving State, County, and City Government Health and Welfare Services for LGBT People

Anthony J. Silvestre
Scott H. Arrowood

INTRODUCTION

Every year billions of dollars are spent to provide government-funded social and health services such as cancer screening, tobacco prevention, foster care, drug and alcohol treatment, and others. There is no reason to believe that lesbian, gay, bisexual, and transgender (LGBT) people are less likely to need these services than non-LGBT people are. Unfortunately, researchers have generated a great deal of evidence showing that despite the need, these programs are not successfully serving the LGBT community (Gay and Lesbian Medical Association [GLMA], 2000).

Government services have increased dramatically over the past 100 years. Generally, members of the executive branch of government have designed services based on political, scientific, and/or social imperatives. Members of the legislative branch influence the design of the programs and services, often resulting in changes in the original design. Funds for these programs are then made available to states for implementation and, in turn, county and local governments are funded to carry out the programs. Theoretically, then, the programs are uniformly administered across the country with the same standards applied and the same goals achieved.

In fact, considerable variation occurs. State political leaders may choose to refuse money for programs that they do not support or they may accept money but interpret the program's goals and standards to conform to their personal beliefs and values. Variations can also arise as programs are imple-

Many thanks to Emilia Lombardi, PhD, of the University of Pittsburgh for her expertise in transgender issues and to Jacquelyn Mitchell, JD, LCISW, of Jackson State University for her expertise in family law and judicial systems.

mented. The implementation of programs is almost always at the county or city level, where local leaders and administrators are in direct contact with people in need. This decentralized approach is also useful to state leaders since it can defuse the inevitable political problems that would arise if one standard was uniformly applied in rural/urban and conservative/liberal areas within one state, not to mention the fact that awarding contracts and programs associated with these programs can win these city, county, and state leaders friends and influence.

According to the National Association of Counties, 3,066 counties are in the United States (National Association of Counties [NACo], 2003). The counties vary greatly in size and population. Some large cities, such as Philadelphia, are also counties. Other cities, such as New York, are composed of a number of counties. Counties range in area from 67 square kilometers (Arlington County, Virginia) to 227,559 square kilometers (North Slope Borough, Alaska). The population of counties varies from Loving County, Texas, with 140 residents, to Los Angeles County, California, which is home to 9.2 million people. Counties provide a wide range of services. The data in Table 12.1, compiled from a study published in 2001, describe the proportion of metropolitan counties, counties adjacent to metropolitan

TABLE 12.1. The Proportion of Metropolitan (Urban), Adjacent (Suburban), and Rural Counties Supervising the Administration of Selected Services in Rank Order (in Percent)

Service	Metropolitan County (Urban)	Adjacent County (Suburban)	Rural County
Law Enforcement	85	79	85
Senior Citizen Programs	68	53	53
Mental Health Services	68	49	47
Health Clinic	66	46	47
Drug and Alcohol Rehabilitation	55	36	27
Emergency Medical Services	48	50	53
Elder Care	43	26	17
Child Care	36	20	15
Shelter for Battered People	34	21	17
Hospital	22	21	21
Homeless Shelter	22	8	4

Source: Kraybill and Lobao, 2001.
Note: Percents are rounded off.

counties, and rural counties offering selected services that have major effects on the lives of LGBT people (Kraybill & Lobao, 2001).

Each of these programs is important to LGBT people. LGBT people, particularly the most vulnerable, desperately need the services that these programs provide and certainly are entitled to receive them in a competent and professional manner. Yet, it is clear that many LGBT-related problems occur in the administration of these programs. For example, many LGBT people fear that law enforcement and emergency medical service (EMS) personnel will be hostile to them and, perhaps, deny them service. Cases have been widely publicized in which the police have refused to investigate domestic violence in gay households and where EMS personnel have refused to transport transgender and HIV-infected people to hospitals. Until the recent Supreme Court ruling overturning sodomy statutes (*Lawrence et al. v. Texas,* 2003), LGBT people in many states could be regarded as criminals because of their choice of sexual partners. Therefore, any interaction with law enforcement or public safety personnel could be dangerous. County and city governments need to train law enforcement and EMS personnel to serve LGBT people competently and effectively. Counties need to hire LGBT personnel and can develop strong liaisons with LGBT communities.

Problems with access to service and care exist in other areas as well. For decades, LGBT people have been reporting that some mental health providers fail to provide adequate care (Cochran & Silvestre, 1979; Garnets, Hancock, Cochran, Goodchilds, & Peplau, 1991; Gonsiorek, 1988). Providers often ignore the problems that patients present, such as depression and relationship issues. Instead, the providers focus on the sexual orientation or gender identity of the client, even though the client has not presented either as a problem. Children and youth workers often do the same thing. They may ignore problems such as bullying of LGBT youth and actually blame the youth for inviting the abuse and violence (Hunter, 1990; Ryan & Futterman, 1997). In our experience running a group home for gay male youth who migrated to the United States from Cuba during the Mariel Boatlift, well-meaning case workers provided some of these boys with female attire. Of course, that made them targets for rape and assaults. Therefore, the focus on the sexual orientation and gender identity resulted in inappropriate support while ignoring needs such as protection from violence and proper health care. Almost all of the boys had untreated STIs on leaving the camps. Cross-dressing U.S. minority youth who later resided in the group home were often allowed to be truant. Teachers and other school staff seemed to have given up hope that these kids could be educated. When these youngsters transferred to a private LGBT school in 1982, they succeeded and were graduated.

In addition to our youth, other LGBT people accessing state and county health and welfare services face similar problems. Many of the most vulnerable members of our community, such as our addicted, disabled, and elderly, live every day at the mercy of government-supported caretakers (GLMA, 2000). Transgendered people using inpatient drug and alcohol clinics often face harassment and even violence at the hands of other patients and staff (Lombardi & van Servellen, 2000). LGBT people who are blind or deaf or live with severe mobility problems often report a deep fear of being identified as LGBT people. They are convinced that they will be victimized by and isolated from the communities that they depend on for many of their needs. In our work with LGBT old people in assisted-living programs, we found that they were afraid to have LGBT newspapers or magazines in their rooms, where cleaning people might find them. They did not allow LGBT friends to visit for fear that their orientation or identity would be discovered. They sat by silently when ministers, priests, and rabbis condemned homosexuality during services at the facilities or when staff told jokes about LGBT people.

The number of LGBT people directly affected by these county-run programs is not insignificant. According to a 1997 analysis of government finances, county governments spent $14.4 billion on health care and $26.7 billion on public welfare (United States Census Bureau, 1997). In the present political climate, it is unlikely that additional funds will be made available for LGBT programs, but strong efforts can be made to assure that current programs serving the general public are effectively serving the LGBT community.

These programs are required to serve all eligible people. Although there appears to be no evidence that any federal or state agency overtly and formally denies services to LGBT people, the question is, are these agencies *adequately* serving LGBT people? State, county, and city bureaucrats often argue that their programs do not discriminate based on sexual orientation or gender identity. Technically, that may be true. However, when programs discourage LGBT people by intimidating them, by urging them to hide their sexual orientation, by allowing untrained staff to act unprofessionally, or by tolerating the bullying of LGBT clients by other clients, those programs are unprofessional and inadequate.

IMPROVING SERVICES

In order to understand how government-funded programs limit services to LGBT people and how to bring about change, it is necessary to understand those who create the rules that regulate the services. The single most important group that influences the actual implementation of policy and programs are the bureaucrats. Although everyone has a tale of horror about a rude, incompetent, or unreasonable bureaucrat, the stereotype is unfair and overdrawn. Bureaucrats generally are trained and committed professionals who derive satisfaction from doing their jobs well and contributing to the health and well-being of society. At the same time, they are often subject to inappropriate political pressures from elected officials.

Bureaucrats see their political bosses come and go. In a normal career, a bureaucrat may serve under a dozen governors, county commissioners, or mayors and even more politically appointed commissioners or secretaries. The bureaucrats learn that program implementation is subject to significant change from one administration to another. Smart bureaucrats who wish to provide the best services possible to the public learn ways to stop or delay changes that they believe will be harmful. They know that the politicians pushing for change may leave office or get distracted so that the changes never occur or are significantly delayed. In one case, a social worker who was ordered to rewrite public assistance regulations to reduce the number of women and children who received benefits wrote the most restrictive regulations that he could imagine, knowing that the courts would throw them out and change would be delayed a few years.

Another strategy often used by bureaucrats is to create an internal task force to study the problem until the administration changes, thus forcing the task force to disband without accomplishing anything. Of course, task forces can also be established to draw up a helpful agenda for change, as will be discussed later. Less ambitious strategies are to discover legal problems that require long evaluations by the administration's attorneys, to assign incompetent or soon-to-retire staff to programs that they want to scuttle, and to simply reinterpret their instructions in ways to minimize what they perceive to be harmful. So, the "faceless" bureaucrat, although not able to create programs, can change them, slow them down, and, sometimes, stop them completely. These tactics are ideology-free and can be used by supporters or opponents of LGBT people.

Thus, LGBT activists who manage to win promises from political leaders running for election often find that the changes they expect to happen do not happen. Because they are frequently unaware of how the system works, activists are often placated with the promise that their goals will be met as soon as funding becomes available or after a task force or council has developed a plan to carry it out. In fact, activists are frequently invited into the process by being offered seats on such task forces. Experienced bureaucrats are well practiced in keeping activists of all kinds engaged in the process while the process actually accomplishes little or nothing. Some ways to derail activists are to set up meetings during daytime hours, when activists

have other work responsibilities. Another is to overwhelm them with diffi-
cult-to-understand stacks of paper dealing with budget, state regulations, or
the law. Another is to fill meeting times with presentations from experts
so that months go by without any discussion other than questions and answers tacked on to complex presentations. An often-used tactic is to listen
intently to the activists, agree with their position, and then ask them to write
up a report with recommendations. If the activists manage to complete the
task, the bureaucrat can easily find many reasons why particular recommendations need to be reconsidered. In one instance, activists were invited to
design an HIV-prevention intervention targeting LGBT youth. The program, which they designed over an eight-month period, was never implemented. The activists were told that the workshops they planned could not
take place in governmental buildings at night or on weekends because of the
union rules regarding maintenance staff. They were also told that they
would need to verify (by checking IDs) that all of the youth coming to the
workshops were sixteen years old or older to avoid violating the law forbid-
ding the corruption of minors. Finally, they were told that they would need
to raise the bulk of the funds for the program because of recent county budget cuts. Clearly, the bureaucrats could have helped design a program that
would work. Denying activists the benefit of meaningful guidance is a way
of occupying them for many months, losing some or all of them to changes
in their lives, and having them create a program that could never work due
to technicalities.

The point is that LGBT people who want to hold government accountable for providing services to all people without prejudice need to understand how to avoid pitfalls by enlisting bureaucrats who can guide them.
The first step in the process of developing or revising a government program is to identify and elicit support from bureaucrats who know the formal
and informal aspects of the particular program being targeted. The best way
to do that is to put out word to LGBT people and allies, telling them about
your need to find insiders who can be of assistance.

It is not enough to find an ally or an LGBT insider. Deeply closeted
LGBT government officials may present their own set of problems. These
bureaucrats may fear being exposed or they may wish to protect their political mentors. High-level, closeted state and federal officials supervising
large bureaucracies may resist supporting any LGBT issues. For whatever
reasons, LGBT activists often give them a free ride by not confronting them
in ways that they otherwise would confront non-LGBT officials.

Activists need to choose LGBT and allied bureaucrats who are not afraid
to go on the record on behalf of LGBT people. They must also know the
system and have significant experience working in it over time. In some
cases, LGBT and other allies may not fully see or understand how the sys-

tem that they are part of is failing LGBT people. LGBT or allied bureaucrats, though sympathetic, may not understand the community needs that
are not being met. One friendly bureaucrat did not understand how lesbians
could be at increased risk of heart disease, despite the health literature
showing that lesbians are at increased risk of smoking and stress, among
other things. If education does not persuade the LGBT and allied bureaucrats about a particular issue, the activists may need to change their agenda
and refocus on one that the bureaucrats support. Finally, the activists must
be prepared to protect the bureaucrats by allowing them to give advice and
input privately. Bureaucrats are by instinct and by training circumspect at
public discussions or meetings. They are expected to represent their agency's official views, even if they personally oppose them. Bureaucrats may reveal
their personal point of view only in private discussion with people whom
they trust.

Choosing Programs to Focus On

We know that the needs of LGBT people receiving services are not being
met in many program areas. Yet, often it is not possible to move ahead in
each area of need at the same time. Change is more likely to succeed in
those areas where the advocates have their strongest LGBT experts, the
most highly placed and sympathetic bureaucrats, and the least politically
charged service. Determining the program or service to be addressed should
be decided with the political and bureaucratic leaders and the insiders who
support the effort. The bureaucrats and politicians should be encouraged to
make it clear where they will support change and where they will not. It is
better to know their areas of support than to spin wheels for a few years
wondering why things are not moving ahead.

It is important that the advocates carefully assess their own and the community's strengths before choosing an arena for action. Can the advocates
marshal more expertise (both professional and consumer) on some LGBT
issues than on others? Are their government allies more powerful in one department than another? Are the midlevel bureaucrats of some agencies
more supportive than others?

Choosing a program area should also include consumers. Once allies
within the bureaucracy have been identified, they need to fully understand
the experience of LGBT people currently served by their agencies. One way
to do this is to set up meetings between the insiders and outside experts, providers, and consumers. These private meetings should be conducted on an
informal level, and those attending them should understand that the meetings are for strategic purposes and not for initiating action. The last thing

needed is for outsiders to begin mucking around with the press or in public forums before a promising strategy can be developed.

Planning Action

Once friendly bureaucrats have been identified, enlisted, and educated and when an area for intervention is selected, the next step is to create a plan of action. The simplest way to do that is to set up a task force.

Although some clever politicians set up task forces in order to sidetrack activists, task forces can also be used to advance change. To be successful such task forces need to be composed of LGBT experts and consumers as well as LGBT activists. Activists who are not also experts in a particular area are sometimes not trained to understand how to design and advance an effective change agenda in a particular program. Activists can provide strong voices, but it is the professional and consumer experts who will ensure that the changes being planned are appropriate. In addition to the experts, consumers, and activists, high-level people from the chosen agency or area of interest must be present as active members of the task force. Too often, low-level bureaucrats are assigned to such task forces. These bureaucrats simply do not have the power to change policy. Many meetings can be spent proposing changes using a low-level bureaucrat as a liaison with the agency head, who will only bounce the propositions back for some clarification or other. This back-and-forth communication can go on for many months. In addition, the governor, county commissioner, or mayor should also be represented by a special assistant, who will ensure that agency personnel support the politician's agenda.

The task force should not have a life longer than six or eight months. This is essential. Commissioners or governors usually serve a term of four or eight years. The first year of their administration is busy with appointing a cabinet or executive staff and learning how to take over the reins of government. The last year is spent doing job searches. Since any substantial change is going to take a few years to implement, it is important that action be initiated as early as possible in any administration. Although a policy can be announced and implemented in weeks, actual change in procedure and program takes years. Bureaucrats need to be thoroughly educated, protocols and regulations need to be instituted, and contracts with agencies need to be rewritten. It is more important that one or two programs be established successfully than that the task force produce a report on all aspects of service change that are needed but which will never occur because of changes in administrations.

The task force should complete its work by drawing up a plan to ensure that services in the chosen area are organized to fully meet the needs of LGBT people. This plan will likely include cultural competency training, policy changes, contract changes, funding of new programs, the identification of private nonprofit agencies that can assist in providing services, and staff- and agency-monitoring processes. An expanded list of possible actions is included on the following pages.

Case Study: Governor Milton Shapp

In Pennsylvania, in 1976, the late Governor Milton Shapp established the Pennsylvania Council for Sexual Minorities. To our knowledge it was the first governmental body charged with ending discrimination against LGBT people in employment and governmental services in the United States, if not the world. In the few years of its active existence it successfully identified changes needed in public welfare, public health, drug- and alcohol-abuse services, mental health, corrections, the attorney general's office, and state police. Unfortunately, only a few changes occurred before Governor Shapp announced his candidacy for president. Once that happened, his top staff and appointees were preoccupied with his election and sexual minority issues (as well as many other progressive issues) were moved to the back burners. More experienced advocates and activists could have moved the agenda more quickly in the early years of his administration and thus it might have had more of an impact on state services.

Building Support

It is most important to understand that a governor, mayor, or county commissioner's policy proclamation supporting one or more LGBT health or social programs is not the final goal but only the first step. Politicians who gain state, county, or city office soon come to realize that the systems they oversee are difficult to change. State laws, complex regulations, union rules, campaign promises, budget constraints, and unexpected occurrences and demands force politicians to pare down their agendas and focus on a few program areas. One governor inherited a few billion dollars' shortfall in his budget. His entire first eighteen months in office was focused on that issue and he had little political capital to spend on controversial social issues. One secretary of welfare hit a roadblock in changing state policy because only one office in the entire state had a complete copy of all state regulations, and it was poorly organized. One county commissioner was warned by a strong union official not to grant domestic benefits to same-sex county workers unless he was also willing to increase other benefits that the union supported.

Early on it is important that the advocates identify allies outside of government who will support their efforts. The first group that needs to be enlisted is state or local LGBT activists. An examination of the political agendas of most national and statewide LGBT groups will reveal that the provision of competent human and health services to LGBT people are not often, if ever, included. LGBT activists commonly work to change laws through the legislative or judicial process. Reforming health and human services is for some reason not on many activists' agendas. It may be that agendas are created, in part, because of the demands of those affected by them. Those receiving government-sponsored services are often in no position to organize themselves into a constituency. LGBT youth in foster care programs, our elderly in assisted-living facilities, and those needing mental health services are much too burdened to organize politically. Also, our activists may not fully understand the problems facing the disadvantaged members of our community who depend on government services. Whatever the reason, serious efforts must be made to educate our political leaders so that they can marshal their forces on behalf of service reform.

Allies could come from state or local professional organizations such as social work, nursing, public health, and medical associations. It may be that their national offices have already issued policies about ending disparities in services based on LGBT status. The state or county affiliate can draw up specific recommendations about how that is to happen at the local level. When a professional association does offer assistance, a representative from that association should also sit on the task force. Other allies could include sympathetic union leaders, religious leaders, highly respected academics from the disciplines related to the chosen area of action, allied business leaders, and foundation board members.

Menus of Goals and Objectives

Governmental health and social programs vary in many ways. Each program has its own regulations established by law, policy, and practice. Each program is funded by one or more sources, each with its own rules and timelines. Each program is governed by different people, targets different people, and has a particular importance assigned to it by the political leadership in the executive and legislative branches. Programs are also under various levels of scrutiny by the media, lobbyists, and other activists. At the same time, most programs have the same underlying structure and function. The following is a description of structural and functional areas in which LGBT interests can be addressed.

Policies

- Strong policies should be established within every agency and in all subcontracts to ensure that discrimination based on sexual orientation and gender identity is forbidden and that mechanisms are established to protect LGBT adults and youth from staff or clients of the agency.
- Sexual orientation and gender identity should be protected categories in nondiscriminatory hiring and promotion policies for the agencies and all agencies with which they contract.
- Policies should guarantee a safe and harassment-free working environment, including provisions supporting employees who form LGBT-interest groups.
- A domestic benefits policy should be enacted.
- Policies establishing review boards, citizen-input committees, or task groups should make clear provisions for participation of LGBT people.
- Confidentiality policies should define the information to be included in records and with whom records may be shared.
- Where relevant, standards of care should include the needs of LGBT populations. Such standards should be prepared with input from experts in LGBT health and psychosocial needs.
- Housing policies, particularly in jails and drug and alcohol treatment programs, should make provisions to provide gender-appropriate and safe housing for LGBT people.
- Policies should ensure that all forms, assessment tools, and research protocols are appropriate for and inclusive of LGBT people.

Training of Staff and Subcontractors

- Cultural competency training that includes sexual orientation and gender identity should be offered for all staff and mandated for staff in agencies subcontracting with the government.
- Because of inadequate college and university training, many health and psychosocial professionals are not prepared to deal with the issues facing LGBT people. Training in health and social issues that particularly concern LGBT populations should be required for all staff for whom it is relevant. Examples are HIV education and training for people working with high-risk populations and LGBT mental health issues for all drug and alcohol counselors, and children and adolescent services staff.

Common Functions of Many Agencies

The actual change agenda will vary program by program. However, many programs share the same characteristics and functions, which should be considered when developing a change agenda. Some of them are

- Routine education and communication by agency directors with legislative bodies, particularly health-and-welfare house and senate committees on LGBT issues
- Subcontracting with competent agencies to provide specific LGBT services and programs
- Appointing LGBT people and allies who have expertise in LGBT needs to state and local positions ranging from secretaries of departments to unpaid members of advisory committees
- Regulating insurance, health maintenance, licensing, and other organizations and services to establish antidiscrimination policies and to mandate competency standards
- Monitoring and evaluation of all programs to see that LGBT needs are being met
- Including LGBT issues in all research programs carried out by state, city, and local agencies
- Placing of job announcements and other relevant ads in LGBT publications
- Including LGBT-capable services on referral pages and Internet links
- Developing regular communication links and partnerships with the LGBT community
- Providing a voice for LGBT needs to the media, professional associations, and public bodies
- Filing court briefs that support LGBT positions

PROGRAM AREAS WITH PARTICULAR RELEVANCE TO LGBT PEOPLE

Policy and training changes should be encouraged for all state employees. However, particular attention should be paid to those programs serving our most vulnerable and needy LGBT community members. These programs include the following:

1. Children and Youth Services
   Group homes
   Foster care

Independent living
Assisted living
Adoption
Teen pregnancy in lesbian, bisexual, and questioning females
Hotlines and referral
2. Public Health Programs
Hepatitis
STI
HIV
Health education
Health communications, including Internet-based programs
Tobacco prevention
Lung, breast, anal, and ovarian cancer-screening programs
Health outreach particularly designed to reach all segments of the
LGBT community
3. Social Welfare Programs
Drug and alcohol treatment and prevention
Mental health
Developmentally disabled assistance
Family assistance
Juvenile detention
Homeless adult and youth
Aging, including assisted living, day care, at home, and nursing home
care
4. Education
HIV education in schools
Sex education in schools
Antibullying programs
Cultural diversity programs
Programs for the homeless and LGBT youth who cannot function in
schools
5. Community colleges and city- or state-run university health and psy-
chosocial services
6. Adult corrections
7. Police
8. Emergency services

PROGRAM MODELS

A number of jurisdictions have taken the lead in reshaping government
programs so that they better serve LGBT people. In 1976, Governor Milton

Shapp of Pennsylvania issued an executive order pledging his administration to work toward ending discrimination based on "sexual preference." He followed up later in 1976 and in 1978, issuing orders to ban discrimination based on "sexual preference" by any state entity (including all agencies that subcontracted with the state) in hiring, crediting, contracting, provision of service, or any other matter whatsoever. He also established the Governor's Council for Sexual Minorities, probably the first such governmental unit in history. The council was directed to work toward ending discrimination in all state policy and practice. During the few years that remained in Governor Shapp's administration, the council trained state employees and the public and published educational materials, including an award-winning booklet by the Pennsylvania Department of Education (1977) titled, *What is a Sexual Minority Anyway?* The council also received complaints of discrimination from citizens and worked with existing state agencies to resolve them. It worked with the American Civil Liberties Union (ACLU) and others to support a successful court challenge to the state's sodomy law.

The council's work provided opportunities for LGBT providers and advocates to work directly with state agencies. Support was generated for licensing two LGBT mental health agencies in the state. A major effort was made to use state resources to educate gay and bisexual men about STIs. When the Mariel Boatlift from Cuba left a dozen young LGBT teens in a state refugee camp, government agencies worked to establish a group home for the youth. Later, local LGBT homeless and needy youth were admitted to the home. A private high school, Byton School, was established for these young people in 1982.

Although the orders against discrimination in state policy continue today, the council has become moribund due to lack of support from the governors who followed Shapp. It is important that activists and advocates move quickly when an opportunity to improve local or state programs is offered and that they move in a way that will make it difficult for future administrations to rescind those policies and programs.

Since the late 1970s, other governmental bodies have moved to respond positively to LGBT issues. In 1983, New York City established an Office of Gay and Lesbian Health Concerns to deal with health issues such as suicide, violence, HIV, and substance abuse. Also in the early 1980s, San Francisco developed a position for a coordinator of lesbian and gay health services. The King's County (Washington State) Department of Health has an LGBT Web page and a number of health-related programs targeting the LGBT population. Boston has moved ahead strongly on the health front. The LGBT Health Office of Boston is collecting data on sexual orientation and health, providing training in a number of health-related arenas, creating culturally competent educational materials, and including LGBT issues in strategic planning processes, among other initiatives. Each of these programs is different.

The actual shape of the body that is reviewing and revising programs will depend on the particular history and practice of each bureaucratic structure as well as the political climate. What is important is that the LGBT community avoids being diverted from their goal of changing programs and policies. The most tempting diversion is to spend an inordinate amount of time focusing on building some kind of structure within government. An ineffectual governmental committee, council, or task force focusing on LGBT issues can be counterproductive. Such a group gives the illusion of power and respect but may never produce anything of importance. A political leader who is pressured to respond to an LGBT issue can simply refer all LGBT matters to the new structure, knowing that people in it do not have the skills or resources to do anything to resolve them. The crafty politician, eager for votes, can claim to be supportive and deserving of support from the LGBT community while avoiding any action that would alienate anti-LGBT supporters. It is a win-win situation—for the politician. The child, prisoner, and senior needing services lose.

The following section describes LGBT interests in the context of a common governmental program, namely, children and youth services. It is offered with the intention to portray the range of issues that will face LGBT health advocates as they work to change health and social services.

CHILDREN AND YOUTH SERVICES

A major problem for LGBT youth and LGBT family members in children and youth services is the assumption that they are nonexistent, invisible, or simply of lower priority. As of September 2001, 542,000 children and youth were in foster care (Children's Bureau, 2003). It is not known how many of these young people are LGBT identified or sexually or gender questioning. Nor is it known how many affected family members, whether birth, foster, or adoptive, are LGBT. Currently, no known attempt has been made to gather national statistics on these populations. Nonetheless, LGBT people are served in all capacities of the system. They may be either parents or youth in families under investigation or already receiving intervention. They may be children already removed from their birth parents and placed in foster care or a group home. They may also be foster or adoptive parents seeking to provide temporary care and/or ultimately to adopt a child. Given the prohibitive costs of private adoption and artificial means of conception, many LGBT people may consider a foster care adoption subsidized by the government. In short, child welfare and the county system have an impact on LGBT youth and LGBT family members.

Before discussing LGBT youth and LGBT family members further, it is important to understand the basics of the child welfare system itself and how families in general become involved. In sanctioning child welfare, the government acknowledges to some degree the paramount concern that the needs of children and youth be met. Families are the primary resource in securing these needs, including but not limited to food, shelter, protection, clothing, discipline, and love. Ordinarily, this primary resource is enough; however, families commonly experience difficulties that threaten their capability to meet even the most basic needs of their children. Such difficulties may include the sudden illness or death of a parent or provider, underemployment or loss of job, domestic violence, loss of property or eviction, parental absence or imprisonment, drug and alcohol abuse, and depression. When such a threat occurs, families primarily turn to informal supports such as extended families, neighbors, friends, religious organizations, and civic associations. At times, they may also turn to other systems, formal or informal, such as drug and alcohol services, private therapy, or mental health services. Ideally, seeking such assistance is enough for families to stabilize their situation and eliminate the threat to the well-being of their children. When its not enough, additional assistance may come formally from the government or private agencies that make up the child welfare system.

Child welfare is a publicly funded, organized system of service delivery designed to assist abused, neglected, or at-risk children and their families. Sanctioned by the federal government and regulated by the states, child welfare is typically administered directly through either county social service departments, private nonprofit agencies contracted by the county, or both. The government and private agencies in this system are designed to

- protect and promote the well-being and safety of all children and intervene in the family, if necessary;
- support the family and seek to prevent problems that may lead to abuse, neglect, and separation; and
- provide responsible and appropriate out-of-home care services for those children who require them.

Primary services in the system are Child Protective Services (CPS), family preservation; out-of-home care (foster care, kinship care, and residential group care), adoption, and independent living.

Children and youth generally enter the child welfare system through CPS. Reports of suspected child abuse and neglect are made by neighbors,

family members, teachers, hospital workers, law enforcement officers, and/or anyone who may have contact with children. CPS agencies respond to these reports and are generally administered by state and/or county government agencies. CPS agencies then conduct investigations, assess degree of harm and continued risk to the child, determine whether a child may remain with the family or be placed into state custody, and work cooperatively with family court. In 2001, 3 million reports concerning the suspected abuse or neglect of approximately 5 million children were made to CPS agencies throughout the United States. Two-thirds of those reports were screened in for investigation and more than a quarter (over 500,000) of the investigations resulted in a finding that one or more children were maltreated or at risk of maltreatment. Approximately 903,000 children were found to be maltreated, which is typically categorized to include neglect, medical neglect, physical abuse, sexual abuse, and psychological maltreatment (Adoption and Foster Care Analysis and Reporting System [AFCARS], 2003). Once again, the numbers of LGBT youth and LGBT family members are not assessed and cannot be known at this time. In cases of physical or sexual abuse, children are generally placed immediately into state custody; however, the majority of investigations generally conclude the child was neglected and every effort is made to preserve the family.

Family preservation services work to support parents in the care of their children through crisis management, educational support, and casework to identify resources and address problems as they arise. Most children in family preservation were identified by CPS, where it was assessed that the children remain in the home with added support in place. Removal from a home, even a neglectful or abusive one, is traumatic for any child, and family preservation seeks to prevent this from happening. For many, family preservation may be the full extent to which they get involved in the system. Once a crisis has been averted or new resources have been identified, the family may no longer require intervention from the county. In some circumstances, however, it may become necessary to intervene for the safety and well-being of the child, in which case they are placed in out-of-home care.

Children and youth in out-of-home care may be in family foster care, kinship care, or residential group care. Family foster care is a temporary resource for children who are best suited for living in a family setting but cannot be cared for by parents or relatives. Children entering foster care have experienced or have been at risk for physical abuse, sexual abuse, or neglect. Many have serious medical or therapeutic needs requiring more intensive levels of foster care. These "special needs" children require experienced and well-trained foster families to adequately address the complexity of need. When at all possible, a child may be placed in kinship care with a relative or other adult with whom the child has an ascribed family relationship. Given the close family ties and preexisting relationship, placement in a kinship home may lessen the trauma of separation experienced by the child. The concerned couple (or individual) becomes certified as foster parents for the expressed purpose of caring for their related child. Some children and youth present such serious emotional and behavioral problems that a family setting may not be appropriate. Residential group care is designed to serve those needs and is generally treatment oriented. Group care may be based in a home out in the community or in a more secured environment such as a facility. Out-of-home care, whichever form it takes, is temporary and ideally serves to provide needed care and support until the birth parent is able to reunite with his or her child. However, family reunification may become unlikely or prolonged and thus may no longer be in the child's best interests. At this point the county may seek to provide a more permanent resolution, such as adoption or independent living.

Adoption and independent living are two other child welfare services and are pursued once the goal of family reunification is no longer considered. Adoption becomes a goal for a child when it is determined that the birth parents can no longer provide care and that a new, permanent family arrangement would be most beneficial. Given the strong ties to the child, the foster or kinship care family is generally considered the first choice for adoption. For older children, neither reunification nor adoption may be possible. Independent living services are provided to young people who must leave foster care when they turn eighteen years of age. Independent living prepares young people with the skills needed for self-sufficiency and competent functioning as adults. Service and support may continue into young adulthood and include educational advancement, career planning, employment maintenance, health care coverage, pregnancy prevention or planning, parenting classes, and assistance in securing adequate housing.

Individuals who provide these services are critical to any success achieved in the child welfare system. Caseworkers practice directly with birth parents, foster parents, and children and youth. They may be professional social workers with formal education or another professional prepared with minimal education in child development and human services. They typically receive clinical supervision on a regular basis and meet regularly with birth parents and the foster family. Caseworkers are heavily relied upon for the information and assessment that is critical for the courts or county department in order to make determinations for a child's permanent family arrangement; therefore, they have considerable influence on the process. Foster and adoptive parents provide the most direct care to the child and are thus critical to ensuring their safety and well-being. Foster parents are engaged in a family relationship with the child and thus are in the ideal position to address sexual concerns and encourage healthy development. Potential foster and adoptive parents are screened and accepted for possible certification. This process typically takes three months or longer and includes home inspection, parent interview assessment, orientation to the agency, and requisite training. Continued training and support may also be provided to help a willing parent take on the added rewards and challenges of caring for children with special needs. Other players in the system include attorneys who may represent the child, birth parent, or county department; judges who make determinations based in part on caseworker assessments and attorney advocacy; clinical staff at group homes or other residential facilities; and the bureaucrats and agency administrators who develop and enforce policy. These individuals will ultimately determine the success of any initiative to serve LGBT people involved in child welfare.

Given that LGBT youth and LGBT family members are served by child welfare, it is important to understand the workings of the system, its inherent problems, its effect on all served, and how it contributes to the existing experiences of many LGBT people. For example, the removal of a child from the only home he or she has ever known, however unstable it may seem to be, is traumatic and can bear considerable consequences on the behavior and emotional well-being of the child. If one separation can cause harm, then multiple placements from one foster home to another serves to increase the lack of stability and attachment experienced by the child. Together, these separations can compound the alienation or isolation already experienced by a sexually or gender-questioning young person.

The invisibility or presumed nonexistence of LGBT youth and LGBT family members in child welfare leads inevitably to what is perhaps the primary problem: institutionalized homophobia and heterosexism in the system. State, county, and private agencies charged with the responsibility of administering child welfare services will inconsistently, if not rarely, take proactive measures to counter such harm experienced by LGBT individuals. Actions such as including sexual orientation in nondiscrimination policies in both employment and service policies vary from state to state. In addition, state or county governments may or may not require such policies in their contracts with private agencies. Even if such a policy is compulsory, exceptions may be made for some. For example, a religious organization may not be allowed for religious reasons to discriminate against people of other religions or based on race; however, a county may allow the organization to discriminate against LGBT people for religious reasons. Such systemic indifference also affects whether adolescent sexuality training, including sexual diversity, is even provided, much less mandated for case- workers, supervisors, attorneys, foster parents, and others in the system with a professional obligation to LGBT youth and LGBT family members.

If these inconsistencies occur at the governmental or agency administrative level, then invariably the same occurrence plays out among workers and foster parents. Individual prejudices or lack of education can have an enormous affect on LGBT youth and family members. An ill-equipped worker or foster parent may cause harm, even when unintentional. For example, a county social service agency placed a transgender girl, who was diagnosed with gender-identity disorder, into state custody because her parents did not force her to conform to male-specific clothing or appearance. Even if education training is mandated, the next question is whether workers or foster parents are held to the expectations put forth in the training. Without appropriate administrative enforcement and supervision, many may disregard such training. For example, if a worker or foster parent refused to work with or otherwise proved to be culturally insensitive to others based on race or ethnicity, then he or she would hardly be allowed to continue practicing as such. In contrast, it is questionable how far an administrator or supervisor would go to prevent such a practice against an LGBT-identified, sexually questioning, or gender-questioning young person. The same question may be even more apparent for foster parents, as they rely on the frontline workers for support, education, and supervision. Even if such a problem is addressed with a foster parent but left unresolved, it is highly unlikely the foster parent would be discharged, given the agency's tremendous need to retain them for either the child already in their home or for future placements.

Others affected by such inconsistencies are LGBT birth, foster, and adoptive parents. County and agency workers, attorneys, and judges all have a tremendous impact on the assessments and decisions made to remove a child from a home, place a child in care, approve or reject a foster parent, and match a child with a family for adoption. Prior to *Lawrence et al. v. Texas,* sodomy laws were sometimes used by judges to criminalize LGBT birth parents and withhold custody of their children for that reason alone. Even if an agency accepts LGBT foster parents, the decisions of which children to place in the home may be inappropriately assessed. For example, an agency may elect to place with the LGBT foster parent only the most medically devastated and needy child, whom no other foster parent may want. This practice was observed to occur particularly when a large number of children with AIDS began entering the system. Another example is rejecting an LGBT adoptive home because the worker involved believed the child was young, new to foster care, and thus still had a chance "to make it" in a "normal" home. Such prejudices speak not only to the negative attitudes and decision making directed toward LGBT individuals and families but also toward all children in the system.

Some issues the child welfare system struggles with in general are with regard to all children under its care. The lack of resources is perhaps the most significant struggle. The increasing number of children in the system coupled with the stagnating numbers of foster homes can place a heavy burden on overworked, and perhaps underpaid, county, agency, and court workers. Increased caseloads for workers and poorly equipped foster parents can lead to clogged court systems, multiple placements in new homes, delayed or abandoned adoptions, and prolonged stays in out-of-care services that were initially intended to be relatively short-term. All of these occurrences undermine the basic goal of providing permanent family arrangements for children and youth. Also, a great need exists for highly experienced and trained foster parents willing to address the special needs of children suffering from medical problems, physical abuse, and sexual abuse. Intensive support from county and agency workers is imperative for retaining these foster parents and ensuring the success of the placement to provide a stable, nurturing environment and to prevent further harm from coming to the child. With such great need and inconsistencies in the system, LGBT concerns will have to compete with other priorities and could easily be dismissed altogether. Ultimately, more resources need to be committed and any activist or policymaker proposing an intervention would have to account for this need when advocating or planning.

An LGBT foster care program was developed in a large urban area in response to a growing number of special needs foster youth already self-identified as LGBT. The program, developed for a private agency contracted by the county, sought to recruit LGBT foster parents to provide temporary homes for these young people. The contracted agency held policies of nondiscrimination based on sexual orientation in both service and employment practices. Although the program was to be staffed by one worker, the agency mandated sexuality diversity training for all staff. The training, provided by an experienced speaker contracted by the county, sought chiefly to educate participants in many of the facts and misconceptions about homosexuality. The agency also hired a sexual-minority foster care program worker experienced in working with the LGBT population. This worker successfully recruited LGBT foster homes through meeting with LGBT community groups, collaborating with community leaders, and advertising in local LGBT-identified publications. The city referred the self-identified youth for placement with these new foster families and the worker assumed caseworker responsibilities for all youth placed in the special program.

Although the program represents a positive step forward on the part of a county service and one agency, several limitations were apparent or became apparent with implementation of the program. The program served only older special-needs youth who had already self-identified as LGBT. As such, it was not a comprehensive program integrated throughout the system for all children and youth but an isolated initiative responding to a small number of special needs cases for whom it appeared the system may be failing. In addition, the changes in agency policies and practices did not include gender identity. The agency training mandated for all staff is a commendable first step toward a more integrated approach; however, it focused primarily on dispelling myths and promoting facts about homosexuality, including a discussion about some of the various experiences of being LGBT. It did not include how to

- Build skills to more effectively work with LGBT youth and family members
- Understand gender-identity issues or the concerns of a gender-questioning young person
- Assess adolescent sexuality and address it with a young person
- Identify sexually and gender-questioning youth
- Educate foster parents and clarify expectations with regard to adolescent sexuality
- Understand the affect of sexual abuse on the sexually questioning young person
- Cultivate a relationship to enable a young person to feel safe coming out

In addition, the training, although clarifying some of the agency expectations on the issue, did not address how workers, particularly those who vocalized opposition, would be managed in relation to LGBT concerns. Some training participants continued to express unfounded prejudicial beliefs about LGBT people (for example, homosexuality is a choice, gay relationships are only about lust, or gay people should be celibate). They stated openly that they believed homosexuality was morally wrong or sinful and some went even further to state that they would never work with an LGBT individual. Some unanswered questions include the following:

- How would this issue be handled in supervision, if at all?
- How will workers be enabled to meet professional obligations if they hold an opposing personal viewpoint?
- What, if any, are the consequences for demonstrating a willful refusal or an incapability to appropriately serve LGBT youth and LGBT family members?

Another limitation that was initially a part of the program was the decision to recruit only LGBT foster parents to work with these special needs youth. The youth generally were perceived as difficult cases, perhaps in the system for some time, who had been through several foster or group homes already. They demonstrated serious emotional and behavioral problems that typically warrant placement in a more experienced foster home; in other words, they had many concerns beyond being LGBT and were not necessarily what the new foster parent should be expected to manage. Targeting the LGBT community for foster parent recruitment was commendable and remains necessary, as the community has historically been an untapped resource for the child welfare system. Time and attention, however, should be taken to properly prepare and support all new foster homes, particularly those with good intentions but limited parenting experience. Also implicit in the initial decision may be the assumption that only LGBT foster parents may be expected or equipped to foster LGBT-identified young people. The extent of this possible assumption is unknown, but the initial decision was later followed by an expanded action to seek out foster parents, regardless of sexual orientation, who could be sensitive to the needs of LGBT young people. The agency also continued to target the gay community and to use LGBT homes as a general resource for foster care and adoption placement. The change was perhaps most suggestive of an increased awareness and expanded understanding of how LGBT people may serve the child welfare community.

In summary, child welfare is a county service largely untapped for advocating for LGBT youth and LGBT family members. Activists and allied bureaucrats have an important opportunity to ensure the protection of gender- and sexually questioning young people and to expand the opportunities for LGBT parenting and service to the community. Individuals interested in serving LGBT children and youth in the child welfare community must be knowledgeable about the various intricacies of how the system operates at all levels, and they must be aware of any variances in their locality.

Recommendations

The following are some recommendations for ensuring the safety and well-being of LGBT young people and enabling LGBT families to foster parent and adopt:

- States and counties should include sexual orientation and gender identity in their antidiscrimination policies and practices for employment and services.

- States and counties should mandate that all contracted agencies include sexual orientation and gender identity in their antidiscrimination policies and practices for employment and services, without exception.
- Counties and private agencies should include LGBT participants on community advisory boards or other community-input mechanisms.
- Counties and private agencies should include the needs of LGBT people in all standards of care, including input from experts who work with LGBT youth and family members.
- Residential placement providers, including group homes and other facilities, should include provisions that provide gender-appropriate and safe housing and facilities for LGBT people, particularly transgendered individuals.
- Activists should seek out advice and support from organizations for the legal profession, including the state Bar Association, to offer LGBT competency training and explore other possible recommendations for family law practitioners.
- Activists should know whether family court judges are elected or appointed in their districts. Political strategies to effectively influence an elected judge may differ from that of an appointed judge.
- Counties and private agencies should recruit and train new staff, foster parents, and adoptive parents to work with LGBT youth and LGBT family members. The following should be considered when recruiting:
  —Recruitment plans, particularly those for foster and adoptive parents, should target the LGBT community.
  —Recruitment plans should include building ties to LGBT community resources and utilizing appropriate media.
  —LGBT issues should be considered when assessing cultural competency in both the hiring of staff and the certification process for foster and adoptive parents.
  —LGBT foster parents should receive placements appropriate to their level of parenting experience and should be nurtured to build capacity for more challenging placements.
  —Foster homes proven most sensitive to LGBT concerns should be considered when placing LGBT-identified young people.
- Counties and private agencies should include LGBTs in mandated cultural competency curricula for training offered to existing staff, foster parents, and adoptive parents. LGBT competency in child welfare should include
  —Education about lesbian, gay, bisexual, and gender-identity (transgender) issues

—Skills building on working with LGBT-identified youth and family members

—Adolescent sexuality and assessment of sexually and gender-questioning young people

—The affect of sexual abuse on the sexual development of adolescents, including LGBT young people

—Working with foster parents who express discomfort with and a lack of capacity to address sexual issues

- County and private-agency administrators should support supervisors to clarify and enforce among workers the professional obligation of cultural competency, including LGBT concerns.
- County and private agency supervisors should support workers to clarify and enforce among foster parents the expectations of cultural competency, including LGBT concerns.

CONCLUSION

Hundreds of thousands and, perhaps, millions of LGBT people receive some health services from county governments across the country. The experiences of the vast majority of LGBT people and the scholarly evidence make it clear that these services are not offered in the most competent way possible. Policies are needed to remedy this situation. Staff training programs, the development of appropriate intake forms, assessments, referral services, and community linkages are just a few of the many changes needed for most government-run or government-funded programs. In addition, it is clear that special programs are needed for particular groups within the LGBT community. Homeless transvestite youth, for example, need safe places to live and special schools or school programs that can effectively educate them. These changes will occur only when our LGBT health advocates and allies begin to effectively articulate the needed changes to the politicians and government officials who are responsible for health programs. It is important to understand and to impress upon them that LGBT people have a right to appropriate services and that the officials are responsible for ensuring this right. LGBT advocates need to learn how health programs are created and implemented. They will need to establish structures for ongoing communication with governmental and agency bureaucrats so that initial changes can be monitored.

Although health services to our most vulnerable LGBT people may not capture the national attention in the same way that other LGBT issues may, they should be at the top of our change agenda. Decades of experience have taught us that unless we take the initiative, change will never happen. The lives of our LGBT youth, elders, addicted, and disabled depend on what we do.

QUESTIONS TO CONSIDER

1. What channels exist in your county for ongoing communication with officials who are responsible for running county health and social welfare programs?
2. What programs does your county have to provide services to LGBT elders and to LGBT people with disabilities?
3. Does your county drug and alcohol program provide appropriate housing for transgendered people seeking inpatient care?
4. What links do you have to professionals who work in county health and social service programs?

REFERENCES

Adoption and Foster Care Analysis and Reporting System (AFCARS). (2003). *The AFCARS report.* Washington, DC: U.S. Department of Health and Human Services.

Children's Bureau, U.S. Department of Health and Human Services. (2003). *Child maltreatment 2001: Summary of key findings.* Washington, DC: National Clearinghouse on Child Abuse and Neglect Information and National Adoption Information Clearinghouse.

Cochran, M., & Silvestre, A. (1979). Mental health for sexual minorities: Walking the straight and narrow. *Currents, 3,* 10-12.

Garnets, L., Hancock, K.A., Cochran, S.D., Goodchilds, J., & Peplau, L.A. (1991). Issues in psychotherapy with lesbians and gay men: A survey of psychologists. *American Psychologist, 46*(9), 964-972.

Gay and Lesbian Medical Association (GLMA) & LGBT Health Experts. (2000). *Healthy people 2010: Companion document for lesbian, gay, bisexual, and transgender (LGBT) health.* San Francisco, CA: Gay and Lesbian Medical Association.

Gonsiorek, J. (1988). Mental health issues of gay and lesbian adolescents. *Journal of Adolescent Health Care, 9,* 114-122.

Hunter, J. (1990). Violence against lesbian and gay male youths. *Journal of Interpersonal Violence, 5*(3), 295-300.

Kraybill, D., & Lobao, L. (2001). *Changes and challenges in the new millennium.* Washington, DC: Rural County Governance Center and Ohio State University, National Association of Counties.

Lombardi, E.L., & van Servellen, G. (2000). Building culturally sensitive substance use prevention and treatment programs for transgendered populations. *Journal of Substance Abuse Treatment 19*(3), 291-296.

National Association of Counties (NACo). (2003). NACo Counties Care for America. Retrieved December 16, 2003, from http://www.naco.org/.

Pennsylvania Department of Education. (1977). *What is a sexual minority anyway?* Harrisburg, PA: Author.

Ryan, C., & Futterman, D. (1997). *Lesbian and gay youth: Care and counseling.* New York: Columbia University Press.

United States Census Bureau. (1997). *Finances of county governments.* Washington, DC: United States Department of Commerce.

Chapter 13

National and Public Infrastructure and Policy: Are We Experiencing Scientific McCarthyism?

Nancy J. Kennedy

INTRODUCTION

Health infrastructure, policies, and laws exist at multiple levels—local, state, federal, and international. Their development and enactment can occur both in public as well as private sectors, often as a by-product of prevailing social policies. Types of health care laws and policies include statutes, regulations, administrative procedures, guidelines, directives, rules, and verdicts. Health laws and policies guide agencies and associations in the organization and financing of services and resources, relevant to the general population and targeted groups. Although this is the allocative function of laws and policies, the dogmatic function can be used to control and possibly eradicate not only defined behavior but also existence of specific groups.

Contributing to the vulnerability of many underserved populations is both the paucity of health laws and policies and also the deleterious intent of extant policies. Although sodomy statutes have been in existence for centuries and other discriminatory laws and policies abound, lesbian, gay, bisexual, and transgender (LGBT) populations have had almost no laws and policies of positive affirmation. Furthermore, as this chapter attempts a historical journey through law and policy at a national level, especially concentrating on the federal bureaucracy, the designations of "lesbian, gay, bisexual, and transgender" are not used initially, as "homosexuality" was the term used to refer to both genders by researchers, policymakers, providers, and others until the 1970s. Furthermore, although the title of this chapter attempts to document federal efforts for all of the populations comprising the acronym LGBT, there is undoubtedly a dearth of information about bisexual and transgender individuals.

Sexual identity is a challenge for individuals who do not choose or self-identify with the monosexual categories of homosexuality or heterosexuality. The discussion of bisexuality has a long history (Fielding, 1932; Garber,

1995) although only recently have scientists and researchers begun an earnest investigation of its parameters, especially within the context of various cultures (Rust, 2001). In the 1970s, and even earlier in entertainment capitals such as Hollywood, Berlin, and Paris, bisexuality was seen as chic because entertainers such as Tallulah Bankhead, Greta Garbo, Josephine Baker, Joan Baez, David Bowie, Andy Warhol, and Marlon Brando did not hesitate to assert themselves as enjoying sexual relations with both sexes. However, the bisexual community did not coalesce in a similar way to the gay and lesbian communities. In fact, the oppression and negative judgment of bisexual individuals emanates from not only heterosexual individuals but also homosexual individuals (Newitz & Sandell, 1994).

The embodiment of the resistance from what seemed to be all sides concentrated on the physicality of sexual behavior, thereby denying the emotionality and spirituality between or among people. Not unlike their gay male counterparts, what impelled bisexual individuals to form a large influential collective and strive for visibility and equal rights was the rapid emergence and spread of HIV/AIDS. In 1984, David Lourea persuaded the San Francisco Department of Public Health to recognize bisexual men in their official AIDS statistics, thereby forcing health care policymakers and providers to recognize the existence of bisexual men (Lourea, 1985). This recognition led to surveys using the terminology "men who have sex with men" (MSM), which continues today and has expanded to include "women who have sex with women" (WSW). As the second epidemic of HIV/AIDS has spread primarily to African-American, Latino, and Native American populations, bisexuality is again emerging not only in professional research efforts but also in the popular press. Unlike the past two census counts, which have provided an estimate, albeit an underestimate, of gay and lesbian individuals living in the same household, no national estimates exist as to the bisexual population. When asked about the number of bisexual men and women who are African American, Dr. Alvin Poussaint, professor of psychiatry at Harvard University said, "If homosexuals are in the closet, then bisexuals are in the closet even more so" (Chappell, 2002, p. 158).

Transgender, an umbrella term that came into common usage during the 1980s, encompasses a variety of people, including transsexuals, cross-dressers, and drag kings and queens, as well as bigender and androgynous individuals (Tewksbury & Gagne, 1996). Transsexual and transvestite are terms deriving from the psychiatric literature; transgender is the term emanating from the transgender community and, therefore, the preferred term (Leslie, Berina, & Maqueda, 2001). Transgender people exhibit the full range of sexual orientations, from homosexual to bisexual to heterosexual (Jamison, 2000). However, no probability studies of transgender people have been reported in the literature and no effort is underway to develop measures for inclusion in federal surveys.

HISTORY OF GAY INDIVIDUALS
AND THE FEDERAL GOVERNMENT

The current federal administration has been likened to the persecution that occurred during the homophobic McCarthy era. A recent book, *The Lavender Scare: The Cold War Persecution of Gays and Lesbians in the Federal Government,* by David Johnson (2004) chronicles the persecution and fear that terrorized gay and lesbian federal employees during the 1950s and the early 1960s. In 1950, a then-obscure, first-term senator from Wisconsin, Joseph R. McCarthy, gave an infamous speech in Wheeling, West Virginia, in which he waved a piece of paper in front of his audience of Republican women and claimed to have the names of slightly over 200 State Department employees who were known communists. Although in subsequent speeches the number of individuals would decrease, with only four individuals positively identified, the fear of the government being permeated with communists became rampant as U.S. troops were deployed into North Korea. Less than three weeks after McCarthy's speech in West Virginia, Deputy Under Secretary of State John Peurifoy testified before a Senate committee investigating the loyalty of government workers. When asked how many State Department employees had resigned while under investigation for being security risks since 1947, Peurifoy answered: "Ninety-one persons in the shady category with most of these being homosexuals" (Johnson, 1994-1995, p. 47). By March 1950 Republicans were calling for an investigation of the problem of the government employing homosexuals. When President Truman's loyalty board refused, newspaper articles and political cartoons accused Truman of protecting "traitors and queers" (Bachelor, 1950).

Senators Styles Bridges and Kenneth Wherry held congressional hearings on the threat posed by homosexuals with such seditious allegations as even one homosexual individual "can pollute an office." Two journalists, Jack Lait and Lee Mortimer (1951), printed repulsive stories about the hearings in an infamous book titled *Washington Confidential.* The attack on homosexual civil servants was a component of the larger attack on the Roosevelt/Truman New Deal. The 1952 presidential election, the first election since the beginning of the lavender scare, saw issues of gender and sexuality permeate the campaign. The Republican campaign slogan "Let's Clean House" alluded to a slew of allegedly immoral behavior in the incumbent Democratic administration, including communism, corruption, and homosexuality (Johnson, 2004). In an Electoral College landslide of 442 versus 89, Dwight David Eisenhower defeated his Democratic challenger Adlai Stevenson (www.ipl.org/div/potus/ddeisenhower.html).

In April 1953 Eisenhower issued Executive Order IO450, revising the loyalty-security program. The campaign to remove homosexual employees from government offices was effective. Under the new policy, "sexual perversion" was sufficient and necessary grounds for exclusion from federal employment (Executive Order, Security Requirements for Government Employment, April 29, 1953). In the first sixteen months of the Eisenhower directive, an average of forty homosexuals were ousted from government positions every month. The number of job applicants who were not hired because of their perceived homosexuality can only be speculated. The civilian purge was reflected in the armed forces as well. In the late 1940s, the U.S. military was discharging homosexuals at the rate of about 1,000 a year. By the early 1950s, the number had jumped to 2,000 a year (D'Emilio, 1998).

Harry Hay founded the Mattachine Society in Los Angeles, the first sustained gay organization in the United States (Johnson, 2004). He was motivated by the rising tide of homophobia emanating from Washington and the fear that, as these federal employment policies spread, homosexuals would find it impossible to find employment. Bruce Scott, a federal employee, was fired in 1956. The next year, 1957, Dr. Frank Kameny, an astronomer with the federal government, was also fired and barred from any future service because of an investigation of immoral conduct outside of work. Kameny sued the government but, in 1961, the Supreme Court refused to hear his case (Marcus, 1992). Given the success of the Mattachine Society in Los Angeles, Kameny founded the Washington, DC, Mattachine Society to confront the federal government actively (Summersgill, 2000). In 1965, the Federal Court of Appeals ruled in *Scott v. Macy* that a vague charge of "homosexuality" was not grounds for disqualification from federal employment. When the government attempted to present more specific charges against Scott, the Court of Appeals in 1968 again found in his favor. In 1975, having lost a number of similar cases, the Civil Service Commission was forced to suspend its discriminatory exclusion of gays and lesbians (Ayyar, 2004).

The functions of the U.S. Civil Service Commission were transferred to the Office of Personnel Management (OPM), pursuant to Executive Order 12107 (December 28, 1978). The Civil Service Reform Act of 1978 prohibits discrimination based on "nonmerit factors," and a 1980 OPM interpretation includes sexual orientation as a nonmerit factor (Hirsch, 1996). The following year, the Office of Special Counsel (OSC) was established on January 1, 1979 (Reorganization Plan No. 2 of 1978, 5 U.S.C. app.).

The president from 1977 through 1981 was Jimmy Carter. In an election win reminiscent of Eisenhower, Ronald Reagan decisively defeated Carter, the incumbent, who captured only 49 electoral votes in comparison to Reagan's 489 votes (Leip, 2001). Critics of President Reagan assert that his homophobia was evident in his slow response to the problems of HIV/AIDS (McCollum, 2003). No definitive answer has been found, and both sides are equally vociferous. After serving the maximum two terms, Reagan's vice president, George H. W. Bush, was successful in defeating the Democratic challenger, Michael Dukakis, with close to 80 percent of the electoral votes (Leip, 2001). The Persian Gulf War was a dilemma for many gay and lesbian members of the military. President George H. W. Bush knew that many openly gay and lesbian military personnel served with distinction during the war. However, the president had instituted a regulation that did permit the dismissal of those same service members for being gay (Lum, 2001). In his bid for reelection George H. W. Bush was defeated by William Clinton, who served two consecutive terms (Leip, 2001).

Clinton began his presidency with the controversial codification of the "don't ask, don't tell" military policy (P.L. 103-160, 1993). To many LGBT individuals, the codification of this policy was seen as a betrayal of campaign promises to allow all able men and women, regardless of sexual orientation, to serve openly and proudly in the nation's armed forces (Belkin, Batemen, & Monks, 2003; Lehring, 2003). Although the issue is still debatable for military personnel, civil servants fared better under Clinton. On May 28, 1998, President Clinton added sexual orientation to the list of discriminatory prohibitions in hiring and firing federal employees (Executive Order 13087) and charged the OSC with enforcement.

Federal employees had little time to celebrate President Clinton's executive order or hope that the Employment Non-Discrimination Act (ENDA) and/or domestic partnership bills introduced by various members of Congress beginning in the early 1990s would ever be passed. The opposition was increasing its power through various advocacy groups that saw Congress as a venue to voice their objections and denials of any rights to sexual minorities. Both the Southern Baptist Convention and the Family Research Council exerted their influence on Congress in opposition to the executive order and their efforts resulted in Representative Joel Hefley's (R-CO) proposed amendment to the Treasury, Postal Service, and General Government Appropriations Act, H.R. 4104, which, if passed, would have prohibited the expenditure of funds to implement, administer, or enforce the president's executive order. (Vote 398, Hefley Amendment, August 5, 1998). Although the amendment was defeated, almost 40 percent of representatives voted in favor of that amendment.

Having served the maximum two terms, the 2000 election matched Vice President Al Gore against Governor George W. Bush, son of the former president. In the closest election ever held, Bush was named president by a Supreme Court decision (Sunstein & Epstein, 2001). Almost immediately, President Bush changed the tenor of the federal government, especially the civil service. Individuals nominated for not only cabinet positions but also the usual thousands of political appointees entered the system with a determination that any rights accorded to specific populations would be reversed and, definitely, no group would be accorded special rights. Another significant change would be that civil servants would no longer make recommendations based on competency, geographic representation, and racial/ethnic diversity to cabinet secretaries for advisory committees and scientific appointees (Union of Concerned Scientists, 2004). All agencies and centers are given the names of the individuals to comprise advisory councils, regulatory boards, and other positions of influence. Numerous instances exist in which nonscientists reside in senior advisory roles and underqualified candidates are now directing agencies and staff who surpass their supervisors relative to experience and education, irrespective of time in government.

Thus, despite the strides that federal employees had made since the homosexual "cold war" of the 1950s, the closet door was far from open. Moreover, the right that President Clinton accorded federal workers in his executive order is now seriously jeopardized as Scott Bloch, director of the OSC, recently removed the categorical protection of "sexual orientation" from not only the OSC Web site but also all OSC printed documents (Chibbaro, 2004). In addition, fundamentalist groups were not satisfied with President Bush's initial actions (or inactions) regarding LGBT federal employees. The Concerned Women for America's (CWA) Culture and Family Institute signaled their disapproval by releasing "The Bush Administration's Republican Homosexual Agenda: The First 100 Days" at the end of May (Knight, LaBarbera, & Ervin, 2001). This document reproached President Bush because he "failed to overturn a single Clinton executive order dealing with homosexuality" and "continued the Clinton policy of issuing U.S. Department of Defense regulations to combat 'anti-gay harassment.'"

The 2004 political race became much more divisive when gay marriage, with all of its attendant issues including hospital visitation rights and other health-related items, became a focal point during the month in which this country celebrates black history. Like most laws and policies, the evolution of gay marriage to the national level came from states such as Vermont, which approved same-sex "civil unions" in 2000 (House Bill 847, 2000) and Massachusetts, whose Supreme Court ruled on November 18, 2003, that gays and lesbians had the right to marry. In San Francisco, California, the newly elected Mayor Gavin Newsom permitted marriage licenses to be issued to same-sex couples beginning February 12, 2004, and within ten days 3,300 couples married, with hundreds more waiting to see the outcome of legal opposition (Gordon & Sebastian, 2004). San Francisco was not the only local jurisdiction to issue licenses; a court clerk in rural Sandoval County, New Mexico, gave marriage licenses to sixty-six same-sex couples before the sheriff's department, on orders from New Mexico's attorney general, moved in and shut down the office (Bryan, 2004).

President George W. Bush, citing an "overwhelming consensus in our country" against same-sex marriage, announced on February 23, 2004, the need for a constitutional amendment banning same-sex marriages (Office of the Press Secretary, 2004). When California governor Arnold Schwarzenegger was asked on the widely watched Sunday-morning NBC news show *Meet the Press* about the almost 3,000 same-sex couples having been granted marriage licenses in San Francisco, he said, "all of a sudden we see riots and we see protests and we see people clashing. The next thing we know is there are injured or there are dead people . . ." (Schwarzenegger, 2004). Despite the governor's portend of potential violence, no adverse circumstances occurred surrounding the marriages, although protesters were omnipresent. At this juncture, the future of same-sex marriage within the United States is undetermined. However, as family and work are inextricably linked to health and well-being (Livingood, 1972), the national debate of this issue is far from over.

FEDERAL AND PROFESSIONAL ASSOCIATION: INSIGHT INTO LGBT HEALTH

In September 1967, a Task Force on Homosexuality was appointed by then-director of the National Institute of Mental Health (NIMH), Dr. Stanley Yolles. The final report was released in 1969 and consisted of recommendations for NIMH as well as seven background papers. Chaired by psychologist Evelyn Hooker and including respected academics such as John Money, Judd Marmor, and Jerome Frank, these papers constituted the knowledge base for the deliberations of the task force. Despite the content of the papers and recommendations for the establishment of a center for the study of sexual behavior, much of the report's language would be considered contemptuous today, as it was to some gay activists at the time. For example, the language within the report articulated that the purpose of primary prevention was to stop homosexuality from developing in children and adolescents. As to treatment, the task force condoned imprisonment and called for rehabilitative measures.

At the 1972 American Psychiatric Association's (APA) convention in Dallas, Texas, another panel on homosexuality included John Fryer, a closeted psychiatrist, who wore a mask for fear of losing his medical license. In 1973, the APA officially removed homosexuality from the DSM following several years of advocacy by gay and lesbian activists and several psychiatrist allies who did not believe that homosexuality was a mental illness. Evelyn Hooker's groundbreaking research on matched samples of homosexual and heterosexual men was used to challenge the widespread belief that homosexuality was a pathology (Hooker, 1957). In the same year that homosexuality was removed from the DSM, gender dysphoria disorder was constructed, and in 1980 that disorder was officially added to the DSM.

During the activism of the 1960s, 1970s, and 1980s, specific national groups formed that assisted in developing health policies and influencing provider training and policies within the major professional associations. These organizations included the Sexuality Information and Education Council of the United States in 1964, the Gay Nurses Alliance in 1972, National Association of Lesbian and Gay Addiction Professionals in 1979, and the American Association of Physicians for Human Rights (AAPHR), founded in 1981, which changed its name to the Gay and Lesbian Medical Association in 1994. In 1975, Walter Lear, MD, and several other members of the American Public Health Association (APHA) founded the Caucus of Gay Public Health Workers (now known as the Lesbian, Gay, Bisexual, and Transgender Caucus of Public Health Workers). Although APHA had been established in the nineteenth century, it was not until the annual meeting in 1976 that included sessions, organized by Lear, acknowledging the existence of public health problems in gay men and lesbians (Fee, Brown, & contributing editors, 2001).

In 1976, Walter Lear convened the National Gay Health Coalition with other early health activists such as Paul Paroski, Frances Hanckel, Bopper Deyton, and Harold Kooden. When Caitlin Ryan was coordinating the 1979 National Gay Health Conference in 1978, she conceived of a national organization that would focus on policy, training, advocacy, research, education, and networking with existing major professional associations. She proposed the idea to Lear and Paroski and found an attorney who would incorporate a gay organization—a significant challenge in the 1970s. Paroski and others established the National Gay Health Education Foundation (later the National Lesbian and Gay Health Foundation) in New York City in 1980, with board members Bernice Goodman, Linda Joseph, and Frank Greenberg, among others (personal communication, Caitlin Ryan, March 31, 2004; Ryan, 2001b). The organization ultimately became known as the National Lesbian and Gay Health Association (NLGHA) and ceased operation in 1998.

During nearly twenty years of operation, the foundation served as a springboard for many important initiatives and groups. In 1979, Caitlin Ryan and Bernice Goodman discussed the need for a major survey to conceptualize lesbian health. They were able to find initial funding, and Ryan initiated the study in 1981, later joining with Judy Bradford in 1984 to conduct the National Lesbian Health Care Survey (NLHCS), the first large-scale health survey of nearly 2,000 lesbians from all fifty states and several U.S. territories (Bradford & Ryan, 1987, 1988; Ryan & Bradford, 1999).

Early organizing activities carried out by NLGHF, AAPHR, and lesbian and gay caucuses within the major professional organizations generated networks of health and mental health providers who would provide a framework for local and, later, national response to the AIDS epidemic. As part of the Federation of AIDS Related Organizations, NLGHF formed and implemented a National AIDS Resource Center that served as a precursor to the National AIDS Network. The National Lesbian and Gay Health Conference (held annually from 1979 to 1998) added an annual AIDS forum in 1982 that provided a nexus for national AIDS policy, prevention strategies, and organized response before the government developed policies or strategies to address the epidemic. In 1983, Caitlin Ryan and Bernice Goodman worked with people living with AIDS in several cities to develop the National Association of People with AIDS, which NLGHF ran from Washington, DC, until a network of people living with AIDS was available to manage the association (Hector & Marston, 2003).

For the twenty years of its existence, NLGHF was the center of attention for providers, researchers, policymakers, and consumers interested initially in lesbian and gay health, but eventually encompassing bisexuality and transgender health and all the various facets associated with the cultures of being lesbian, gay, bisexual, and transgender (Shernoff & Scott, 1988). Each year, NLGHF convened the national conference and published important networking materials such as the *National Gay Health Directory* (Ryan & Brossart, 1979) and the *Sourcebook on Lesbian/Gay Health Care* (Shernoff & Scott, 1988). The foundation also provided venues for forming other national groups, such as the National Association of Lesbian and Gay Community Centers (History of the Community Center Movement, www.lgbtcenters.org) or facilitating networking and training for other groups, such as the National Association for Lesbian and Gay Addiction Professionals (NALGAP). Joyce Hunter, DSW, a long-time activist, especially with LGBT communities of color, and a former president of NLGHA, recalls how the Women's Caucus of NLGHA met in 1989-1990 in New Orleans to identify strategies to advance the lesbian health movement (Drabble, 2000). In the late 1980s, Ellen Ratner, then president of NLGHA, worked with Damien Martin, Gabe Kruks, and others to form a network for organizations that worked with LGBT youth (Ryan, personal communication, March 31, 2004).

The discovery of AIDS in the early 1980s in the United States provided the impetus for the U.S. Department of Health and Human Services (DHHS) and its many operating divisions to become united in addressing a public health problem that could no longer be ignored, despite the reluctance by many of having the federal government inquire about sexual behavior. It was understood that HIV was transmitted from one person to another by three means: sexual contact, sharing needles in intravenous drug use, and blood transfusion. By far, the most frequent mode of transmission was sexual contact. In 1988, DHHS National Institute of Child Health and Human Development (NICHD) issued a contract to the National Opinion Research Center (NORC) to design a national survey of adult sexual behaviors (Laumann, Michael, & Gagnon, 1994). NICHD and NORC tried for four years to obtain approval for the survey from the Office of Management and Budget, which must approve all surveys using federal funds (Solarz, 1999). With the federal government's unwillingness to fund a study of adult sexual behavior, the primary researchers from NORC (Laumann et al., 1994) received funding in 1991 from the Robert Wood Johnson Foundation for a scaled-back version of the study—still the largest sexuality study since Kinsey (Michael, 1997). Still today, the National Health and Social Life Survey, called by some "The Sex Survey," provides the data indicating that 2.8 percent of men and 1.4 percent of women identify as gay or lesbian, while 7.7 percent of men and 7.5 percent of women reported homosexual desire (Laumann, Gagnon, Michael, & Michaels, 1994).

In 1998, when it became clear that NLGHA would close due to significant funding problems, Eric Rofes, a former NLGHA conference organizer and a member of what is now the collective organizing the Gay Men's Health Summit, began investigating ways to revive the conference. Rofes vigorously contacted numerous sources including federal officials, the Gay and Lesbian Medical Association, the National Gay and Lesbian Task Force, and several LGBT community centers about assuming sponsorship of the event (Rofes, 2005). Unfortunately, although most individuals wanted to continue conferences and were interested in expanding gay men's health beyond issues of HIV/AIDS, Rofes did not succeed in receiving fiscal resources from those he contacted. Undeterred, he and several other organizers, including Mark Beyer, Matt Brown, and Kirk Read, under the fiscal sponsorship of the Boulder County AIDS Project (BCAP), held the first Gay Men's Health Summit in 1999 in Boulder, Colorado (E. Rofes, personal communication, September 9, 2005). The success of the conference was measured by the participation of close to 500 individuals, comprising physicians, other clinicians and health care providers, researchers, policymakers, activists, and community leaders.

With the exception of the NLHCS and a few other researchers, lesbian health took a backseat to AIDS and gay male health issues until the 1990s. The first policy breakthrough came in February 1994 with the Lesbian Health Roundtable. More than sixty lesbian and bisexual women health activists met in Washington, DC, to develop recommendations for the DHHS to establish a lesbian health agenda (Solarz, 1999). Lesbian health advocates met with federal health officials at several key agencies. A community letter-writing campaign generated by the Mauntner Project for Lesbians with Cancer (founded by Susan Hester in 1990), GLMA, the Lesbian Health Fund (founded by Kate O'Hanlan and other lesbian physicians in 1992), the National Center for Lesbian Rights, and many lesbians across the country urged NIH to include lesbians and bisexual women and questions on sexual orientation in the Women's Health Initiative and other key studies (Ryan, 2001a). Eventual inclusion of lesbian and bisexual women in the Women's Health Initiative, a large longitudinal study and randomized clinical trial of women's health, led to the publication of critical articles describing possible health disparities among lesbians and bisexual women and heterosexual women (Valanis et al., 2000).

The Centers for Disease Control and Prevention (CDC) established in 1997 a cooperative agreement with the Mautner Project for Lesbians with Cancer, a project called Removing the Barriers, which is a training program targeted at increasing clinicians' skills in proving culturally relevant health care to lesbians of all races and ethnicities (Scout, Bradford, & Fields, 2001).

In 1997, with funding by NIH's Office of Research on Women's Health and the CDC, the Institute of Medicine (IOM) convened the investigation of lesbian health, which led to the publication of the landmark IOM report on lesbian health. After listening to twenty-one invited speakers, public testimony from more than a dozen presenters, and approximately fifty interested members of the public who participated in the discussion, the committee reached the following three conclusions:

1. Additional data are required to determine if lesbians may be at higher risk for certain health problems. Further research is needed to determine the absolute and relative magnitudes of such risk and to better understand the risk and protective factors that influence lesbian health.
2. There are significant barriers to conducting research on lesbian health, including lack of funding, which have limited the development of more sophisticated studies, data analyses, and the publication of results.
3. Research on lesbian health, especially the development of more sophisticated methodologies to conduct such research, will help ad-

vance scientific knowledge that is also of benefit to other population groups, including rare or hard-to-identify population subgroups and women in general. (Reprinted with permission from *Lesbian Health: Assessment and Directions for the Future.* © 1999 by the National Academy of Sciences, courtesy of the National Academies Press, Washington, DC.)

After the publication of the IOM report, Suzanne Haynes, PhD, assistant director of science at the Office on Women's Health, was the impetus for organizing in March 2000 a two-day public-private collaboration, the Scientific Workshop on Lesbian Health. At this workshop, more than 100 invited experts in lesbian research worked with DHHS representatives in addressing the conclusion from the IOM report (Bradford, Ryan, Honnold, & Rothblum, 2001).

HEALTHY PEOPLE

The federal government began the Healthy People initiative in 1979, focusing on the diseases and disorders that need to be addressed and encouraging state and local communities to develop similar plans. The document was amended each decade. Not until *Healthy People 2010* (USDHHS, 2000a), did the DHHS officially identify sexual orientation as a U.S. subpopulation that experiences significant health disparities. (Gender identity was not included in the document.) For persons defined by sexual orientation, *Healthy People 2010* includes twenty-nine specific objectives for which sexual orientation is included in the data templates (USDHHS, 2000a). These objectives occur with ten of the twenty-eight focus areas. Those ten areas are:

1. Access to quality health services
2. Educational and community-based programs
3. Family planning
4. HIV
5. Immunizations and infectious diseases
6. Injury and violence prevention
7. Mental health and mental disorders
8. Sexually transmitted diseases
9. Substance abuse
10. Tobacco use

However, for almost every one of the twenty-nine objectives, the abbreviation "DNC" appears in the data templates. DNC means that data specific to sexual orientation are not currently collected by the data system used to track the objective (USDHHS, 2000b). Approximately 200 national data sets monitor *Healthy People 2010* objectives. Of the twenty-nine objectives, twelve data sets are involved. Six systems have had some experience in measuring some aspect of sexual orientation (Sell & Becker, 2001). One system, the National Household Survey on Drug Abuse, now known as the National Survey on Drug Use and Health, included in 1996 a twenty-five question supplement, of which only one question dealt with the gender of the partner(s) with whom the respondent had sexual relations (Anderson et al., 1999). The National Crime Victimization Survey (NCVS), administered by the U.S. Department of Justice, has been asking one question, since 1995, of perceived sexual orientation (U.S. Department of Justice, 2000). The CDC's HIV/AIDS Surveillance system distributes cases into categories, including MSM, a category that is inclusive only of sexual behavior, not necessarily sexual orientation. However, since 1990, the CDC has included a supplement to the case reports that is population based and includes measures of sexual orientation as well as same-sex behavior (Sell & Becker, 2001).

From January 22, 1993, until January 20, 2001, Donna E. Shalala served as President Clinton's secretary of DHHS. Since the formation of DHHS in 1979, previously part of the Department of Health, Education, and Welfare (DHEW), Shalala has had the longest tenure of any secretary. Secretary Shalala hired Marty Rouse as director of the Office of Scheduling and Advance. In addition, the secretary asked Rouse to "conduct outreach to the lesbian and gay community, to inform [her] of some of the Department's recent activity on issues related to sexual orientation and to make recommendations" (Rouse, 2000, p. 1). Beginning in 1999, Rouse convened informal internal meetings in the department for DHHS employees interested in or already working on issues related to sexual orientation. Rouse's travels outside of the Department were sparked by an article in the *Washington Blade* criticizing the department about *Healthy People 2010,* despite its seminal inclusion of lesbian and gay populations (Smith, 2000). In July 1999 Rouse and several other federal officials attended the first Gay Men's Health Summit, held in Boulder, Colorado. Despite strident complaints about the department's failure to be more inclusive of LGBT populations, Rouse continued to travel the country and coordinated first-ever meetings between public health officials and LGBT providers and activists. His insights and recommendations undoubtedly led to the next unprecedented interagency committee.

In May 2000, Surgeon General and Assistant Secretary for Health David Satcher created an interagency steering committee within DHHS to develop a strategic plan for addressing research and health needs related to sexual orientation (Satcher, 2000). The committee coleads were Christopher Bates, Office of HIV/AIDS Policy; Suzanne Haynes, Office on Women's Health; and Adolfo Mata, Health Resources and Services Administration (HRSA) (USDHHS, 2001). All DHHS operating divisions were represented on the committee and completed an inventory of DHHS activities among sexual orientation (SO) and gender identity (GI) populations. The activities were indexed according to the following goals of the strategic plan:

- Increase access to quality health care for SO/GI populations (forty-six activities)
- Improve the quality of care and services for SO/GI populations (forty activities)
- Increase our understanding of health disparities related to SO/GI (fifty-two activities)
- Strengthen health-promotion and disease-prevention programs serving SO/GI populations (thirty-three activities)
- Improve the federal policy and work environment for SO/GI populations (nine activities)

The actual number of activities was an undercount, as the inventory did not contain any grants or contracts funded by the National Institutes of Health (NIH), which comprised twenty-seven separate institutes and centers. A search of the NIH's Computer Retrieval of Information on Scientific Projects (CRISP) reveals a large portfolio of extramural projects, grants, contracts, and cooperative agreements conducted primarily by universities, hospitals, and other research institutions related to sexual orientation and gender identity.

HRSA, one of the operating divisions of DHHS, began the unprecedented agencywide focus on LGBT health. C. Earl Fox, MD, MPH, administrator of HRSA, the highest-ranking openly gay official within DHHS, established an HRSA steering committee on LGBT health disparities in 2000. The steering committee collaborated with nongovernmental organizations to identify health disparities among LGBT persons and to implement solutions that are truly responsive to their needs. In October 2000 Fox appointed Nancy Kennedy, DrPH, as HRSA's intra-agency liaison for LGBT issues. Reporting directly to him, Kennedy was the first federal DHHS employee to work full-time on LGBT populations.

Kennedy and the HRSA Steering Committee on LGBT Health Disparities worked with GLMA and other federal agencies to produce a companion
document to *Healthy People 2010* that focused exclusively on LGBT health
concerns. *Healthy People 2010: Companion Document for Lesbian, Gay,
Bisexual, and Transgender (LGBT) Health* (GLMA & LGBT Health Experts, 2001) built on the knowledge base generated by a previous HRSA-
funded white paper: *Lesbian, Gay, Bisexual, and Transgender Health:
Findings and Concerns* (Dean et al., 2000). This particular paper, the first
federally funded paper on LGBT health, was a collaboration between
GLMA and academicians/researchers at Columbia University, Joseph L.
Mailman School of Public Health, Center for Lesbian, Gay, Bisexual, and
Transgender Health.

This companion document addressed thirteen areas of health where disparities were shown to exist through published research and/or ethnographic studies. As a result of all of these activities, the National Coalition
for LGBT Health was initiated in October 2000. Comprised of representatives from national and local health-related organizations, LGBT advocates, researchers, academicians, health care professionals, and other representatives of the LGBT community, the coalition offers opportunities to
work together to address the health needs of all four communities comprising sexual minorities (Bradford et al., 2001). The coalition is committed to
improving the health and well-being of lesbian, gay, bisexual, and transgender individuals through federal advocacy that is focused on research,
policy, education, and training (www.lgbtheath.net). Because the coalition
is an advocacy organization, LGBT federal health employees cannot, by
law, participate actively in the leadership of the organization. Both the coalition and GayHealth.com provide weekly newsletters to assist in assem-
bling the resources and information to address the diverse needs of the multifaceted communities. In June 2001 the *American Journal of Public Health*
released the first issue, in its ninety-one years of publication, on lesbian, gay,
bisexual, and transgender health. Without even a call for papers, the journal's
editor received more than 100 submissions (Northridge, 2001).

THE PRESENT:
THE THREAT OF SCIENTIFIC McCARTHYISM

The nearly 500-page companion document generated hope that LGBT
health issues would finally be incorporated into the nation's health care
agenda. However, that hope dissipated as the administration changed from
Clinton to Bush, and leaders such as Dr. Fox were summarily dismissed.
The LGBT liaison position created by Fox was immediately abolished and

DHHS refused to publish the companion document. Support and hope for the future has been kept alive by outside organizations, not just LGBT groups such as the National Coalition for LGBT Health, but allied organizations such as the National Mental Health Association. The Internet has made it possible for the companion document to be downloaded from numerous Web sites and sent to every possible city, town, county, university, and municipality looking for information and strategies to address the disparities of LGBT populations.

For many sexual minorities working for DHHS, the change in administration meant a "return to the closet." The military's "don't ask, don't tell" refrain was mimicked within DHHS. Some agencies within the operating divisions of DHHS dismantled their internal workgroups addressing the concerns of not only LGBT employees but also LGBT populations served by the agency. A notable exception has been NIH's group Salutaris— among the first, if not the first, gay and lesbian employee group to form within the federal government. Two National Library of Medicine employees, Joe Pagano and Paul Weiss, started the group in 1991, and the group continues to not only represent LGBT employees at NIH but also to serve as a resource on LGBT issues for NIH (http://www.recgov.org/glef).

As the antipathy toward LGBT health issues increased within the administration, federal health officials at NIH and CDC began to warn potential grant applicants not to use specific terminology such as condom effectiveness, needle exchange, abortion, commercial sex workers, transgender, and men who have sex with men when applying for federal funding, especially for HIV/AIDS grants (Goode, 2003; Kaiser, 2003b). Federal Web sites were changed dramatically. For example, a fact sheet about condoms, including not only the proper use but also the research studies about the efficacy of condom use, on CDC's Web site was replaced in October 2002 with a document describing the failure rates associated with condom use and the efficacy of abstinence (Clymer, 2002). In addition, CDC discontinued a project titled Programs That Work, which identified evidence-based sex-education programs that were considered comprehensive programs for teenagers. The implication for discontinuing this CDC program is that President Bush favors abstinence-only programs despite the evidence that they don't work (Union of Concerned Scientists, 2004).

Beginning in 1998 and culminating in 2003, the Traditional Values Coalition (TVC), using the CRISP online public research database, generated a list of almost 200 "questionable" NIH grants addressing sexual orientation, gender identity, HIV/AIDS, and other related topics (Gallagher, 2003). However, information was included in their list that is not accessible to the public, such as the amount of each grant and whether grants were funded for a particular investigator, leading Representative Waxman (2003, p. 2) to conclude that "officials within HHS itself appear to have been directly involved with the creation of this list." As a result of the list, Representative Patrick Toomey of Pennsylvania proposed an amendment on July 10, 2003, to defund five specific NIH grants (House Amendment 221 to H.R. 2660). Despite broad awareness among many researchers and civil servants of the scientific rigor of NIH reviews, Toomey's amendment was barely defeated 210-212 (House of Representatives, Roll No. 352, July 10, 2003).

Even with this vote, the matter was not finished. The TVC list was widely disseminated to not only Congress and the press but also to federal officials and researchers. At professional meetings, such as the American Public Health Association, American Medical Association, American Psychological Association, and the like, participants scrutinized the registry of names, which had become a "hit list" that many saw as a right-wing agenda to rid the government, inside and outside, of not only sexual minorities but also any heterosexual individuals who were conducting or requesting such research. More than 250 grants involving more than 150 senior investigators comprise the list, and the sponsoring colleges and universities include Baylor, Emory, Harvard, Johns Hopkins, Miami, Penn State, the University of Wyoming, the University of Kentucky, and the University of Washington. Quite naturally, many federal project officers at NIH called their grantees to apprise them of their status on this list to prepare them for any future scrutiny as to the public health value of their research (Agres, 2003). The result of questioning and overturning the NIH scientific peer review process has been to intimidate many public health bureaucrats and scientists, particularly those affiliated with academic institutions whose livelihood is often dependent on federal funding.

On October 2, 2003, the Senate's Committee on Health, Education, Labor and Pensions and the House's Committee on Energy and Commerce held a joint hearing on the future of NIH during which the current NIH director, Elias Zerhouni, MD, was repeatedly asked about the controversial grants funded by NIH (Varmus, 2003). Congressman Henry Waxman, House Government Reform ranking minority member, reported that he had received many telephone calls and written complaints, especially from the Web site (democrats.reform.house.gov/features/politics_and_science) maintained by the minority staff of the Committee on Government Reform. In an October 27, 2003, letter to Secretary Tommy Thompson, Representative Waxman decried the "scientific McCarthyism" that was occurring at NIH and asked the secretary both to denounce the attacks on science and affirm support for the NIH review process (Waxman, 2003). Two days later, Andrea Lafferty, TVC executive director, wrote and posted on TVC's Web site (www.traditionalvalues.org) her response to Congressman Waxman's letter, taking full credit for the generation of the list and suggesting that the review process at NIH be investigated by the Justice Department (Kaiser, 2003a).

The following thirty-six scientific organizations issued statements in defense of the targeted peer-review research funded by NIH (democrats. reform.house.gov/features/politics_and_science/nih_support.htm):

    Academy of Behavioral Medicine Research
    Ambulatory Pediatric Association
    American Academy of Nursing
    American Academy of Pediatrics
    American Association for the Advancement of Science
    American Association of Medical Colleges
    American College of Obstetricians and Gynecologists
    American Foundation for AIDS Research
    American Medical Association
    American Pediatric Society
    American Psychiatric Association
    American Psychological Association
    American Psychological Society
    American Public Health Association
    American Sociological Association
    Association of American Universities
    Association of Medical School Pediatric Department Chairs
    Association of Population Centers
    Association of Reproductive Health Professionals
    Association of Schools of Public Health
    Association of Teachers of Preventive Medicine
    Center for the Advancement of Health
    Consortium of Social Science Associations
    Federation of Behavioral, Psychological and Cognitive Sciences
    Federation of American Societies for Experimental Biology
    HIV Medicine Association
    Infectious Diseases Society of America
    Institute for the Advancement of Social Work Research
    Population Association of America
    Society for Adolescent Medicine
    Society for Pediatric Research
    Society for Research in Child Development
    Society for Research on Adolescence
    Society for Women's Health Research
    Society of Behavioral Medicine
    University of California

On February 18, 2004, the Union of Concerned Scientists, an independent, nonprofit alliance of more than 100,000 scientists and concerned citizens, launched a grassroots campaign to halt the misuse of science by the Bush administration, noting the interference with independent scientific inquiry at the Environmental Protection Agency, the Food and Drug Administration, and the Departments of Health and Human Services, Agriculture, Interior, and Defense (Union of Concerned Scientists, 2004).

CONCLUSION

Those who do not know the past are, as the saying goes, destined to repeat it. Given the passage of the Patriot Act that erodes civil liberties, the president's proposed constitutional amendment against same-sex marriage, and the encasement of politics within a fundamentalist Christian framework that uses a literal interpretation of the Bible to rally against the "immoralities" of homosexuality, the federal government is, once again, not a safe work environment for individuals who are sexual minorities. As long as we can keep the door ajar and see the light, then we are not again closeted or, worse yet, institutionalized. Those of us who have lived at least five decades understand the pendulum of change; after the oppression, constraint, and separatism of the 1950s came the 1960s celebration of diversity and merging of cultures and disciplines. Scientific McCarthyism is a preventable condition. We know the risk factors and, even more important, we have the resiliency to withstand the stressors and live life one day at a time.

People comprise bureaucracies, and people are the infrastructure of change. Federal GLOBE, the Gay, Lesbian, Bisexual, Transgender Employees of the Federal Government, began in 1992. As a voluntary, nonprofit 501C (3) organization, GLOBE's chartered purpose is

> to eliminate prejudice and discrimination in the federal government based on sexual orientation by (1) developing and providing educational programs, materials, and assistance mechanisms which address the distinctive concerns and problems of lesbians, gay men, and bisexuals in the federal government and (2) educating the general public, policy makers, and federal employees about issues of concern to lesbians, gay men, and bisexuals. (www.fedglobe.org)

Federal GLOBE's quarterly newsletter, *globalview,* is direct-mailed to 800 dues-paying members, not just in Washington but throughout the various duty stations. Total readership among federal employees is estimated at approximately 2,000, although many more access the Web site (www. fedglobe.org).

Through that Web site federal employees can "come out" through self-identification and serve as role models. Scientific terrorism is defeated when people speak up and acknowledge that no one can strip another of self-dignity. As civil servants and health advocates, we can model the behavior that we wish to see in our elected officials and put forth the laws and policies for those who have no voice or are invisible.

Four decades after the McCarthy era, following a period of increasing public awareness and acceptance of homosexuality and visibility of LGBT persons in the media, the clock has been turned back by the Bush administration. These actions have caused fear among federal employees and some grantees, trepidation among potential grant applicants, and, in the words of Representative Henry Waxman, they have "manipulated the scientific process and distorted or suppressed scientific findings" (Malakoff, 2003, p. 901). Support for the president's proposed amendment to prevent same-sex marriage and the framing of social and health policy from the perspective of a literal interpretation of the Bible endangers the many gains earned by LGBT Americans since Evelyn Hooker demonstrated in the late 1950s that there were no discernable differences in psychological health between homosexual and heterosexual men. The beginning of this new century is foreboding for individuals who are sexual minorities as the "current Bush administration has suppressed or distorted scientific analysis of federal agencies" (Union of Concerned Scientists, 2004, p. 1). To what extent will the lessons learned during the illustrious past shape the policies and practices of this new century?

REFERENCES

Agres, T. (2003, November). Sex, drugs, and NIH. *The Scientist*. Retrieved November 3, 2003, from www.the-scientist.com.

Anderson, J. E., Wilson, R. W., Barker, P., Doll, L., Jones, T. S., & Holtgrave, D. (1999). Prevalence of sexual and drug-related HIV risk behaviors in the U.S. adult population: Results of the 1996 National Household Survey on Drug Use. *Journal of Acquired Immune Deficiency Syndromes and Human Retrovirology, 21,*148-156.

Ayyar, R. (2004, March 22). Interview: Historian David K. Johnson exposes the U.S. government's anti-gay crusades. *Gay Today, 8,* 26.

Bachelor, C. D. (1950). Political cartoon. *Washington Times Herald,* March 31 (c) New York Daily News, L.P.

Belkin, A., Bateman, G., & Monks, N. (Eds.). (2003). *Don't ask, don't tell: Debating the gay ban in the military.* Boulder, CO: Lynne Rienner Pubs.

Bradford, J., & Ryan, C. (1987). *National Lesbian Health Care Survey: Mental health implications for lesbians.* National Institute of Mental Health, National Technical Information Service, PB88-201496/AS.

Bradford, J., & Ryan, C. (1988). *The National Lesbian Health Care Survey: Final report.* Washington, DC: National Lesbian and Gay Health Foundation.

Bradford, J., Ryan, C., Honnold, J., & Rothblum, E. (2001). Expanding the research infrastructure for lesbian health. *American Journal of Public Health, 91*(7), 1029-1032.

Bryan, S. M. (2004, February 21). License about-face in New Mexico. *San Francisco Chronicle,* p. A4.

Chappell, K. (2002, August). The truth about bisexuality in black America: AIDS epidemic and social problems create explosive situation–lifestyle. *Ebony, 57.* Retrieved July 15, 2005, from http://www.findarticles.com/p/articles/mi_m 1077/is_10_57/ai97997636.

Chibbaro, L. (2004, March 14). Bush's special counsel tied to anti-gay groups. *Washington Blade.* Retrieved July 15, 2005, from http://www.washblade.com/ 2004/3-19/news/national/council.cfm.

Clymer, A. (2002, December 27). U.S. revises sex information and a fight goes on. *The New York Times,* A15.

Dean, L., Meyer, I. H., Robinson, K., Sell, R. L., Sember, R., Selenzio, V. M. B., Bowen, D. J., Bradford, J., Rothblum, E., Scout, et al. (2000). Lesbian, gay, bisexual, and transgender health: Findings and concerns. *Journal of the Gay and Lesbian Medical Association, 4*(3), 101-151.

D'Emilio, J. (1998). *Sexual politics, sexual communities: The making of a homosexual minority in the United States, 1940-1970.* Chicago: University of Chicago Press.

Drabble, L. (2000). *Advancing gay and lesbian health: A report from the Gay and Lesbian Health Roundtable.* Los Angeles: L.A. Gay and Lesbian Center.

Fee, E., Brown, T. M., & contributing editors. (2001). Voices from the past: Editor's note. *American Journal of Public Health, 91*(6), 901.

Fielding, W. (1932). *Love and the sex emotions.* New York: Donn, Mead & Company.

Gallagher, R. (2003). No sex research please: We're American. *The Scientist, 17*(23), 6.

Garber, M. (1995). *Vice versa: Bisexuality and the eroticism of everyday life.* New York: Simon & Schuster.

Gay and Lesbian Medical Association & LGBT Health Experts. (2001). *Healthy people 2010: Companion document for lesbian, gay, bisexual, and transgender (LGBT) health.* San Francisco, CA: GLMA.

Goode, E. (2003, April 18). Certain words can trip up AIDS grants, scientists say. *New York Times,* A10.

Gordon, R., & Sebastian, S. (2004, February 25). Same-sex marriage ban of "national importance." *San Francisco Chronicle,* p. A1.

Hecktor, A., & Marston, B. (2003). Guide to the National Lesbian and Gay Health Association Records, 1983-1992, Collection No. 7613, Division of Rare and Manuscript Collections, Cornell University Library.

Hirsch, L. P. (1996). Welcome and state of Federal GLOBE. *Globalview, 5*(1), 2.

Hooker, E. (1957). The adjustment of the male overt homosexual. *Journal of Projective Techniques, 21*, 18-31.

Jamison, G. (2000). Introduction to transgender issues. In *Transgender equality: A handbook for activists and policymakers* (p. 7). New York: Policy Institute, National Gay and Lesbian Task Force, and the National Center for Lesbian Rights.

Johnson, D. J. (2004). *The lavender scare: The cold war persecution of gays and lesbians in the federal government.* Chicago: University of Chicago Press.

Johnson, D. K. (1994-1995). Homosexual citizens: Washington's gay community confronts the civil service. *Washington History, 6*, 44-63.

Kaiser, J. (2003a). NIH roiled by inquiries over grants hit list. *Science, 302*(5646), 758.

Kaiser, J. (2003b). Studies of gay men, prostitutes come under scrutiny. *Science, 18*, 403.

Knight, R., LaBarbera, P., & Ervin, K. (2001). The Bush administration's Republican homosexual agenda: The first 100 days. Retrieved July 15, 2005, from http://www.cultureandfamily.org/articledisplay.asp?id/2574&department/CFI&categoryid/papers.

Lait, J., & Mortimer, L. (1951). *Washington confidential.* New York: Dell Publishing.

Laumann, E. O., Gagnon, J. H., Michael, R. T., & Michaels, S. (1994). *The social organization of sexuality: Sexual practices in the United States.* Chicago: University of Chicago Press.

Laumann, E. O., Michael, R. T., & Gagnon, J. H. (1994). A political history of the national sex survey of adults. *Family Planning Perspectives, 26*(1), 34-38.

Lehring, G. (2003) *Officially gay: The political construction of sexuality by the U.S. military.* Queer Politics, Queer Theories. Philadelphia, PA: Temple University Press.

Leip, D. (2001). Atlas of U.S. presidential elections. Retrieved July 15, 2005, from http://www.uselectionatlas.org.

Lesbian and Gay Rights. (2000). *AIDS/HIV 2000.* An ACLU Report.

Leslie, D. R., Berina, B. A., & Maqueda, M. C. (2001). Clinical issues with transgender individuals. In U.S. Department of Health and Human Services, SAMHSA, CSAT, *A provider's introduction to substance abuse treatment for lesbian, gay, bisexual and transgender individuals,* DHHS Pub. No. (SMA) 01-3498, 91-98.

Livingood, J. M. (Ed.). (1972). *Task force on homosexuality: Final report and background papers.* DHEW Pub. No. (HSM) 72-9119. Rockville, MD: National Institute of Mental Health.

Lourea, D. N. (1985). Psycho-social issues related to counseling bisexuals. *Journal of Homosexuality, 11*(1-2), 51-62.

Lum, M. (2001, September 20). Gays could serve in war, be discharged in peace. *TexasTriangle.* Available at www.mattlum.com/journalism/fom.htm.

Malakoff, D. (2003). Democrats accuse Bush of letting politics distort science. *Science, 301*(5635), 901.

Marcus, E. (1992). *Making history: The struggle for gay and lesbian equal rights, 1945-1990.* New York: HarperCollins.

McCollum, C. (2003, November 4). Controversial mini-series on Reagans to air November 30. (San Jose) *Mercurynews.com.*

Michael, R. T. (1997). The National Health and Social Life Survey: Public health findings and their implications In S. L. Isaacs & J. R. Knickman (Eds.), *To improve health and health care, 1997: The Robert Wood Johnson anthology* (pp. 232-249). San Francisco: Jossey-Bass.

National Defense Authorization Act of 1994, Public Law 103-160, 107 Statute 1670, November 30, 1993.

Newitz, A., & Sandell, J. (1994). Bisexuality and how to use it: Toward a coalitional identity politics. *Bad Subjects, 16.* Retrieved April 2, 2001, from http://eserver.org/bs/16/Sandell.html.

Northridge, M. E. (2001). Editors note: Advancing lesbian, gay, bisexual and transgender health. *American Journal of Public Health, 91*(6), 855-856.

Office of the Press Secretary, White House, for George W. Bush. (2004). Presidential call for constitutional amendment protecting marriage, February 21.

Rofes, E. (2005). Gay bodies, gay selves: Understanding the gay men's health movement. *White Crane Journal,* Fall, 1-9.

Rouse, M. (2000). Memorandum to the secretary, Lesbian and gay community outreach.

Rust, P. (2001). Too many and not enough: The meaning of bisexual identities. *Journal of Bisexuality, 1*(1), 33-70.

Ryan, C. (2001a). Lesbian health—Looking back, looking ahead. Plenary Address. Lesbian Health Conference, San Francisco, June 22.

Ryan, C. (2001b). My roots as an activist. *Journal of Lesbian Studies, 5*(3), 141-149.

Ryan, C., & Bradford, J. (1999). Conducting the National Lesbian Health Care Survey: First of its kind. *Journal of the Gay and Lesbian Medical Association, 3*(3), 87-93.

Ryan, C., & Brossart, J. (1979). *National gay health directory: A compendium of services for lesbians and gay men.* New York: National Gay Health Coalition.

Satcher, D. (2000, March 8). Memorandum to deputy secretary of Health Kevin Thurm. Sexual orientation issues and Healthy People 2010: Briefing.

Schwarzenegger, A. (2004). Interview by Tim Russert, *Meet the Press,* NBC, February 22.

Scout, Bradford, J., & Fields, C. (2001). Removing the barriers: Improving practitioners' skills in providing health care to lesbians and women who partner with women. *American Journal of Public Health, 91*(6), 989.

Sell, R. L., & Becker, J. B. (2001). Sexual orientation data collection and progress toward Healthy People 2010. *American Journal of Public Health, 91*(6), 876-882.

Shernoff, M., & Scott, W. (Eds.). (1988). *The sourcebook on lesbian/gay health care* (2nd ed.). Washington, DC: The National Lesbian/Gay Health Foundation.

Smith, R. (2000, February 25). Healthy criticism: Activists complain report omits gays. *The Washington Blade.*

Solarz, A. L. (Ed.). (1999). *Committee on Lesbian Health Research Priorities, Neuroscience and Behavioral Health Program and Health Sciences Policy Program, Institute of Medicine, lesbian health.* Washington, DC: National Academy Press.

Summersgill, B. (2000). 75th birthday tribute to Franklin E. Kameny GLAA 29th Anniversary Reception, Doyle Washington Hotel, Washington, DC, April 27.

Sunstein, C. R., & Epstein, R. A. (2001). *The vote: Bush, Gore and the Supreme Court.* Chicago, IL: University of Chicago Press.

Tewksbury, R., & Gagne, P. (1996). Transgenderists: Products of non-normative intersection of sex, gender, and sexuality. *Journal of Men's Studies, 5,* 105-129.

Union of Concerned Scientists. (2004). *Scientific integrity in policymaking: An investigation into the Bush administration's misuse of science.* Cambridge, MA: Union of Concerned Scientists.

U.S. Department of Health & Human Services. (2000a). *Healthy people 2010, Understanding and improving health and objectives for improving health* (2nd ed.) (2 volumes). Washington, DC: GPO.

U.S. Department of Health & Human Services. (2000b). *Tracking Healthy People 2010.* Washington, DC: U.S. Government Printing Office (GPO).

U.S. Department of Health & Human Services. (2001). Strategic plan on addressing health disparities related to sexual orientation. Steering committee on health disparities related to sexual orientation. Unpublished draft.

U.S. Department of Justice. (2000). *Bureau of Justice Statistics, National Crime Victimization Survey, NCVSI—basic screen questionnaire.* Washington, DC: U.S. Department of Justice.

Valanis, B. G., Bowen, D. J., Bassford, T., Whitlock, E., Charney, P., & Carter, R. A. (2000). Sexual orientation and health: Comparisons in the Women's Health Initiative sample. *Archives of Family Medicine, 9,* 843-853.

Varmus, H. (2003). Managing biomedical research to prevent and cure disease in the 21st century: Matching NIH policy with science. Washington, DC: The House Committee on Energy and Commerce, the Senate Committee on Health, Education, Labor and Pensions.

Waxman, H., to the Honorable Tommy G. Thompson, October 27, 2003, p. 4.

PART VI:
EMPLOYERS AND BUSINESS

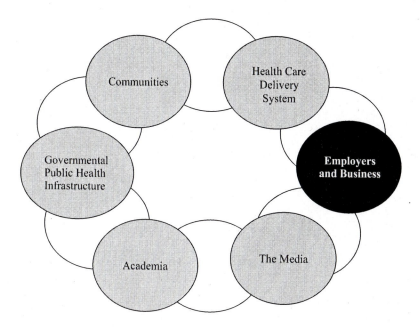

PART VI:
EMPLOYERS AND BUSINESS

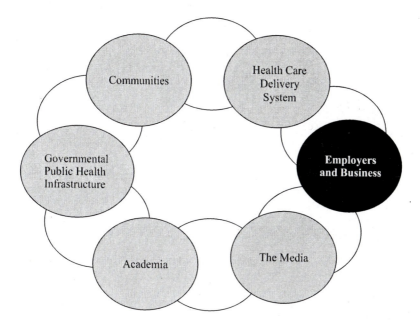

315

Chapter 14

The Need for Change:
Bridging Employers and Business

Robert C. Preston Jr.
Rob J. Fredericksen
Daryl Herrschaft

INTRODUCTION

LGBT-friendly workplace policies are increasingly becoming a common business practice. As of April 2004 a total of 377 companies in the Fortune 500, or 75 percent, include sexual orientation in their equal employment opportunity (EEO) policies. The closer a company is to the top of the Fortune list the more likely it is to have an inclusive EEO policy. Ninety-eight percent, or 49, of the Fortune 50 companies include sexual orientation in their EEO policy.

Similarly, 212 companies in the Fortune 500, or 42 percent, provide domestic partner benefits. In 1998, just 13 percent of Fortune 500 companies offered domestic partner benefits. Further, not having LGBT-friendly policies in place ignores a large and recently more visible proportion of the workforce. The 2000 U.S. Census found that same-sex-couple households exist in more than 99 percent of counties in the United States (Human Rights Campaign [HRC], 2004d).

Employers are finding that creating a workforce climate that fosters the inclusiveness of LGBT employees and equalizing benefits improves overall health, productivity, and the bottom line. Subtle discrimination impacts LGBT people disproportionately. Those who try to hide their sexual orientation may find that simple discussions, for example, about summer vacations or weekend activities, can lead to stress, a modifiable risk factor. Harassment, hostile work environments, and the threat of violence may also lead to increased risk behaviors. Employers with proactive policies can reduce the risk of increased health care expenditures and potential harassment or discrimination litigation. Cost savings are also achieved through increased productivity because healthy employees are more productive employees. Maintaining inclusive workplace policies improves corporate reputation and can provide a competitive advantage in the labor and consumer markets. Popular regard as an employer of choice can also lead to lower turnover and higher recruitment potential.

So why is everyone not on board? To most it would be relatively clear that the road is paved for LGBT-friendly work environments. Whether cultural, rooted in religious beliefs, or simply a lack of knowledge where the senior leadership team is concerned, this is not the case with many. This chapter will look at some of the implications of not offering comprehensive benefits packages, discuss recent updates, and leave the reader with the resources and framework from which to ensure an LGBT-friendly work environment exists in their own workplace.

LINKING LGBT HEALTH AND EMPLOYMENT

So, how is employment linked to LGBT health? To address this, we must consider the magnitude of inequities that still exist for many LGBT people on the job. Some workplaces do not include sexual orientation in their antidiscrimination policy. Some workplaces do not have same-sex domestic partner benefits. Predominately, this is the case with smaller businesses. Of course, having these policies and benefits is no guarantee that a workplace climate will be welcoming or equitable to LGBT people. Countless ways exist to consciously, yet covertly, exclude and discriminate without the appearance of explicitly violating the terms of an antidiscrimination policy. Exclusion and discrimination on the basis of sexual orientation and/or gender identity is also a subconscious process that even well-meaning colleagues can unknowingly stride. The result is a spectrum of workplace climates that vary greatly in their true level of comfort with openly LGBT employees, regardless of policy or institutional intent (Community-University Institute for Social Research, 2003).

How does this spectrum of workplace climates, lack of protective policies, and lack of domestic partner benefits adversely affect the health of LGBT workers? Stress is caused by marginalization, social isolation, and discrimination. This poses serious short- and long-term effects on one's physical and mental health. Both chronic and short-term stress have been shown to result in poor immune functioning, slower healing time, and susceptibility to viral infection. Stress also has been found to increase the risk of cardiovascular disease, as well as the development of back and upper-extremity musculoskeletal disorders (Wein, 2000).

Work, of course, implies a degree of stress by definition. We are paid to apply our skills to a set of tasks and issues that must be completed within a certain time frame. Adverse working conditions, such as a lack of job security or overload of responsibility, are common stressors.

For LGBT individuals in an unwelcoming work environment, another layer of stress is added at the level of social interaction, greatly increasing the psychological demand of returning to a workplace each day. Persons who feel pressure in the workplace to conform to heterosexual norms and gender roles may opt to conceal their orientation and identity, which in itself has been found to negatively affect physical health, specifically, a higher incidence of cancers and of infectious diseases such as pneumonia, sinusitis, and bronchitis (Sauter et al., 1990).

Lack of domestic partner benefits is another mechanism that links employment and LGBT health. Partners of LGBT workers may lack their own health benefits for a number of reasons, including unemployment, working for a company that does not offer medical coverage, or because of financial reasons. Lack of health insurance results in the uninsured or underinsured individual avoiding primary care, which limits the opportunity for routine health screenings and prevention education. Many medical problems remain undiagnosed and can become permanently disabling or potentially life threatening without appropriate intervention. When a health problem finally becomes detectable, painful, or otherwise impairing, it is generally far more expensive to treat and results in a lower chance of a positive outcome. Without prescription drug insurance, regular access to medications in order to manage health conditions may be interrupted. Finally, the National Academy of Science's Institute of Medicine (IOM, 2002a) reported that those without insurance receive fewer diagnostic and treatment services after traumatic injuries or heart attacks, resulting in an increased risk of death, even when in the hospital. A meta-analysis of health access studies showed that among working-age Americans, those without health insurance are more likely to be sicker and die sooner. Further, an employee with an ailing and uninsured partner is likely to be under a considerable degree of psychological distress, especially if the illness or injury is severe. Last, financial stress placed on LGBT workers from helping pay out-of-pocket for a domestic partner's care can be overwhelming and financially devastating.

The World Health Organization (WHO) defines health as a state of complete physical, mental, and social well-being, and not merely the absence of disease or infirmity (World Health Organization, 1948). Work acts as a defining characteristic of most of our lives and is, at the very least, a tremendous time and energy commitment. For many of us, our identities and well-being are intimately linked with our work lives: our careers have the potential to contribute to or to erode our overall health. Supportive workplace climates, protective policies, and fair benefits help generate the sense of well-being that WHO defines as central to the very definition of health. The economic benefits of higher productivity, increased retention, and a harmonious work environment show that investing not only in preventive and curative health care but also the well-being of LGBT employees and their domestic partners is indeed a win-win situation.

EMPLOYMENT DECISIONS AND THEIR EFFECTS ON LGBT WORKERS

Hiring decisions, personnel policy administration, and bias on behalf of the employer can cause a dysfunctional work environment. LGBT workers are entitled to the same privileges as heterosexual workers, including a workplace free from harassment, cultural barriers, or ignorance. With this said, it is amazing how even today, many LGBT workers do not share this experience. It is also important to note that when making hiring decisions, the organization must select senior leadership that will embrace diversity and include sexual orientation.

In 1999, in the southeast, a governor appointed a known conservative to head the Department of Health. The appointee made known his belief that the LGBT lifestyle was immoral through his work in the legislature. In a letter to the CFO of an international entertainment and theme-park giant, which was signed by fourteen other lawmakers, he stated that offering domestic partner benefits to same-sex couples was a big mistake, both morally and financially ("Bush appointee in Florida grilled," 1999). Imagine that you are a tenured employee with the Department of Health, openly gay, and perhaps well respected. How would you feel about your job security under this new leadership? One might also feel unable to continue being open about his or her sexuality with co-workers, for fear of retaliation. Over time this stress could potentially lead to physical aliments.

In the Midwest, a health care worker who was openly gay was terminated, in her opinion, because she did not have the protection of the Family and Medical Leave Act (FMLA). In a relationship with her partner of eighteen years, she was in a precarious situation when she needed to take time off to care for her partner. Had she been legally married, she would have simply filed for leave under FMLA. However, because the federal government does not recognize domestic partnerships, the legal protection of FMLA was not available to her. According to the hospital, she was fired for performance issues. However, over fifty supporters came forward to attest to their belief that it was because of her sexual orientation. In an interview the health care worker stated that she was struggling, trying to balance work and the love of her life. She would not let her life partner suffer and die alone.

Ultimately, when her partner became very sick, she used all of her remaining vacation days up until the day her partner died. The only reason she was able to attend the funeral was due to the generosity of her fellow employees, who were allowed to donate their sick days to her. The expectation, however, where the hospital was concerned, was that she would be back at work the following day.

According to the health care worker, exactly 160 days after she came out to her boss, she was fired. Keep in mind that during this period, according to her, she received a good evaluation after her ninety-day probation.

At the point of termination, and with the obligation of having to support eight children, five of her partner's and three of her own, and fourteen grandchildren, she pleaded with the hospital to allow her to work in other departments, such as neonatal and obstetrics, which would have allowed for the work/life balance necessary to maintain her salary while caring for her family. The request was denied (Napier, 2002).

Now imagine that you were an employee in the previous examples. If you worked for the Department of Health in that southeastern state, do you feel you could continue to add value to your position knowing the views of the appointee? Would you feel motivated to stay in a helping profession, if you knew in your greatest time of need, your employer would not support you? These are critical questions, as labor shortages abound in helping professions, including public health. Many workers cannot risk losing their livelihood, so instead they choose to remain closeted. This lack of equality fosters an environment of closed minds and closets.

THE STATE OF THE WORKPLACE
AND RECOMMENDATIONS FOR EMPLOYERS

No federal law protects LGBT employees from workplace discrimination based on sexual orientation or gender identity or expression. As of September 2005, workplace discrimination based on sexual orientation is illegal in fourteen states, and in four of those states on the basis of gender identity or expression. Legislation has been introduced in the U.S. Congress to address some of these inequities (see Exhibit 14.1 for information on tracking such legislation). For example, the Employment Nondiscrimination Act (ENDA) would outlaw job discrimination on the basis of sexual orientation. As of January 2004, more than 100 businesses publicly supported passage of ENDA, including more than forty major corporations (HRC, 2004d). Likewise, federal law does not recognize same-sex relationships for federal tax purposes or for employment benefits. For example, FMLA, tax-preferred plans, and the continuation of health care benefits fol-

---

EXHIBIT 14.1. The Human Rights Campaign Foundation's WorkNet
http://www.hrc.org/worknet

One comprehensive, national source of information on workplace policies and laws surrounding sexual orientation and gender identity is HRC WorkNet. It is home to the nation's most comprehensive and regularly updated database of workplace policies at thousands of corporations, businesses, colleges and universities, and public employers.

HRC WorkNet continually monitors and reports on federal, state, and local legislative, judicial, and corporate activities that affect the LGBT community in the workplace. HRC WorkNet provides essential guidance, "how-to" tools, and individual consultation to individuals and groups in an effort to bring more inclusive policies and programs to more workplaces.

---

lowing employment (Consolidated Omnibus Budget Reconciliation Act [COBRA]) do not automatically extend to gay and lesbian couples as they do to heterosexual married couples.

At the state and local level, some limited recognition of gay and lesbian relationships exists. Vermont's civil union law, enacted in 2000, entitles same-sex couples to the more than 300 state-level rights and responsibilities extended to opposite-sex spouses. In 2003, the Massachusetts Supreme Judicial Court ruled that under that state's constitution same-sex couples could not be denied marriage licenses. Although that decision sparked several other communities—most notably San Francisco—to begin issuing marriage licenses for same-sex couples, licenses issued in Massachusetts beginning in May 2004 will carry the full weight of state law (San Francisco Human Rights Commission, 1998).

Employers that have already implemented domestic partner benefits programs are prepared for many of the contingencies that the advent of legal marriage for same-sex couples raises. Forward-looking employers will also realize that the recognition of committed same-sex relationships on par with opposite-sex married relationships across the United States—and around the world—is better for business.

On February 24, 2004, President George W. Bush said he supports an amendment to the U.S. Constitution that would limit marriage to one man and one woman. The proposed changes to the constitution could have antibusiness and antihealth ramifications. For instance, the availability of domestic partner health insurance benefits through state-regulated plans could end. In addition, health care benefits for public employees' partners are unlikely to be considered constitutional, leading to more uninsured people and higher health insurance costs for everyone.

Domestic partnership laws in the states of California, Hawaii, and New Jersey provide some legal rights to gay and lesbian couples in registered relationships. Although these laws are a first step in ensuring equality, these state-level legal protections do not address more than 1,100 rights, benefits, and protections that are provided to heterosexual, married couples by the federal government.

As of January 2004 one state, California, and nine cities and counties have passed equal benefits ordinances, which require that contractors with state and local governments offer equal benefits to their employees' domestic partners. To get a contract with these governments, a contractor who already offers an employee benefits package that includes spousal coverage must offer an equivalent benefits package to employees with domestic partners.

WHAT EMPLOYERS AND BUSINESSES ARE DOING

In response to the patchwork of legal protections that exist in the United States, employers across the country are implementing policies and benefits that address the needs of LGBT employees. In many cases, state and federal law set forth minimum benefits requirements, and employers are free to go beyond what is required. Public health employers are uniquely situated to receive multiple gains by addressing LGBT issues in the workplace. As both employers and providers of health care services, public health organizations not only experience work-force benefits, such as improved productivity, recruitment, and retention, but also can deliver improved quality of care with a staff that is culturally sensitive regarding LGBT issues.

A nondiscrimination or equal employment opportunity policy that includes the terms sexual orientation and gender identity or expression is the cornerstone of a fair and equitable workplace for LGBT employees. Without such a policy, LGBT employees may have well-grounded fears about coming out as LGBT, because in most places they can be terminated without any legal recourse. Explicitly including these terms in nondiscrimination and antiharassment policies may help ensure that all employees will be judged based on performance rather than on sexual orientation.

Domestic partner benefits, particularly health benefits, make good business and public health sense and have become an essential part of many benefits packages. LGBT people are more likely than their heterosexual counterparts to be uninsured or underinsured. Further, 60 percent of employees rank health insurance as the number-one employer benefit. Thus, employers that offer health insurance benefits to domestic partners can increase the proportion of the LGBT population that receives adequate medical insurance and secure benefits in the workforce such as improved employee morale and productivity (U.S. Department of Health and Human Services, 2000).

Domestic partner health care benefits are easy to administer. Because the benefits are simply an extension of eligibility for existing benefits programs, implementation is usually simple. Many insurance carriers provide standard domestic partner policies, though some employers will have to negotiate for the coverage. Insurance companies in most states will write policies covering domestic partners and, in several other locations, laws either compel them to (Maine and Vermont) or provide significant incentives to do so (Employee Benefits Research Institute, 2002). The San Francisco Human Rights Commission maintains a database of insurance companies that write domestic partnership policies in all fifty states (San Francisco Human Rights Commission, 1998).

One common argument employers have raised against extending domestic partner benefits has been cost. In fact, more than two decades of employer experience in offering domestic partner health benefits have proven that the overall cost is quite low. Numerous empirical studies, as well as the testimonials of human resource professionals who have implemented domestic partner benefits programs, have shown this to be the case (HRC, 2004b).

The benefits do not add a significant amount to overall health care costs of employers because many may choose to stay away from these plans. For example, domestic partners may be offered insurance through their own employer or the taxation of the benefits is too costly to the employee (see Exhibit 14.2). Low enrollment rates should not be used as an excuse to not offer the coverage, however. Usually, the costliest component is time spent negotiating with insurance providers. The commitment to diversity that offering domestic partner benefits shows to LGBT and heterosexual employees alike, however, outweighs the administrative burden and cost.

Many employers that provide domestic partner benefits require the employee and his or her domestic partner to sign an affidavit of domestic partnership or to register with a state or municipality that recognizes domestic partnerships to obtain coverage. As of January 2004, more than sixty such jurisdictions in the United States allowed such registration, some of which have residency requirements. A multitude of sample policies are available on the Internet from various types of employers.

Many more employers are going beyond health insurance to include domestic partners in FMLA and COBRA coverage, bereavement leave, adoption assistance, and retirement and pension benefits. According to a recent survey of Fortune 500 and Forbes 200 companies, 66 percent of employers that offer domestic partner health coverage also extend family medical

EXHIBIT 14.2. Taxation of Domestic Partner Benefits

Unless the domestic partner qualifies as a dependent, the Internal Revenue Service has ruled that domestic partners cannot be considered spouses for tax purposes. Thus, employers are obligated to report and withhold taxes on the fair market value of the domestic partner coverage. The fair market value of the domestic partner coverage is usually the amount the employer contributes to a health plan to cover the domestic partner, over and above the amount contributed for single and/or dependent coverage. Both the employee and the employer must pay income taxes on the value of the benefits. The same is true for state tax everywhere except Vermont, Massachusetts, and California. The proposed changes to the federal constitution would force the federal government to continue to unfairly tax companies and employees on health insurance purchased for domestic partners and may negatively impact equal tax treatment of benefits in states.

leave to employees to care for domestic partners. Similarly, 79 percent of employers that offer health coverage provide COBRA-like benefits continuation to domestic partners and 72 percent provide bereavement leave (HRC, 2004e).

Savvy organizations embrace their LGBT employees as an integral part of their business model. By establishing and supporting LGBT employee resources groups, employers can integrate their unique experiences into business planning and decision making. LGBT employee groups act as conduits of information from management to employees on LGBT issues and can alert management to developing concerns. Supporting LGBT employee groups can lead to improvements in delivery of services to the LGBT population, LGBT marketing opportunities, outreach efforts, and community goodwill.

Cultural competency training will help ensure that LGBT and non-LGBT employees work effectively together and that all LGBT clients or patients receive the best care. Such training might include learning exercises to understand how sexual orientation is a workplace issue, to give examples of effective means of communication between co-workers, and to make employees comfortable with LGBT employees and the needs of their LGBT clients. Sometimes LGBT issues in the workplace are covered in general diversity training curricula that are available. Ideally, all employees should attend such training. Depending on the type of employer, such training may be required, for example, frontline medical practitioners or all managerial staff. Cultural competency and diversity training on LGBT issues should be repeated routinely to ensure that new employees have basic competencies and provide additional professional development opportunities for more senior staff.

TRANSGENDER ISSUES IN THE WORKPLACE

Someone is termed transgender if his or her personal identity or gender expression falls outside of stereotypical gender norms. Whether a person is transgender has no direct or predictable connection to his or her sexual orientation. Being transgender can be understood as a form of gender nonconformity that includes people who transition from one biological sex to another as well as women who are perceived by some as too masculine and men who are perceived by some as too feminine. Discrimination against transgender people is often rooted in stereotypes about what are appropriate masculine and feminine behaviors and presentations (The Harry Benjamin International Gender Dysphoria Association, 2001).

Transgender or transitioning employees can present new challenges in many workplaces, particularly around sensitive issues such as restroom access. No single solution will work in every workplace. As a result, employers handle restroom access issues in a variety of ways.

It is the employer's responsibility to provide access to restroom facilities for all employees under Occupational Safety and Health Administration guidelines (HRC, 2004a). At the same time, employers must permit use of facilities by any individual without infringing on the privacy of other users. Restroom stalls with locking doors generally fulfill this requirement. Some employers choose to provide a nearby unisex restroom, if one is available and reasonably accessible, that a transitioning employee may agree to use for some period during the process of transition.

Many employers will set their company's policy to address permanent personal and public redefinition of one's gender. Predicating a policy on such a concept eliminates concerns that employees will change their gender regularly, even though standards of care make hasty decision unlikely. Ultimately, employers should allow employees to use restrooms that correspond with the employees' permanent presentation as either female or male.

Generally speaking, employers have a right to regulate employee appearance and behavior in the workplace for reasonable business purposes. Requiring conformity to accepted community standards of dress and behavior arguably serves the business purpose of promoting an orderly workplace and making employees and customers comfortable. Dress codes based on business-related rationales that are applied consistently are generally acceptable to most employees and legally defensible.

The transitioning process involves several steps which may or may not occur with the assistance of numerous health and mental health professionals. These steps may include psychological testing, psychiatric monitoring and counseling to assess an understanding of consequences and obstacles of transitioning, administration of sexual hormones, and a trial period of at least one year of living in the desired gender. It is usually at this stage that the employer is given notice of the employee's intentions and begins the planning process of implementation, including measures such as changing e-mails, business cards, personnel records, and security identification.

In the health care industry specific employees are required to obtain official certification in order to do their jobs. Some transsexuals find that they are unable to change their gender markers on their government-issued identification documents. Some states will not change the sex or name on birth certificates. Companies that are committed to comprehensive nondiscrimination policies should be sensitive to the issues of identity and documentation that many transgender and transitioning individuals experience. Some companies have gone to great lengths in support of their transgender employees, including lobbying federal agencies to modify their rules to accommodate the realities of transition.

The Harry Benjamin International Gender Dysphoria Association's *Standards of Care for Gender Identity Disorders* provides guidance on what is considered "medically indicated and medically necessary" treatment for transgender people. For that reason, wherever possible, employers should remove exclusions for medically necessary treatments and procedures, as defined by the HBIGDA, from company-provided health care coverage (The Harry Benjamin International Gender Dysphoria Association, 2001).

Effectively supporting transgender employees is also good for business. The investment an employer makes in an employee is significant. Improved job satisfaction, employee morale, productivity, retention, and being established as an employer of choice are all good for the bottom line (see Exhibit 14.3).

RECOMMENDATIONS FOR U.S. BUSINESSES AND EMPLOYERS

1. Include the terms "sexual orientation" and "gender identity or expression" in the primary nondiscrimination or equal employment opportunity policy.
2. Provide equal benefits to employees' same-sex domestic partners as is provided to opposite-sex, married couples.

3. Remove coverage exclusions for medically necessary procedures for transgender employees.
4. Conduct routine LGBT diversity training. Require managers and supervisors to attend, at a minimum.
5. Sanction official LGBT employee resource groups and support them organizationally and financially.
6. Engage in appropriate and respectful LGBT advertising, if applicable.
7. Engage in ongoing, substantive philanthropy to LGBT political, health, education, or community events or organizations.
8. Disclose LGBT-related workplace policies to the public and participate in awards and recognition programs that celebrate positive LGBT workplace policies.
9. Respect employees' right to collectively bargain for antidiscrimination language and equal benefits. Because legal rights are so limited in many locations, a collective bargaining agreement or union is the only legal protection available to some LGBT workers.
10. Actively support federal, state, and local antidiscrimination and equal taxation legislation. Oppose measures that seek to limit legal rights, benefits, and obligations of LGBT people and their relationships.

EXHIBIT 14.3. Recognition for Best Practices
http://www.hrc.org/worknet

The Institute of Medicine's publication *The Future of Public Health in the 21st Century* (IOM, 2002b) recommends that recognition be given to high performers in all areas of public health, including employer and business policies. The Human Rights Campaign Foundation Corporate Equality Index provides a clear comparison of corporate policies in many industries, including health care and insurance.

The index rates corporations on a scale from 0 to 100 percent based on several key criteria that define corporate responsibility toward lesbian, gay, bisexual, and transgender employees, consumers, and investors. The index covers workplace criteria such as inclusive nondiscrimination policies, equal benefits, diversity training, and support of LGBT employee resource groups. It also recognizes advertising to the LGBT community that is appropriate and respectful and community partnerships and philanthropy that advance LGBT public health.

HOW TO EFFECT CHANGE

The following steps are designed to help individuals achieve LGBT-friendly workplace policies. They are provided by the Human Rights Campaign Foundation workplace project, HRC WorkNet (HRC, 2004e).*

1. Understand your employer's decision-making process and structure and utilize it to make a strong business case for change. Who in management will be supportive? Who will not? Who will need to sign off on the new policy? Does your company have a LGBT employee group or union?
2. Identify your company's competitors—by industry or geography—that already offer LGBT-friendly policies.
3. Talk to your supervisor about what you are trying to accomplish. Make sure he or she understands what you are doing and why it is so important to you.
4. Research the topic thoroughly and write a proposal.
5. Follow up.

RESPONDING TO CULTURAL AND COMMUNITY RESISTANCE

Historically, employers initially cautious about implementing LGBT-friendly policy revisions have raised common concerns. One common belief is that discrimination is not a problem, and employers often claim that they do not discriminate against anyone. However, LGBT people have historically been singled out for discrimination based on who they are. Federal law requires employers to include only race, religion, national origin, sex, age, and disability in their EEO policies. By not adding the terms sexual orientation and gender identity or expression to the written EEO policy, a company sends a clear signal that sexual orientation discrimination is not on the same footing as these other types of discrimination. Although discrimination based on sexual orientation may not be a current problem, many forward-thinking employers will plan for future problems.

Often, an employer's EEO policy is designed to comply with federal law, and traditional wisdom holds that going beyond that will open up an employer to increased liability. However, having internal procedures to deal with discrimination and harassment is superior to confronting outside legal

---

*Reprinted with permission from the Human Rights Campaign Foundation, WorkNet Project, Washington, DC.

action. In the event of a legal action, an employer's previous attempts to diminish discriminatory practices can bode well in those proceedings.

Employers that encounter resistance based on religious and moral grounds should be careful to frame their arguments for policy change in business terms. LGBT workplace policies are not designed to change personal values; they are designed to foster an inclusive work environment where employees from differing backgrounds can work together to get the job done. Last, some religious political organizations have attempted to damage companies' reputations because of their LGBT-friendly policies. For example, the Southern Baptist Convention announced a boycott of Disney in 1997, and others banded together in an attempt to drive customers away from American Airlines in the late 1990s (HRC, 2004c). These efforts failed and have not made a dent in the bottom line of corporate America.

CONCLUSION

It is not as simple as making one change or adding one policy to cover all of the needs of LGBT workers. However, as demonstrated in this chapter, it starts with a fundamental understanding of the challenges that face workers. From here, you can begin as an employer to build a framework from which to build LGBT-friendly policies, procedures, and benefit packages. Ultimately, this will help employers with one of their biggest challenges in the new millennium—to attract and retain dedicated and motivated employees.

EMPLOYMENT AND BUSINESS: SELECTED RESOURCES

Gay Financial Network
www.gfn.com

Business and financial news for GLBT Americans.

Gender Public Advocacy Coalition (GenderPAC)
www.gpac.org

A national advocacy organization working to ensure every American's right to his or her gender, free from stereotypes, discrimination, and violence, regardless of how they look, act, or dress or how others perceive their sex or sexual orientation.

Harry Benjamin International Gender Dysphoria Association, Inc.
www.hbigda.org

Human Rights Campaign Foundation's WorkNet Project
www.hrc.org/worknet

The nation's largest LGBT advocacy organization provides a host of resources and contacts for employees and employers on LGBT issues.

Out & Equal Workplace Advocates
www.outandequal.org

A national nonprofit devoted to the LGBT community in workplace settings. Hosts an annual workplace summit.

San Francisco Human Rights Commission
http://www.sfgov.org/site/sfhumanrights_index.asp?id=4560

Transgender at Work
www.tgender.net/taw/

Useful resources for handling transgender issues in the workplace.

QUESTIONS TO CONSIDER

1. Do you know any openly gay LGBT co-workers or managers? If not, chances are your workplace has someone who is LGBT. How will you reach out to them?
2. What would your gay or lesbian co-worker do if his or her partner died and the human resources bereavement-leave policy did not include domestic partners?
3. Does your company offer a comprehensive benefits package to its LGBT employees, including FMLA and COBRA? What can you do to make this a priority for your company?
4. Have you ever heard an antigay joke or stereotype mentioned at work? What was your response? Did you challenge it?
5. How would you feel if your marriage was not recognized simply because you had moved to another state? Would you be worried about tax, insurance, and estate benefits and rights?
6. If you were a member of the LGBT public health community, would you be comfortable being open about your orientation at work? If not, why? What can you do to change this?

REFERENCES

Bush appointee in Florida grilled on anti-gay views. (1999, February 9). *Orlando Sentinel.*

Community-University Institute for Social Research. (2003). *The cost of homophobia: Literature review on the human impact of homophobia on Canada.* Saskatoon, SK: University of Saskatchewan.

Employee Benefits Research Institute. (2002). Value of benefits survey. *EBRI Notes, 23*(3), 23.

The Harry Benjamin International Gender Dysphoria Association. (2001). *Standards of care for gender identity disorders,* 6th version. Retrieved August 22, 2004, from www.hbigda.org/socv6.html#10.

Human Rights Campaign Foundation. (2004a). *Corporate equality index survey.* Retrieved August 22, 2004, from www.hrc.org/Template.cfm?Section=Corporate_Equality_Index&Template=/TaggedPage/TaggedPageDisplay.cfm&TPLID=23&ContentID=16051.

Human Rights Campaign Foundation. (2004b). *Cost of domestic partner benefits.* Retrieved August 22, 2004, from www.hrc.org/Content/NavigationMenu/Work_Life/Get_Informed2/The_Issues/Cost/Cost.htm.

Human Rights Campaign Foundation. (2004c). *Equal benefits ordinances.* Retrieved August 22, 2004, from www.hrc.org/worknet.

Human Rights Campaign Foundation. (2004d). *Organization database.* Retrieved August 22, 2004, from www.hrc.org/Template.cfm?Section=Get_Informed2&Template=/CustomSource/Agency/AgencySearch.cfm.

Human Rights Campaign Foundation. (2004e). WorkNet Project. Retrieved August 22, 2004, from www.hrc.org/worknet.

Institute of Medicine. (2002a). *Care without coverage: Too little, too late.* Washington, DC: National Academy Press.

Institute of Medicine. (2002b). *Future of the public's health in the 21st century.* Washington, DC: National Academy of Science.

Napier, C. (2002). Protesters rally at Carle for fired lesbian worker. *The Daily Illinois.*

San Francisco Human Rights Commission. (1998). Equal benefits for domestic partners and spouses: Insurance providers list—all states. Retrieved August 5, 2004, from www.ci.sf.ca.us/site/uploadfiles/sfhumanrights/.

Sauter, S., Murphy, L., Colligan, M., Swanson, N., Hurrell, J., Jr., Scharf, F., Jr., Sinclair, R., Grubb, P., Goldenhar, L., Alterman, T., et al. (1990). *Stress at work.* National Institute of Occupational Safety and Health. Publication no. 99-101. Retrieved July 17, 2004, from www.cdc.gov/niosh/stresswk.html.

U.S. Department of Health and Human Services. (2000). *Healthy People 2010* (2nd edition). Washington, DC: GPO.

Wein, H. (2000). *Stress and disease: New perspectives.* Retrieved August 22, 2004, from www.nih.gov/news/wordonhealth/oct2000/story01.htm.

World Health Organization. (1948). Preamble to the constitution of the World Health Organization. *Official Records of the World Health Organization,* Number 2 (p. 100).

PART VII:
THE MEDIA

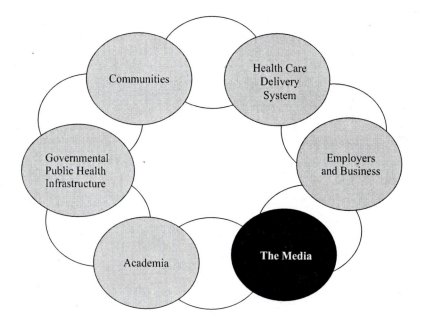

Chapter 15

Media Strategies for Advancing Health in Lesbian, Gay, Bisexual, and Transgender Communities

Laurie Drabble
JoAnne G. Keatley
George Marcelle

INTRODUCTION

Mainstream media sources including newspapers, radio, television, and advertising have long since expanded to include numerous alternative communications including a wide range of LGBT media venues. The Internet and the Web have given birth to new media formats *and* equipped their users to create, or even become, media themselves. In all its forms, the media is a powerful mechanism for advancing public health in LGBT communities. The mass media can also be a source of misleading messages about health, sexuality, and risky behavior; a conduit for marketing of harmful products for corporate profit; and even a tool for an ideological agenda that is harmful to LGBT communities. This chapter will focus on several dimensions of media and their intersections with LGBT health, including influencing mainstream media, addressing health in LGBT media, challenging target marketing, and navigating through the evolving world of LGBT Internet resources.

MAINSTREAM MEDIA AND LGBT HEALTH

Media and Coverage of LGBT Health Issues

Substantial movement in coverage of LGBT issues has recently occurred, including LGBT health, in mainstream media sources. LGBT issues are discussed by mainstream media sources at greater rates than ever before. Although media coverage of LGBT health, social, and political issues has increased and objectivity in reporting LGBT issues has improved, reports by the media on some segments of LGBT communities are still skewed by oversimplification, generalization, and prejudice.

Bennett (1998) conducted an analysis of five decades of reporting on gays and lesbians in two major U.S. weekly news magazines and found that coverage of gay and lesbian issues grew from two articles in the 1940s to 151 in the 1990s. At the same time, problems with fairness and accuracy in reporting on LGBT issues, including health and mental health topics, persisted over the decades. The study found that beginning in the 1940s and continuing well into the 1990s, journalists disproportionately focused on pathology and stereotypically negative portrayals while failing to focus on issues of substance to the LGBT community. For example, the removal of homosexuality from the *Diagnostic and Statistical Manual of Mental Disorders* during the 1970s was not generally considered newsworthy by mainstream media, although journalists had, prior to the removal, reported on homosexuality as an illness and often quoted psychiatrists and psychologists when referring to gays and lesbians. During the 1980s, the weekly news magazines published twenty-two stories on AIDS, and most of those stories linked the disease to stereotypical depictions of a "promiscuous homosexual lifestyle," a depiction that was grounded in a history of stereotyping gays and lesbians as sexual predators. This depiction represented "a misleading generalization based on one subsection of a very diverse population, and one that implicitly suggested that the gay and lesbian campaign for civil rights was based on little more than hedonistic self-interest" (Bennett, 1998, p. 8). Gay men with HIV/AIDS were portrayed as vectors of infection rather than victims of the epidemic. Mainstream media, both in the past and present, have not recognized the difference between sexual identity and behavior and have tended to vilify bisexual men while minimizing the importance of safer-sex practices regardless of sexual orientation (Miller, 2002). The advent of the AIDS epidemic instilled fear in the LGBT community, not only of the disease itself but also because it was used as a pretext to advance anti-LGBT public opinion and policy rather than public health solutions, often with the complicity of mainstream media.

Problems with fair and accurate coverage of LGBT communities persist. Coverage disproportionately focuses on gay, white men to the exclusion of other segments of LGBT communities. Lesbians are underrepresented and bisexuals are virtually invisible in mainstream media coverage. The media rarely presents communities of color objectively, and depictions of transgender people are plagued by inaccuracy and sensationalism. Until all segments of the LGBT community are objectively covered in mainstream media, the entire community will continue to struggle with the stigmatizing consequences of misrepresentation. Community members often challenge mainstream media to improve accuracy and sensitivity in coverage (see case example).

Several "fair practices" described by Bennett (1998), if adopted more broadly in mainstream media, would strengthen coverage of LGBT health issues. First, journalists can respond to derogatory comments about LGBT individuals or issues by questioning sources directly about such statements and avoiding prejudicial language and perspectives. Second, journalists can counter the continuing problem of unfounded allegations against LGBT populations (e.g., that LGBT individuals are hedonistic and irresponsible) by insisting upon evidence from sources rather than accepting unsubstantiated anecdotal information or relying on the authority of highly visible spokespersons. Journalists should be willing to challenge assertions from powerful sources of information, such as celebrities, religious leaders, physicians, politicians, and psychiatrists. Finally, media professionals should apply the same rigorous standards in their coverage of LGBT subjects as would be expected of them in reporting on other important social and health issues.

Case Study: Transforming Media Coverage of Violence Against Transgender Individuals

On October 16, 2002, the body of Gwen Araujo, a young transgender teen, was discovered buried in Northern California. Gwen had been brutally beaten and murdered by four young men after attending a house party in Newark, California. Initially, news reports reported her death as one involving a young man who had lived as a woman. Most news reports referred to Gwen as "he" and avoided the word "transgender." The Bay Area transgender community was outraged at what they perceived as insensitive coverage and dismayed that news organizations would ignore Associated Press guidelines for reporting on transgender individuals.

In response to this community outrage, on October 24, 2002, the Transgender Resources and Neighborhood Space (TRANS) Project, Gay Straight Alliance (GSA) Network, Asociación Gay Unida Impactando Latinos/Latinas A Superarse (AGUILAS), the National Center for Lesbian Rights, the Transgender Law Center, and the Gay and Lesbian Alliance Against Defamation (GLAAD) called a news conference to call for more sensitive reporting by the news media. Many local and national news organizations attended the press conference and candlelight walk held immediately afterward. This event, attended by several hundred members of the transgender community, was widely reported by print and electronic media. Soon after the press conference, some news organizations started reporting Gwen's murder and developments in the investigation with more sensitive and accurate use of pronouns and use of the word "transgender." However, others did not, and several journalists actually began a discourse over the use of pronouns and Araujo's family's preferences. In fact, the discourse itself became newsworthy, with several local reporters taking sides on what pronouns to use when referring to Gwen.

The discourse, although not always pretty, did lead to changes on the part of reporters and news organizations. Ultimately, on December 22, GLAAD released an e-newsletter that praised the Associated Press as an organization that has been "receptive to evolving terminology issues in the past and continues to make changes that reflect more fair and inclusive coverage of transgender issues." This example demonstrates how community involvement can influence not only what is covered in the media but also the editorial policies and practices of the media itself.

Guidelines from the Associated Press

Use the pronoun preferred by the individuals who have acquired the physical characteristics (by hormone therapy, body modification, or surgery) of the opposite sex and present themselves in a way that does not correspond with their sex at birth. If that preference is not expressed, use the pronoun consistent with the way the individuals live publicly. (The Associated Press, 2002, p. 231)

Influencing Media Coverage of LGBT Health Issues

Numerous organizations have been formed over the past several decades to advocate for LGBT communities and have devoted substantial time and effort to educating the media on LGBT social, health, and political issues. There are far too many organizations to list here; however, a few prominent examples include GLAAD, the AIDS Coalition to Unleash Power (ACT UP), the Gender Public Advocacy Coalition (GenderPAC), and the Human Rights Campaign.

GLAAD is a national organization dedicated to changing public attitudes toward LGBT populations by serving as a watchdog and advocate in relation to print, television, and film media (Vaid, 1995). Among other activities, GLAAD offers online resources (at www.glaad.org) including media resource kits, a media resource guide (with LGBT Directory of Community Resources, LGB Glossary of terms, Transgender Glossary of terms), scholarly work about LGBT-oriented media trends and issues, recent news of importance to LGBT communities, and reports on the status of LGBT people in television, film, and print media.

A diverse array of LGBT organizations, from grassroots advocacy groups, to health coalitions, to formal nonprofit and advocacy organizations, have learned that informing and influencing the media is a critical strategy in overall efforts to effect policy, practice, and public perceptions related to LGBT health issues. The success of AIDS activists in developing relationships with medical and science reporters to strengthen and broaden coverage of HIV/AIDS illustrates the kind of strategies that have been adopted in improving coverage of broader LGBT health and political issues. Vaid (1995) describes such an effort targeted to a specific newspaper:

> We assembled a cross-section of gay organizational and constituency representatives to talk to editors about the important stories they were missing. We presented lists of story ideas, and a contact sheet so that they could get in touch with gay people who had different kinds of expertise. At the meeting, it was clear the editorial staff was eager to hear our suggestions and had very little idea about what the gay and lesbian community was, who its leaders were, and what political issues it was concerned with. At a follow-up briefing, attended by nearly twenty-five reporters and editors, the need for information exchange became even clearer. (p. 201)

Public health advocates are faced with a growing battle to advance evidence-based health prevention and intervention efforts in the context of ideological forces that would marginalize rather than advance LGBT health. In the early fight against HIV/AIDS, "the right characterized AIDS as God's punishment for the sin of homosexuality" (Vaid, 1995, p. 327). More recently, major federal health institutions such as the Centers for Disease Control and Prevention (CDC) and the National Institutes of Health (NIH) have been besieged by demands to challenge or eliminate research and prevention efforts related to sexual orientation or sexual behavior (Goode, 2003; Kaiser, 2003). In this context, it is important to recognize that media messages related to health in marginalized communities, particularly LGBT communities, may be driven more by ideology than science. LGBT public health advocates and allies must recognize that efforts to advance LGBT disease-prevention and health policy messages require a parallel process of organizing to defuse potential attempts by anti-LGBT groups to silence or distort these messages.

Media advocacy, using the media to strategically apply pressure for policy change (Jernigan & Wright, 1996; Wallack & Dorfman, 1996), is a powerful tool for shaping the social and policy environment that affects LGBT communities. Using media advocacy to advance policy changes also applies to LGBT media markets (see Exhibits 15.1 and 15.2).

Public health researchers, practitioners, and policy advocates all share a responsibility to advance LGBT health through various media outlets. In addition, foundations have an important role in funding LGBT health initiatives, including efforts to advocate for policy change and social justice

EXHIBIT 15.1. Tips for Media Advocacy: Developing Media Relationships and Supporting Journalists

1. *Build relationships with journalists.* Montor local media and collect clippings of reporters who cover health and LGBT issues. Acknowledge appropriate, balanced, and supportive media presentations of LGBT health issues and information.
2. *Prepare your "pitch."* Prepare for initial contact with a journalist. Be prepared to establish your credibility and the importance of your story.
3. *Be sensitive to deadlines.* If you need preparation time to talk to a reporter, always ask about and meet his or her deadline. Press conferences should be held in the morning to allow reporters to make afternoon deadlines.
4. *Create media kits.* For press conferences or contacts with multiple reporters, it will be important to create a media packet that should include a news release with a catchy headline, strong opening, background information, and, if possible, a quote from a reliable source. The packet should also include fact sheets (facts on front and references from credible sources on the back), a brochure or one-page description of your organization, and news clippings related to your topic and/or organization.
5. *Respond to requests for information.* If you are contacted by a reporter, the key questions to ask are as follows. "What is your story? Who else have you talked to? What do you need? What is your deadline?"

Source: Summarized from Wallack, Dorfman, Jernigan, & Themba. (1993). *Media advocacy and public health.* Newbury Park, CA: Sage Publications.

through the media. Conservative foundations have been extremely successful in promoting a national policy agenda through generous funding of right-wing think tanks, political groups, and media groups (Callahan, 1999; Covington, 1997), including efforts to depict LGBT civil rights and LGBT people as dangerous to the well-being of the population as a whole. Progressive and mainstream foundations have been more hesitant to fund organizations engaged in policy change, including health policy, that affects marginalized groups such as communities of color and LGBT communities. At the same time, foundations that do support community-based organizations committed to equity and to addressing health disparities report positive outcomes (Drabble, 2000b).

**EXHIBIT 15.2. Tips for Media Advocacy:
Preparing for Doing Media Advocacy**

1. *Plan the initiative.* Planning involves identifying your goals, developing messages, determining your target audience, and identifying what media strategies will best work for this audience.
2. *Frame for media access.* Strategies for attracting media include finding a local angle for national stories, creating news (e.g., through public release of a report or a public demonstration), piggybacking on hot stories, highlighting controversy or injustice, and promoting attention to new breakthroughs.
3. *Frame for content.* Frame issues to shift the focus from the individual to a public health perspective and clearly assign responsibility for the problem to a specific industry or other environmental factor. Make statistics more meaningful by stressing the impact on your community or comparing numbers with something that is identifiable and that directly affects the audience. Develop specific media bites, visuals, and symbols.
4. *Select spokespersons carefully.* Even experts are not always the best spokespersons for the media. Ensure selection of someone with credibility, the capacity to speak clearly to the issue, and the ability to get back on track when asked questions unrelated to the main focus of the primary health issue or policy concern.

Source: Summarized from Wallack, Dorfman, Jernigan, & Themba. (1993). *Media advocacy and public health.* Newbury Park, CA: Sage Publications.

LGBT MEDIA

Over the past fifty years, a wide range of LGBT publications have emerged and given voice to diverse segments of LGBT communities. Given the barriers to LGBT content in the broadcast media in the early decades of the modern LGBT rights movement and emergence of an LGBT media market, it is not surprising that members of this growing "community" used print as their primary, dominant vehicle for communicating about their lives and interests. Traditionally, open LGBT socializing has centered on LGBT-welcoming bars, a tradition that continues outside of the larger metropolitan areas, with bars and dance clubs still a major force in the culture, even in the largest cities. Hence, one of the first LGBT media venues was the "bar rag," a cheaply produced periodical heavily promoting bar activities, light on editorial content, and sometimes including paid personal ads. Bar rags were often published by a particular bar or a particular area's group of LGBT bars and served as the closest thing available at the time to a directory of whatever LGBT communities, organizations, or activities existed. LGBT travelers often looked for the local bar rag as their entrée into a new locale and a means of making contact with other LGBT people and LGBT-safe environments.

Local community papers were one example of a wide array of expanding alternative media sources that offered a venue and a voice for the political and social concerns of the marginalized groups. Because these concerns were often invisible or distorted in mainstream media, the LGBT community, like other marginalized groups, created their own alternatives through print media and, to a lesser extent, radio and other electronic media. In contrast to large, mainstream corporate media organizations, alternative media was created by, reflective of, and embedded in the communities from which they emerged. At the same time, a majority of these early alternative media were not reflective of the diversity of the LGBT community and were frequently weighted to the interests and concerns of white gay men. Streitmatter (1995) conducted an extensive analysis of the development of LGBT media and observed that a wide range of publications speaking to the concerns of different segments of LGBT communities evolved during the 1970s and 1980s. Some LGBT publications published key health information that was largely ignored in mainstream media, including explicit information about safer sex practices, breaking news on HIV/AIDS treatment, and discussion of risks for sexually transmitted diseases among lesbians (Streitmatter, 1995). During this era, many of these grassroots publications emphasized political and social change. Population-specific publications for lesbians, bisexuals, transgender communities, and LGBT communities of color evolved to advance the concerns of groups that were often marginalized by both mainstream media and gay media.

By the mid-1990s, a new generation of publications evolved that differed from the grassroots publications of the earlier decades of LGBT movement. These publications were generally glossier and less radical than the earlier LGBT movement publications. Examples of the new generation of publications include *The Advocate, Out, Genre, 10 Percent, Deneuve* (for lesbians, now *Curve*), *Square Peg* (for lesbians, out of print), *POZ* (for HIV-positive individuals), and *BLK* (for gay African Americans). Streitmatter (1995) notes, "the glossy magazines increased the total number of gay and lesbian publications only slightly, to about 850 . . . but they caused the total circulation to explode" (p. 311). Though explicitly political publications still thrive, the new genre of LGBT magazines are different in tone and content than their predecessors. This new generation of publications grew by attracting mainstream advertisers who perceived the lesbian and gay community as a market with substantial disposable income and, as such, "the driving force was not providing timely information but attracting more ads" (Streitmatter, 1995, p. 313). Added to these are a few other widely circulated newspapers with reputations as voices for the liberal establishment at large, which in recent years have evolved into what might be called "gay-friendly," or even "LGBT-supportive," media outlets such as *The Village Voice,* founded in New York City in 1955, and its Los Angeles counterpart, *LA Weekly.*

Increasingly, LGBT media has expanded into other venues. *Bi Cities!* a cable show by and about bisexuals in the Minneapolis/St. Paul area, reflects the myriad of venues for communication and community emerging in LGBT communities. Technological advances allow for LGBT public health advocates and health providers to develop and market their own media products for dissemination into mainstream audiences such as a video, discussion guide, and optimal care kit on "Tools for Caring about Lesbian Health" (a Mautner Project order form is available at http://www.mautner project.org/images/form.pdf) developed by the Mautner Project for Lesbians with Cancer (Washington, DC). Access to technology also allows for creating population-specific media tools to augment specific health interventions, such as a video clip developed to personalize perceptions of HIV/AIDS as a tool in implementing a community-based prevention intervention for transgender individuals (Bockting, Rosser, & Coleman, 2001).

LGBT media sources, from bar rags to professionally produced cable shows, provide a rich venue for communicating public health messages and policy agendas. At the same time, LGBT public health advocates and allies must navigate through potential barriers to accessing LGBT media, including editorial policies or practices that may reject strong public health content for fear of offending potential advertisers. Entertainment media is receiving increased attention as a major source of public health communication as well as being powerful purveyors of unhealthy norms. For example, government and private organizations have published research findings relating to the frequency and nature of tobacco, alcohol, and drug references in popular movies, television, and music (Christenson, Henrisken, & Roberts, 2000). Research on the possible influence of entertainment media on specific populations is scarce and opportunities for infusing public health messages into LGBT entertainment media are relatively unexplored.

TARGET MARKETING TO LGBT COMMUNITIES

From the Margins to a "Market":
Healthy Profits or Healthy People?

Inclusion in the economic marketplace is perceived as symbolic of progress toward social acceptance for many LGBT individuals and communities (Penaloza, 1996). The increased focus on lesbian and gay consumers is reflected in research exploring how best to reach these populations through advertising (Burnett, 2000; Grier & Brumbaugh, 1999). In addition to advertising, corporate sponsorship of cultural events and direct donations to national and local nonprofit organizations have become common strategies for promoting products and increasing consumer goodwill (Stewart & Rice, 1995). LGBT media, community organizations, and leaders need to critically consider the environmental impact of advertising, sponsorship, and promotions by corporations whose products affect LGBT health and whose motives may be driven more by profit than public health.

Marketing of alcoholic beverages and tobacco products is often targeted to specific communities based on geography, age, culture, gender, and lifestyle (Cummings, 1999; Hill & Caswell, 2001). LGBT communities have been increasingly targeted with specialized marketing from alcohol and tobacco businesses, even while research suggests that alcohol, tobacco, and drug-related problems may be higher in the LGBT community than the population as a whole (Drabble, 2000a). Target marketing may undermine the health of individuals through provision of biased information (Drabble, 2000a) and may indirectly influence the degree to which community organizations challenge corporate messages (Mosher & Frank, 1994; Rahn, 1994). Despite health concerns, long-term social and financial marginalization may leave LGBT communities particularly vulnerable to the influence of corporate philanthropy, such as funding from tobacco companies (Offen, Smith, & Malone, 2003).

LGBT publications have also been targeted with advertising from businesses interested in reaching HIV-positive populations. Some health advocates have questioned whether the profits garnered by corporations far outweigh possible benefits to consumers in the case of ads for nutritional supplements that may have limited or no evidence regarding their effectiveness and for companies that offer cash in exchange for being listed as life insurance beneficiaries of people with HIV/AIDS (Streitmatter, 1995). Pharmaceutical industries also target HIV-positive populations within LGBT communities. Although some of the information provided through pharmaceutical industry sponsorship, such as communicating about the efficacy of various medications in the gay press, may prove informative to LGBT consumers, these strategies are ultimately about market competition and commercial success for companies. In this context, LGBT media outlets and organizations accepting pharmaceutical industry funds are placed in a position of balancing the interests of their constituents and consumers with those of their corporate sponsors.

Responding to Target Marketing

In response to increased target marketing, LGBT organizations and media entities can adopt policies (e.g., prohibiting or limiting certain promotions or advertising) to affirm the value that they place on LGBT health and to ensure their independence from profit-making influences in the pursuit of their mission (Drabble, 2000a). In an analysis of one tobacco company campaign to target gay men, Smith and Malone (2003) observe that the relationship between the tobacco industry and the gay community is relatively undeveloped. To the degree that target-marketing efforts are still evolving, public health advocates and LGBT advocates have an opportunity to work together to forge policies to protect the public health of LGBT communities (see Exhibit 15.3).

Counterads are also a valuable tool for contextualizing health problems, focusing attention on the misinformation promoted by specific corporations, such as the alcohol or tobacco industry, and generating support for change in policy (Dorfman & Wallack, 1993). Counteradvertising strategies are effective, and messages focusing on industry manipulation and secondhand smoke appear to be the most useful for reducing tobacco consumption and challenging cultural norms that enable smoking (Golfman & Glantz, 1998). Communities have also been successful in organizing to reduce point-of-purchase advertising, such as store window and sidewalk tobacco promotions designed to target specific populations and increase tobacco purchases (Rogers, Feighery, Tencati, Butler, & Weiner, 1995). LGBT health advocacy groups have used these same strategies, including placement of counterads in LGBT media venues and organizing a community-based campaign that successfully reduced tobacco point-of-sale advertising among stores in one LGBT neighborhood (the Castro area in San Francisco) (Drabble & Soliz, 1996).

BEYOND MASS MEDIA: THE INTERNET AND LGBT HEALTH

For a media-savvy U.S. population of LGBT women and men in desperate need of community, visibility, and safe ways to self-identify and connect with others like themselves, the Internet has become a powerful nexus for

---

**EXHIBIT 15.3. LGBT Media and Health Organizations:
Developing Guidelines for Ethical Funding**

- Plan a discussion with your organization's editorial board, board of directors, steering committee, or other policymaking body about the issue of corporate donations. Ground this discussion in the context of your overall funding plan and organizational mission. Discuss concerns about funding, issues about community health, and potential conflict, real or perceived, with your mission.
- Discuss perceived advantages and disadvantages of accepting sponsorship from corporations that profit from products that impact LGBT health. Identify sources of alternative funding.
- Review policy options from other organizations (e.g., prohibiting sponsorship/funding, limiting promotions, ensuring freedom from influence in content of publications or programming).
- Select elements of a written policy statement that match the purpose of your publication or organization and your long-term vision for your community.
- If your organization is reluctant to eliminate specific funding sources such as tobacco, alcohol, or pharmaceutical corporate funding, be prepared to discuss how corporate influence within your organization can be limited (e.g., ensuring that media content or educational program content is independent of the marketing interests of donors, limiting promotions allowable by corporate funders of a special event).

Source: Adapted from Drabble, L. (2001). Ethical funding: The ethics of tobacco, alcohol & pharmaceutical funding—A practical guide for LGBT organizations. See this publication for sample policy options. Available from the Tobacco Education Clearinghouse of California at 831-438-4822.

---

communication (Finlon, 2002b; Haag & Chang, 1997; Highleyman, 2002; Weinrich, 1997). Lesbians, gay men, bisexual people, and transgender individuals and groups have seized the opportunity with such speed and imagination that gay content is not only a significant presence on the Web, its presence is all but unavoidable. This phenomenon may be one important factor in recent demands for software designed to block access to Web sites whose content is deemed unsuitable for children and teens and receipt of e-mail containing similarly objectionable images, language, or information.

The results of Internet access for the health of LGBT people themselves are decidedly mixed, with greatly increased access to health information and resources accompanied by a still-proliferating cornucopia of opportunities for LGBT people to engage in behaviors that may undermine their health or place them at increased risk for disease and other harms. For example, the trend of men who have sex with men searching for sex over the Internet appears to be associated with increased risk for sexually transmitted disease, including syphilis and HIV. In response, a number of community-based organizations are beginning to use the same technology to conduct online outreach to men at risk (AIDS Alert, 2003).

Financially struggling nonprofit groups attempting to meet LGBT health needs are greatly aided by use of Web sites and other electronic media in their ability to organize and educate members and constituencies, as evidenced by a growing number of Web sites dedicated to addressing LGBT health and substance abuse (Finlon, 2002a,c; Highleyman, 2002). Even smaller groups that have struggled for over a quarter of a century to reach large numbers of LGBT individuals, such as the National Association of Lesbian and Gay Addiction Professionals (NALGAP, www.nalgap.org), now have Web sites and are able to reach a larger audience than would be possible through newsletters and other traditional media. Even organizational Web sites (such as www.nalgap.org) that offer only minimal information and that operate without resources for sophisticated content and Web marketing have dramatically increased communication with LGBT communities and health professionals. Although NALGAP is not yet widely known outside of LGBT substance-abuse professional circles, the NALGAP site is visited hundreds of times monthly, as compared to the pre-Web handful of written and telephone queries the group's unstaffed office once received.

Examples of LGBT organizations that have leveraged communication with constituents and consumers include the Gay and Lesbian Medical Association (www. glma.org), the Mautner Project for Lesbians with Cancer (www.mautnerproject. org), Bisexual Resource Center (www.biresource.org/health), and the National Transgender Advocacy Coalition (www.ntac.org).

Commercially, the Internet has also increased access to LGBT health, with GayHealth.com serving as an illustration of the value, limitations, and economic fragility of such an enterprise. The Web site (www.gayhealth. com) offers a wealth of consumer-friendly information about common and uncommon health topics affecting the lives of LGBT individuals. GayHealth.com appears to have had considerably less success at generating a stable base of revenues to support itself and its small staff than it has at presenting balanced gay health information in an appealing and user-friendly format. However, the site is valuable for its daily news updates, archived articles about alcohol and drug use among LGBT individuals, and clear and nonjudgmental responses to medical questions submitted to its "Ask the Doctors" feature.

Searching for information on gay health at commercial Web sites sponsored by profit-making businesses rather than government or nonprofit public health organizations makes clear how rare, and therefore precious, a resource such as GayHealth.com may be. For example, of 182 links under one randomly selected commercial health Web site, many more offer penis enlargement, body building, and marketing of commercial "health" products than access to quality information about lesbian risks for cancer, possible causes of bloody semen, risks of substance abuse, and hormone issues for transgender people.

On the whole, governments have presented little LGBT-specific information on the Web. One laudable exception is the GLBT health pages of the Seattle and King County Public Health Department's Web site (http://www.metrokc.gov/health/glbt/). Another is an extensive section of information about LGBT substance abuse within the primary site of the Substance Abuse and Mental Health Service Administration's (SAMHSA) National Clearinghouse for Alcohol and Drug Information (http://ncadi.samhsa.gov). At this Web site, users can locate the LGBT pages via an "Audience" drop-down menu. However, changing political winds can easily blow away such scarce and important resources or render them of less value to LGBT seekers of health information. HIV/AIDS and LGBT health researchers were among the first of those to witness the quiet removal and alteration of content at some government Web sites in the wake of new federal guidelines regarding HIV prevention.

Beyond enhancing the visibility and communication options of LGBT agencies and public health organizations, the Web has also provided a nexus for essential organizing and advocacy. The National Coalition for LGBT Health is a model for utilization of Web-based technology to organize, communicate, and advocate. The coalition's site (www.lgbthealth.net) lists dozens of member organizations and even more participating organizations, signaling a rallying point for diverse LGBT groups and an opportunity to create consensus and an increasingly powerful policy voice. Many of these groups would otherwise lack the capacity to be heard by policymakers. In yet another cost-effective realization of Internet opportunity, the coalition circulates a weekly summary of news and announcements relating to gay health to its membership electronic mailing list.

CONCLUSION

Mainstream media, LGBT media, and the Internet all offer critical opportunities to promote LGBT public health. Key opportunities include (1) campaigns, events, and media advocacy to increase media coverage of LGBT health and policy issues in mainstream media and to support accurate, sensitive, and fair reporting of LGBT issues; (2) creative initiatives to use diverse LGBT media venues to mobilize awareness of and support for public health goals; (3) adoption of written guidelines for ethical funding on the part of LGBT media and community-based organizations; and (4) expanded development and dissemination of accessible and high-quality Internet sites and alternative media related to specific LGBT health issues. Sophisticated use of media as a tool for increasing healthy and safe behaviors within LGBT communities and for organizing and advocating for policy change is crucial in the context of pressing LGBT health needs and a political environment that is largely indifferent or hostile to LGBT public health service, research, and advocacy.

QUESTIONS TO CONSIDER

1. Do you have a written communications and, as needed, media advocacy plan with a goal reflecting your group's mission and achievable objectives, a primary audience, key message(s), and methods for measuring effectiveness?

2. Do you provide opportunities for staff, members, and/or constituents to develop media advocacy skills and do you actively engage in media advocacy to influence policies related to LGBT health?

3. Do you have written policies that guide fund-raising and promotional activities from corporate entities whose products affect LGBT health and who seek access to your constituents/consumers as a target market (e.g., prohibiting sponsorship/funding, limiting promotions, ensuring freedom from influence in content of publications or programming)?

4. Do you provide media outlets with stories that present a positive view of LGBT culture, highlight LGBT achievements and contributions, and create a health-promoting LGBT image for LGBT audience members, particularly coming-out youth?

5. Can you provide published references and expert contacts to back up facts about LGBT health and positively influence coverage related to LGBT health and policies that affect LGBT health?

6. When information about LGBT life is presented in a negative way, do you look for ways to reframe the discussion (e.g., if a study concludes that 20 percent of gay men engage in some harmful behavior, this means that 80 percent do not do so) and to propose LGBT-positive public health policy solutions?

7. Do you have working partnerships with other groups who can add to your communications resources, add credibility to your voice and message, support your efforts to get a particular message or piece of information to audiences you need to reach, or collaborate in your ef-

forts to advance public health policies related to LGBT health through the media?

8. Do you keep media contacts, your members, constituents, supporters, and allies fully informed and current about your group's activities and issues?

9. Does your group send messages of appreciation, present awards, or acknowledge in other ways when media professionals present positive information about LGBT issues, public health policies that impact LGBT health, your work, and so on?

REFERENCES

AIDS Alert. (2003, October 1). *The Internet's role as modern bathhouse is being scrubbed: On-line hookups increasingly popular among MSM.* Atlanta, GA: Thompson American Health Consultants.

The Associated Press. (2002). *Stylebook and briefing on media law.* Cambridge, MA: Perseus Publishing.

Bennett, L. (1998). *The perpetuation of prejudice in reporting on gays and lesbians—Time and Newsweek: The first fifty years.* Cambridge, MA: Joan Shorenstein Center on Press Politics and Public Policy, John F. Kennedy School of Government, Harvard University.

Bockting, W., Rosser, B. R. S., & Coleman, E. (2001). Transgender HIV prevention: Community involvement and empowerment. In W. Bockting, E. Kirk, & E. Sheila (Eds.), *Transgender and HIV: Risks, prevention, and care* (pp. 119-144). Binghamton, NY: The Haworth Press.

Burnett, J. J. (2000). Gays: Feelings about advertising and media used. *Journal of Advertising Research, 40*(1-2), 75-84.

Callahan, D. (1999). *$1 billion for ideas: Conservative think tanks in the 1990s.* Washington, DC: National Committee for Responsive Philanthropy.

Christenson, P. G., Henrisken, L., & Roberts, D. F. (2000). *Substance use in popular prime time television.* Washington, DC: Office of National Drug Control Policy.

Covington, S. (1997). *Moving a public policy agenda: The strategic philanthropy of conservative foundations.* Washington, DC: National Committee for Responsive Philanthropy.

Cummings, M. K. (1999). Community-wide interventions for tobacco control. *Nicotine & Tobacco Research, 1,* S113-S116.

Dorfman, L., & Wallack, L. (1993). Advertising health: The case for counter-ads. *Public Health Reports, 108*(6), 716-726.

Drabble, L. (2000a). Alcohol, tobacco, and pharmaceutical industry funding: Considerations for organizations serving lesbian, gay, bisexual and transgender communities. *Journal of Gay & Lesbian Social Services, 11*(1), 1-26.

Drabble, L. (2000b). *A democratic landscape: Funding social change in California.* Washington, DC: National Committee for Responsive Philanthropy.

Drabble, L. (2001). *Ethical funding: The ethics of tobacco, alcohol, and pharmaceutical funding—A practical guide for LGBT organizations.* Scotts Valley, CA: Tobacco Education Clearinghouse of California.

Drabble, L., & Soliz, G. (1996). *Final report—Alive with pleasure: Prevention of tobacco and alcohol problems in lesbian, gay, bisexual and transgender communities.* Oakland, CA: Progressive Research and Training for Action.

Finlon, C. (2002a). Health care for all lesbian, gay, bisexual and transgender populations. *Journal of Gay & Lesbian Social Services, 14*(3), 109-116.

Finlon, C. (2002b). Internet resources. *Journal of Gay & Lesbian Social Services, 14*(1), 99-107.

Finlon, C. (2002c). Substance abuse in lesbian, gay, bisexual and transgender communities. *Journal of Gay & Lesbian Social Services, 14*(4), 109-116.

Goldman, L. K., & Glantz, S. A. (1998). Evaluation of antismoking advertising campaigns. *Journal of the American Medical Association, 279*(10), 772-777.

Goode, E. (2003, April 18). Certain words can trip up AIDS grants, scientists say. *The New York Times,* p. 10, Health.

Grier, S. A., & Brumbaugh, A. M. (1999). Noticing cultural differences: Ad meanings created by target and non-target markets. *Journal of Advertising, 28*(1), 79-93.

Haag, A. M., & Chang, F. K. (1997). The impact of electronic networking on the lesbian and gay community. *Journal of Gay & Lesbian Social Services, 7*(3), 83-94.

Highleyman, L. (2002). Health and medicine. In A. Ellis, L. Highleyman, K. Schaub, & M. White (Eds.), *The Harvey Milk Institute guide to lesbian, gay, bisexual, transgender, and queer Internet research* (pp. 131-146). Binghamton, NY: The Haworth Press.

Hill, L., & Casswell, S. (2001). Alcohol advertising and sponsorship: Commercial freedom or control in the public interest? In T. Stockwell (Ed.), *International handbook of alcohol dependence and problems* (pp. 823-846). New York: John Wiley & Sons.

Jernigan, D. H., & Wright, P. A. (1996). Media advocacy: Lessons from community experiences. *Journal of Public Health Policy, 17*(3), 306-329.

Kaiser, J. (2003, April 18). Studies of gay men, prostitutes come under scrutiny. *Science, 300,* 393.

Miller, M. (2002). "Ethically questionable?" Popular media reports on bisexual men and AIDS. *Journal of Bisexuality, 2*(1), 95-112.

Mosher, J., & Frank, E. (1994). Reaching consensus: Assessing support for national alcohol policies. Paper presented at the 122nd Annual Meeting of the American Public Health Association, Washington, DC, November.

Offen, N., Smith, E. A., & Malone, R. E. (2003). From adversary to target market: The ACT-UP boycott of Philip Morris. *Tobacco Control, 12,* 203-207.

Penaloza, L. (1996). We're here, we're queer, and we're going shopping! A critical perspective on the accommodation of gays and lesbians in the U.S. marketplace. *Journal of Homosexuality, 31*(1/2), 9-41.

Rahn, P. (1994). Alcohol marketing to the gay community. *Prevention Pipeline, 7*(6), 30-31.

Rogers, T., Feighery, E. C., Tencati, E. M., Butler, J. L., & Weiner, L. (1995). Community mobilization to reduce point-of-purchase advertising of tobacco projects. *Health Education Quarterly, 22*(4), 427-442.

Smith, E. A., & Malone, R. E. (2003). The outing of Philip Morris: Advertising tobacco to gay men. *American Journal of Public Health, 93*(6), 988-993.

Stewart, D. W., & Rice, R. (1995). Nontraditional media and promotions in the marketing of alcoholic beverages. In S. E. Martin (Ed.), *The effects of the mass media on the use and abuse of alcohol* (Research Monograph 28, NIH Publication No 95-3743, pp. 209-238). Rockville, MD: National Institute of Alcohol Abuse and Alcoholism.

Streitmatter, R. (1995). *Unspeakable: The rise of the gay and lesbian press in America.* Boston: Faber and Faber.

Vaid, U. (1995). *Virtual equality: The mainstreaming of gay & lesbian liberation.* New York: Anchor Books.

Wallack, L., & Dorfman, L. (1996). Media advocacy: A strategy for advancing policy and promoting health. *Health Education Quarterly, 23*(3), 293-317.

Wallack, L., Dorfman, L., Jernigan, D. H., & Themba, M. (1993). *Media advocacy and public health.* Newbury Park, CA: Sage Publications.

Weinrich, J. D. (1997). Strange bedfellows: Homosexuality, gay liberation, and the Internet. *Journal of Sex Education and Therapy, 22*(1), 58-66.

Afterword

Members of the LGBT community are in every town, city, state, and country in the world. We come into contact, often unknowingly, with members of the LGBT community in our practices. The preceding pages have outlined numerous new dimensions of improving the health and well-being of the LGBT community. Good health and access to quality health services should not be a privilege of a few, but the right of all individuals, including the LGBT community. Homophobia, miscommunication, and lack of quality health services are unacceptable components of public health and the health care delivery system. Again, this book is not to be assumed to be an all-encompassing treatment of the public health issues affecting the LGBT community, but rather a starting point for creating conditions for optimal LGBT health. Hopefully, the knowledge and resources provided by the contributors will assist in building agency capacity and knowledge in the public health community.

Change will take time and effort on the part of all members of the public health community. We must make concerted and collaborative efforts to include all members of the LGBT community in our public health practice and health services. It is not the responsibility of the LGBT community to educate researchers, policymakers, and practitioners in recognizing their community's needs. We, as public health practitioners, must create accountability and partnerships with our own practices and agencies to address the special health needs of the LGBT community. Success starts by eliminating institutional barriers and homophobic beliefs and by educating ourselves about our deficiency in meeting the needs of this community.

We have the ability to be a beacon of knowledge, resources, and skills for the LGBT community in our often overwhelming and complex public health and health care delivery system. We need to utilize our skills effectively to navigate and to overcome the limitations to achieving optimal LGBT health. It is time we light the path for others to follow and work together on illuminating the many roads ahead.

Index

Page numbers followed by the letter "f" indicate figures; those followed by the letter "t" indicate tables; and those followed by the letter "e" indicate exhibits.

Marijuana use
bisexual men, 204
FTMs, 205
gay men, 202, 204
lesbians/bisexual women, 202
LGBT youth, 207
MTFs, 205
national population, 205
transgender persons, 205
transgender women, 204
Marmor, Judd, 17, 297
Martin, Damien, 299-300
Mass media, LGBT health issues coverage, 335
Massachusetts, gay marriage, 296
Massachusetts Youth Risk Behavior Survey (MYRBS)
drug use, 207
sexual orientation, 38
Mastery, cultural competence, 62, 62f
Mata, Adolfo, 304
Matex, Stan, 19
Mattachine Society, founding of, 294
Mauntner Project for Lesbians with Cancer, 25, 99, 301, 343, 347
Mazzoni Center, 25, 190
McCarthy, Joseph, 293
Media
and alcohol/tobacco use, 209-210
LGBT coverage, 336-338
LGBT health coverage, 336, 338-341
sources of, 335
Media advocacy, 339, 340e, 341e
Media kits, 340e
Medical records, 179-180
Medical schools, sensitivity training, 187-188
MEDLINE, LGBT topics, 177, 250
Men
alcohol use patterns, 205
homosexual contacts, 121
sexual orientation assessment, 30t
sexual orientation survey, 37
"Men who have sex with men" (MSM), 121, 231, 292
Mental health, HP2010, 302
Mental health services
county services, 264t
lesbian battering, 108-109
lesbians use of, 96

Mental health services *(continued)*
service reform target, 275
and transsexuals, 157-158
Methamphetamine use
MTF, 205
transgender women, 204
Metoidioplasty, 166
Metropolitan counties, selected services, 264-265, 264t
Millennium March, substance abuse survey, 206e
Money, John, 297
Mortimer, Lee, 293
Multipurpose sampling, 47
Mycobacterium avium complex (MAC), 122
Mycobacterium avium intracellulare (MAI), 122

National AIDS Network, 299
National AIDS Resource Center, 299
National Association of Alcohol and Drug Abuse Counselors, 212
National Association of Counties, 264
National Association of Lesbian and Gay Addiction Professionals, 197, 216, 298, 299, 347
National Association of LGBT Community Centers, 98-99, 299
National Association of People with AIDS, 299
National Association of Social Workers
Committee on Lesbian and Gay Issues, 197
gay/lesbian caucuses, 15t
National Center for Health Statistics, 51
National Center for Lesbian Rights, 301, 337
National Clearinghouse for Alcohol and Drug Information, 348
National Coalition for LGBT Health, 305, 306, 348
National Crime Victimization Survey, 303
National Gay and Lesbian Health Foundation, 27

"Unsafe sex," 44
U.S. Public Health Service (USPHS)
    and NGHC, 20
    reorganization of, 27
    research activities, 13

Vaccinations, hepatitis, 124-125, 135
Values clarification, sensitivity
        training, 75-76
Vermont, civil unions, 296
Vermont Youth Risk Behavior Survey
        (YRBS), drug use, 207
Village Voice, The, 343
Vinette, transgender youth, 238-239
Violence
    FTMs, 169
    lesbian relationships, 105-106
    MTFs, 165
Violence prevention, HP2010, 302
Viral hepatitis, gay/bisexual men, 123
Vital statistics, health data, 13
Volkow, Nora, 213
Vulvar warts, 92

Waldren, David, 15t, 17-18
Warhol, Andy, 292
Warner, Michael, 5
Washington
    LGBT health care Web site, 193
    public health services, 12
Washington Blade, 303
Washington Confidential, 293
Waxman, Henry, 306, 307-308, 310
Web, media source, 335
Weight, 13, 101, 104
Weiss, Paul, 306
West Hollywood, gay neighborhood, 7
What is a Sexual Minority Anyway?,
        276
Wherry, Kenneth, 293
Whitman-Walker Clinic, 25, 190
Will & Grace, 4, 248
Wisconsin Youth Risk Behavior Survey
        (YRBS), drug use, 207

Women
    alcohol use patterns, 205
    chronic diseases, 99-100
    CVD deaths, 99
    HIV infections, 90-91
    sexual orientation survey, 37
Women for Sobriety, 216
"Women who have sex with women"
        (WSW), 292
Women's Health Initiative (WHI)
    lesbian inclusion, 301
    lesbian obesity, 101
    lesbian tobacco use, 101
    physical activity, 102
WorkNet project, HRC, 322e, 331
Workplace
    discriminatory/exclusionary
        practices, 318
    effecting change, 329
    employment decisions, 320-321
    equal benefits law, 323
    LGBT friendly, 317-318, 330
    LGBT protection, 321-323
    transgender issues, 326-327
World Health Organization (WHO),
        definition of health, 319

Yolles, Stanley, 297
Young men who have sex with men
        (YMSM), 223, 231
Youth
    alcohol use, 211
    LGBT health barriers, 180-181
    LGBT health services, 221-223, 224
    LGBT research, 29
    service recommendations, 285-287
    substance abuse, 206-207
Youth Risk Behavior Survey (YRBS),
        43, 51

Zerhouni, Elias, 307

Order a copy of this book with this form or online at:
http://www.haworthpress.com/store/product.asp?sku=5557

THE HANDBOOK OF LESBIAN, GAY, BISEXUAL, AND TRANSGENDER PUBLIC HEALTH
A Practitioner's Guide to Service

_____in hardbound at $69.95 (ISBN-13: 978-1-56023-495-1; ISBN-10: 1-56023-495-4)

_____in softbound at $39.95 (ISBN-13: 978-1-56023-496-8; ISBN-10: 1-56023-496-2)

Or order online and use special offer code HEC25 in the shopping cart.

COST OF BOOKS_____

POSTAGE & HANDLING_____
(US: $4.00 for first book & $1.50
for each additional book)
(Outside US: $5.00 for first book
& $2.00 for each additional book)

SUBTOTAL_____

IN CANADA: ADD 7% GST_____

STATE TAX_____
(NJ, NY, OH, MN, CA, IL, IN, PA, & SD
residents, add appropriate local sales tax)

FINAL TOTAL_____
(If paying in Canadian funds,
convert using the current
exchange rate, UNESCO
coupons welcome)

☐ **BILL ME LATER:** (Bill-me option is good on
US/Canada/Mexico orders only; not good to
jobbers, wholesalers, or subscription agencies.)

☐ Check here if billing address is different from
shipping address and attach purchase order and
billing address information.

Signature_____

☐ **PAYMENT ENCLOSED: $**_____

☐ **PLEASE CHARGE TO MY CREDIT CARD.**

☐ Visa ☐ MasterCard ☐ AmEx ☐ Discover
☐ Diner's Club ☐ Eurocard ☐ JCB

Account # _____

Exp. Date_____

Signature_____

Prices in US dollars and subject to change without notice.

NAME_____

INSTITUTION_____

ADDRESS_____

CITY_____

STATE/ZIP_____

COUNTRY_____ COUNTY (NY residents only)_____

TEL_____ FAX_____

E-MAIL_____

May we use your e-mail address for confirmations and other types of information? ☐ Yes ☐ No
We appreciate receiving your e-mail address and fax number. Haworth would like to e-mail or fax special
discount offers to you, as a preferred customer. **We will never share, rent, or exchange your e-mail address
or fax number.** We regard such actions as an invasion of your privacy.

Order From Your Local Bookstore or Directly From
The Haworth Press, Inc.
10 Alice Street, Binghamton, New York 13904-1580 • USA
TELEPHONE: 1-800-HAWORTH (1-800-429-6784) / Outside US/Canada: (607) 722-5857
FAX: 1-800-895-0582 / Outside US/Canada: (607) 771-0012
E-mail to: orders@haworthpress.com

For orders outside US and Canada, you may wish to order through your local
sales representative, distributor, or bookseller.
For information, see http://haworthpress.com/distributors

(Discounts are available for individual orders in US and Canada only, not booksellers/distributors.)
PLEASE PHOTOCOPY THIS FORM FOR YOUR PERSONAL USE.
http://www.HaworthPress.com

BOF06